Teaching Atlas
of Breast Ultrasound

Teaching Atlas of Breast Ultrasound

Wolfgang Leucht

in collaboration
with Dagmar Leucht

Foreword
by Elizabeth Kelly-Fry

299 illustrations

1992
Georg Thieme Verlag
Stuttgart · New York

Thieme Medical Publishers, Inc.,
New York

Wolfgang Leucht, M. D.
Attending Physician, Heidelberg University
Gynecological Clinic
Voss Strasse 9

6900 Heidelberg
Germany

Dagmar Leucht, M. D.
Attending Physician, Heidelberg University
Gynecological Clinic
Voss Strasse 9

6900 Heidelberg
Germany

Prof. Elizabeth Kelly-Fry, M. D.
Department of Radiology
Wishard Memorial Hospital
1001 West 10th Street
Indianapolis, IN 46202
USA

Library of Congress Cataloging-in-Publication Data
[Lehratlas der Mammasonographie. English]
Teaching atlas of breast ultrasound / Wolfgang Leucht in collaboration with Dagmar Leucht ; foreword by Elizabeth Kelly-Fry ; translated by Terry C. Telger.
p. cm.
Translation of: Lehratlas der Mammasonographie.
Includes bibliographical references and index.
ISBN 3-13-774101-7. – ISBN 0-86577-415-3
1. Breast – Ultrasonic imaging – Atlases.
2. Breast – Diaseases – Diagnosis – Atlases.
3. Breast – Tumors – Diagnosis – Atlases.
I. Leucht, Dagmar. II. Title.
[DNLM: 1. Breast Diseases – diagnosis – atlases.
2. Mamography – atlases. 3. Ultrasonography – atlases.]
RG493.5.U47L4813 1991
618.1'907543 – dc20
DNLM/DLC
for Library of Congress 91-36872
CIP

This book is an authorized translation of the German edition, published and copyrighted 1989 by Georg Thieme Verlag, Stuttgart, Germany.
Title of the German edition: Lehratlas der Mammasonographie.

Translated by Terry C. Telger

Rüdigerstraße 14, 7000 Stuttgart 30, Germany
Thieme Medical Publishers, Inc., 381 Park Avenue South, New York, N.Y. 10016

Typesetting by R. Hurler, D-7311 Notzingen,
Printed in Germany by K. Grammlich, D-7401 Pliezhausen

ISBN 3-13-774101-7 (GTV, Stuttgart)
ISBN 0-86577-415-3 (TMP, New York)

Important Note: Medicine is an ever-changing science undergoing continual development. Research and clinical experience are continually expanding our knowledge, in particular our knowledge of proper treatment and drug therapy. Insofar as this book mentions any dosage or application, readers may rest assured that the authors, editors and publishers have made every effort to ensure that such references are in accordance with the state of knowledge at the time of production of the book.

Nevertheless this does not involve, imply, or express any guarantee or responsibility on the part of the publishers in respect of any dosage instructions and forms of application stated in the book. Every user is requested to examine carefully the manufacturers' leaflets accompanying each drug and to check, if necessary in consultation with a physician or specialist, whether the dosage schedules mentioned therein or the contraindications stated by the manufacturers differ from the statements made in the present book. Such examination is particularly important with drugs that are either rarely used or have been newly released on the market. Every dosage schedule or every form of application used is entirely at the user's own risk and responsibility. The authors and publishers request every user to report to the publishers any discrepancies or inaccuracies noticed.

To my academic teachers,
Professor Emeritus Karl Knörr, M. D.
and
Professor Fred Kubli, M. D. (1930–1987).

Foreword

For women living in this last decade of the twentieth century, breast cancer remains a devastating, fatal disease. Early detection of this pathology, which offers the best hope for long-term patient survival, is a universal goal. With some exceptions—such as Japan, where manual examination and ultrasound mammography are widely applied—X-ray mammography is the primary imaging technique used to achieve this goal of early detection. However, radiologists routinely encounter cases in with an X-ray image is noninformative with respect to whether a dense or semidense breast is normal. Additionally, in some cases, X-ray images are equivocal regarding the benign or malignant nature of a detected breast mass. As indicated by Dr. Wolfgang Leucht in the text of this Teaching Atlas, ultrasound imaging can provide the correct diagnosis in a majority of these equivocal X-ray images and thus is an invaluable partner of X-ray mammography.

It is significant that Dr. Leucht recommends ultrasound imaging as the initial examination for all patients with a palpable mass. This is a distinct departure from the clinical protocoll for such patients in the United States, where ultrasound mammography is the initial examination only if the patient is young, pregnant, or lactating. Dr. Leucht and colleagues have had the unique opportunity of carrying out thousands of X-ray and ultrasound breast examinations. On the basis of that vast experience, they are able to clearly demonstrate that ultrasound mammography has a diagnostic capability that is beyond the simple ability to differentiate between a solid and cystic mass. Increased application of ultrasound mammography, along with continued improvement of image quality, should advance the diagnostic capabilities of this technique even further than those so well described in this Atlas.

Elizabeth Kelly-Fry
Professor of Radiology
Indiana University School of Medicine

Preface

Breast ultrasound is gaining increasing importance as a diagnostic modality. Yet in contrast to the great, number of competent examiners who practice X-ray mammography, relatively few have adequate experience with breast ultrasound, and most of these have had to acquire their knowledge through laborious self-teaching. We have been in the fortunate position of being able to gain our experience at a hospital where large numbers of breast operations are performed. In this setting we have conducted more than 5000 breast ultrasound examinations, the most informative of which were some 1500 preoperative cases in which we were able to compare sonographic findings with the postoperative pathology report.

In this book we attempt to respond to the wishes of our many colleagues whom we have introduced to breast ultrasound and who seek to further their education by having "something written or in pictures" that they can take home as a reference. Our intent is to provide them and all interested professionals with a learning tool and memory aid that will benefit their daily practice.

I am deeply grateful to our late chief of staff, Prof. Fred Kubli, who did much to support and advance breast sonography while also taking a productively critical stance toward the method and its limitations. I thank Prof. W. Schmidt for giving me the opportunity to perform so many examinations and for constantly encouraging me to record my experience in written form. Prof. D. von Fournier, through his critical discussions, motivated me constantly to reappraise the value of the method; his help is gratefully acknowledged.

I thank my tireless colleague, doctoral candidate Klaus-Dieter Humbert, for his constant willingness to help with important work and questions. I acknowledge the skill and great personal commitment with which Mr. Manfred Liedtke handled the photographic reproductions. I also thank Mrs. Christine Hellwig for typing the manuscript and the staff of the Ultrasound Department for their kind cooperation.

Finally I wish to thank Prof. Elizabeth Kelly-Fry, who provided invaluable advice on the translation and who so kindly agreed to write the Foreword for this book.

Heidelberg, October, 1991 *Wolfgang Leucht*

Table of Contents

Introduction

A teaching atlas can replace a textbook only to a degree. To the reader not well versed in the subject matter, illustrations may not be informative enough. It is assumed that the user of this atlas possesses a basic knowledge of the breast and its disorders and of the sonographic technique. Unlike a textbook, which typically begins with diagnosis and proceeds from there, this atlas seeks to demonstrate how a diagnosis can be arrived at through image analysis. It is based on the principle of learning from illustrative case material. Chapters 1 through 5 provide the reader with a concise "basic skills review." The terminology is our own, but it is comprehensible to all. The bulk of the atlas, presented in chapter 6, is devoted to illustrative cases and their interpretation. The cases are arranged according to the indications that prompted ultrasonography. We selected cases that were both representative and instructive by virtue of their clarity. The case presentations cover the entire spectrum of sonographically detectable breast lesions. The detection of these lesions is trained by analyzing images in terms of specific criteria for diagnosis a sonographic abnormality and predicting its benignancy or malignancy. Reference to differential diagnosis is made where appropriate.

In the search for images that would satisfy both critical and aesthetic demands, we decided to use photographic reproductions and enlarged the original Polaroid pictures so that they approximately matched the format of a large monitor image. The examiner utilized images of this size and quality when making his evaluation. The text portion of the atlas was kept brief. We hope that readers experienced in sonography will excuse the repetitions included to aid the beginner. Modifications of the usual examination technique (e.g., a 7.5-MHz transducer with a standoff) are noted where they occur. Marking symbols are used in figures only where deemed necessary for clarification.

This atlas is not a substitute for personal experience frame of reference.

1 Historical Development of Breast Ultrasound, Basic Equipment Requirements

The history of breast ultrasound began in the early 1950s, when Wild and Reid (1952) performed sonographic examinations of the female breast on an experimental basis. The low technical standard at that time did not permit clinical application of the method. The introduction of gray-scale imaging (Kossoff 1972) was the breakthrough that permitted the detailed visualization of the complex tissue structures of the breast.

Further advances, relating mainly to clinical implementation, took place in Japan (Kobayashi et al. 1974, Kobayashi 1977, Wagai and Tsutsumi 1977, Wagai et al. 1977), in Australia (Jellins et al. 1975, 1982), and in the United States (Cole-Beuglet et al. 1975, Kelly-Fry et al. 1977, Kelly-Fry 1983). Researchers took two basic approaches to instrument design, according to their goals. The concept of using ultrasound as a basic screening examination for early breast cancer detection, perhaps as a substitute for X-ray mammography, led to the development of *automated* systems for whole-breast examination. The best-known devices of this kind are the Octoson immersion scanner, the Japanese automated scanners, and the multifrequency automated scanner based on the research of E. Kelly-Fry. To date, however, with the exception of Japan, the whole-breast system has not gained wide acceptance as a screening tool, and rightly so.

The other goal, that of using breast ultrasound as an adjunctive procedure for special inquiries as well as a primary modality in selected patients, was realized through the development of advanced *manual* scanning techniques in which hand-held transducers are used. The indications and contraindications for manual scanning derive from its *advantages* (direct characterization of a palpable mass, better image detail, dynamic examination, capability for ultrasound-guided aspiration) and its *disadvantages* (incomplete image documentation, examination cannot be delegated to assistants).

The use of manually controlled high-resolution real-time scanners, operating at frequencies of 5–10 MHz with a penetration depth of about 6 cm, has become fairly standard among practitioners today. An additional advantage, which will contribute to the further expansion of manual real-time scanning, is the fact that an existing ultrasound system can be supplemented at any time by a higher-frequency transducer for breast imaging. To ensure a certain quality standard in breast ultrasound, the German Association of National Health Service Physicians issued guidelines on Dec. 7, 1985 (valid as of April 1, 1986), which establish quality criteria for personnel and instrumentation. The most important equipment requirement is a transducer with an operating frequency of at least 5 MHz. This also appears to be an adequate ultrasound frequency. Higher frequencies are still being tested.

2 Manual Real-Time Examination Technique

For manual real-time scanning, the patient is placed in the supine position. The ipsilateral arm is extended above the head to stabilize the breast and flatten it against the chest wall. A sitting position may be necessary in rare cases, e.g., when a mass is accessible to palpation only when the patient is sitting. Where possible, it is advantageous to follow the same sequence of steps in all examinations. For example, scanning may begin in the upper inner quadrant of the breast and proceed slowly to the outer quadrant to obtain a series of sagittal images. The transducer is then moved lower on the breast and the scanning action repeated until the whole breast has been examined. At that point the transducer ist rotated 90°, and transverse scans are taken proceeding from the inner to the outer quadrants. Longitudinal scans are best for examination of the axillary region.

It is important to apply moderate tissue compression when performing the scans. In areas where shadowing or attenuation is a problem, this can often be eliminated by applying greater pressure. This may be necessary to obtain an image of acceptable quality (Fig. 2.**1**). The experienced examiner will match the tissue compression to the image displayed on the monitor. To obtain an optimum image, it is essential that the time gain compensation (TGC) controls (gain, near gain, far gain) be properly matched and adjusted. TGC evens out echo amplitudes from different depths by attenuating reflections from near structures and amplifying echoes from more distant structures. The gain setting should be adjusted so that contrasts are balanced throughout the image area. No structural details should be lost as a result of under- or overamplification. A "standard" gain setting cannot be used due to interindividual and intraindividual variations. Near-field focusing should be employed.

A standoff should alway be used in breast examinations with a sector scanner. Linear scanners with good near-field focusing generally do not require a standoff. However, if one is used (advantageous for imaging superficial lesions), it must be considered that the ultrasound image characteristics, and thus some of the diagnostic criteria, will be altered in relation to scanning without a standoff.

A focal sonographic abnormality should be analyzed in terms of all static and dynamic diagnostic criteria (see p. 20ff.). The dynamic part of the examination consists in evaluating the focal abnormality under increasing tissue compression, which is applied under sonographic viewing, using either the transducer or the palpating finger. Any abnormalities that are found should be documented on two planes (Polaroid, video printer, multiformat camera, video cassette), indicating the plane and direction of the scan on the documented image. The absence of abnormalities cannot be definitively documented in a manual real-time examination. A standard ultrasound report form is filled out for each examination (p. 19).

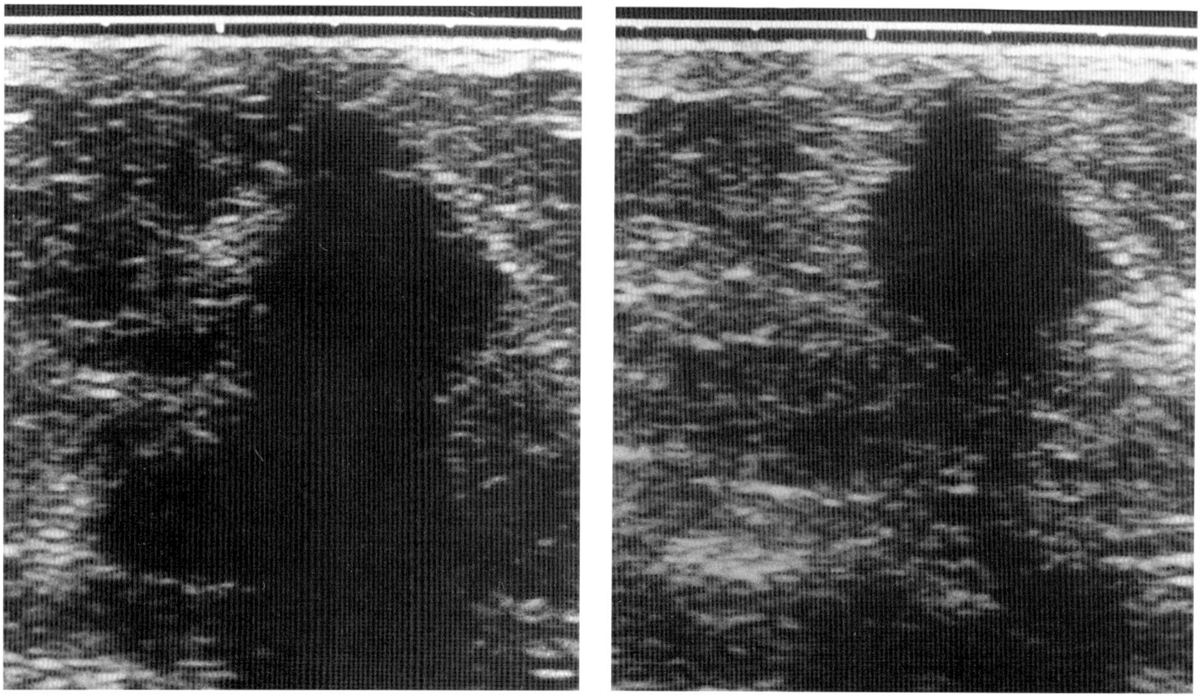

a b

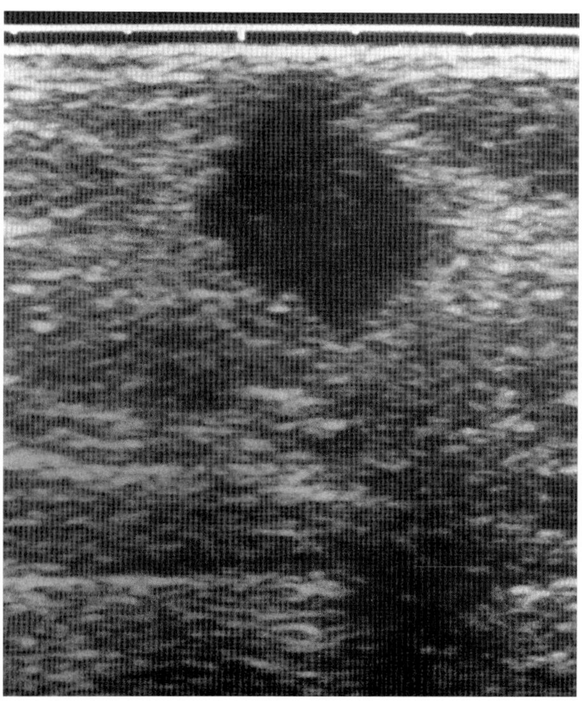

c

Fig. 2.**1** Focal sonographic lesion seen with an infiltrating ductal carcinoma, 30×23 mm
a Extensive acoustic shadow (without compression)
b Same view as **a** with slight compression
c Same view as **a** with strong compression

3 Sonographic Anatomy of the Female Breast

Major Tissue Types and Structures

The female breast is composed of four major types of tissue: fat, parenchyma (alveoli and lactiferous ducts), dense collagenous connective tissue (supports the parenchyma), and loose intralobular connective tissue. This complex tissue composition is reflected in the alternating high- and low-level echo patterns that appear within the breast. A structure appears strongly echogenic on sonograms if it has a nonhomogeneous composition that contains numerous reflective interfaces ("acoustic jumps") like that between collagenous and noncollagenous connective tissue. If a structure has a homogenous composition with few jumps, it will appear hypoechoic. The following structures generally can be seen on the breast sonogram of a sexually mature woman (Figs. 3.**1**, 3.**2**):

1. Skin
2. Subcutaneous fat
3. Breast parenchyma (glandular tissue)
4. Cooper ligaments
5. Retromammary fat (not obligatory)
6. Pectoralis muscle and fascia
7. Ribs
8. Pleura

a
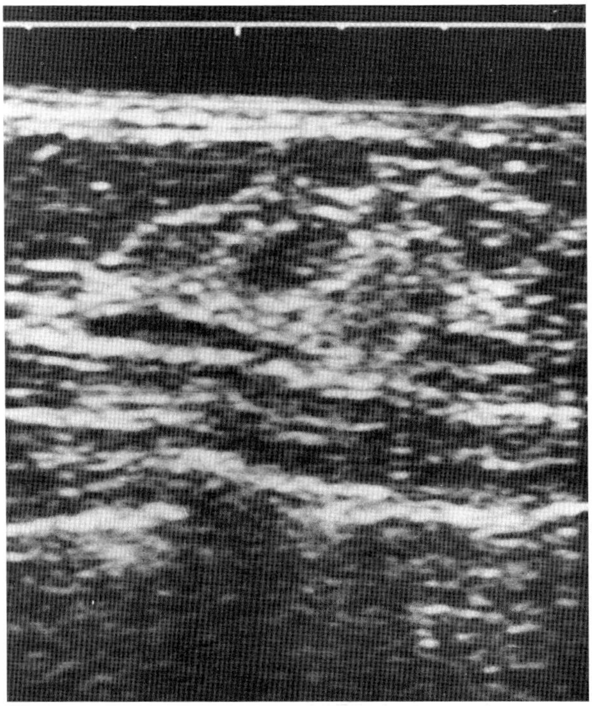

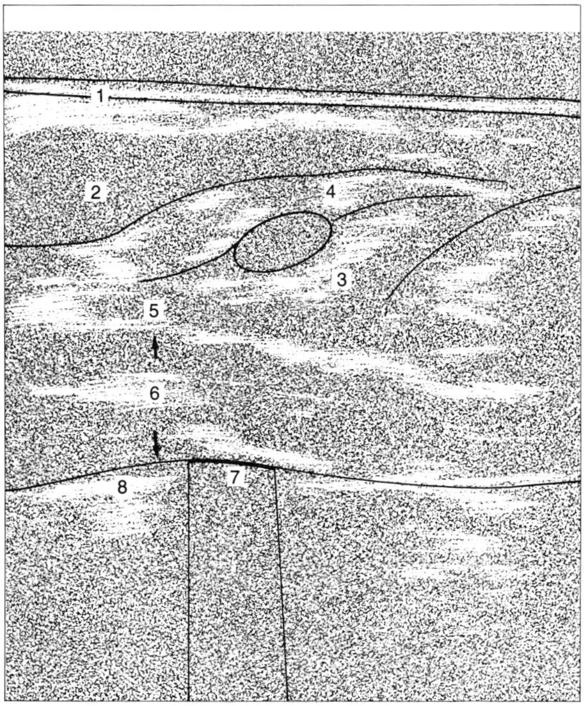

b

Fig. 3.**1** Woman, 33 years of age
a Normal sonogram (with water path)
b Schematic drawing: 1-skin, 2-subcutaneous fat, 3-glandular region, 4-Cooper ligaments, 5-retromammary fat, 6-pectoral muscle and fascia (arrows), 7-rib with shadow, 8-pleura

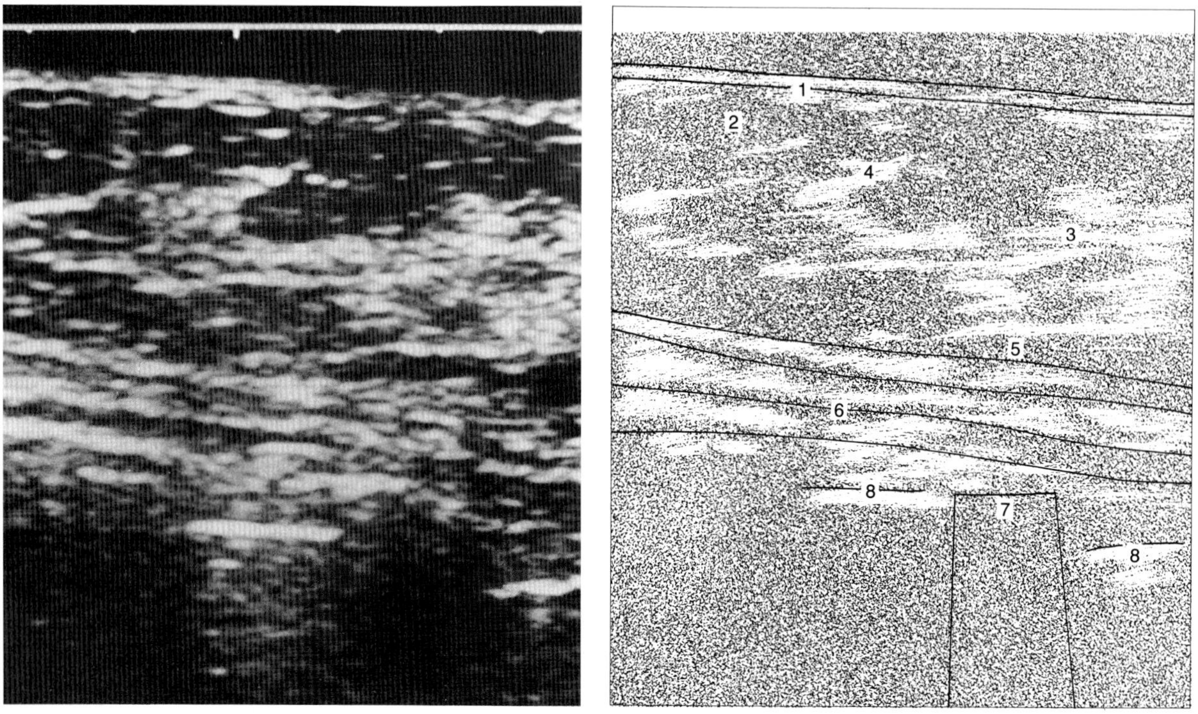

Fig. 3.**2** Woman, 47 years of age
a Normal sonogram (with water path)
b Schematic drawing: 1-skin, 2-subcutaneous fat, 3-glandular region, 4-Cooper ligaments, 5-retromammary fat, 6-pectoral muscle and fascia, 7-rib with shadow, 8-pleura

Skin

The skin appears as a bright linear echo near the top of the image. As greater pressure is applied with the transducer, the apparent thickness of the skin increases. This should not be mistaken for cutaneous edema.

Subcutaneous Fat

The quantity of subcutaneous fat varies considerably with age and parity. Little or no subcutaneous fat may be seen in young women, and large interindividual variations occur. As it is structurally homogeneous, subcutaneous fat appears hypoechoic. Only the Cooper ligaments traversing the fat provide echogenic contrast. Blood vessels coursing through the fat are sometimes visible as tubular structures (Fig. 3.**3**).

Cooper Ligaments

Cooper ligaments appear as septumlike (Fig. 3.**4**) or tentlike structures (Fig. 3.**5**) that arise from the surface of the breast parenchyma and taper to their sites of insertion in the corium. Anatomically they represent planes of fibrous tissue. Shadowing may occur behind the apices of the Cooper ligaments (Fig. 3.**6**) or behind the sawtoothlike extensions of breast parenchyma with which they are continuous (Fig. 3.**7**). These shadows should not be confused with retrotumoral shadowing and will disappear at once if the transducer angle is changed.

a 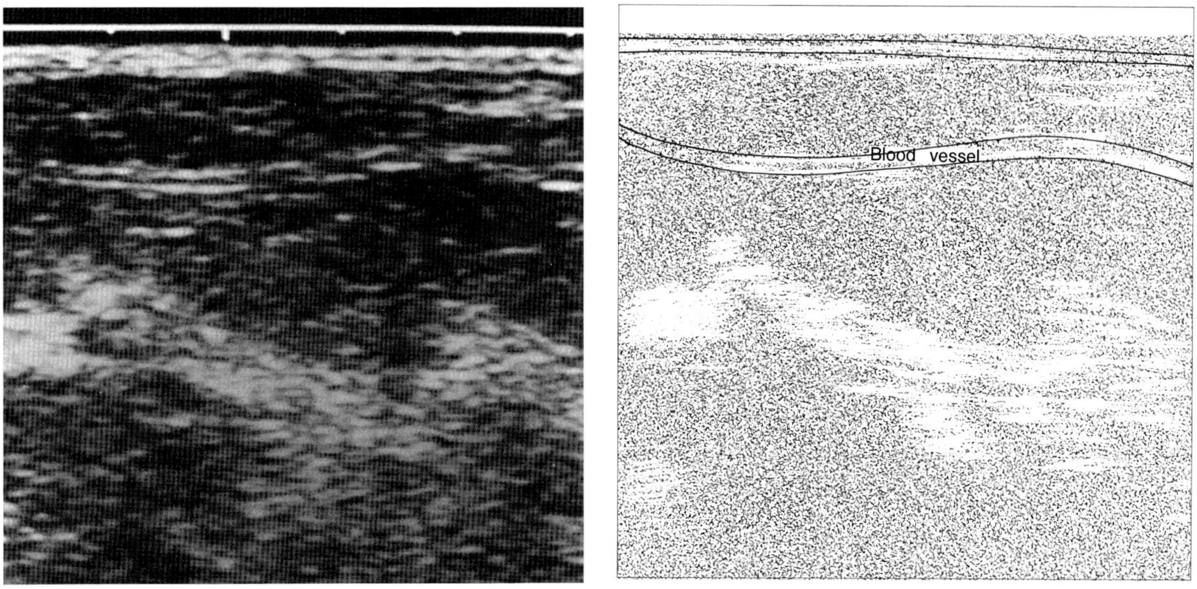 b

Fig. 3.**3** Abundant subcutaneous fat in a largely involuted breast
a Sonogram. The fat is traversed by two echogenic lines representing a blood vessel
b Schematic drawing

a 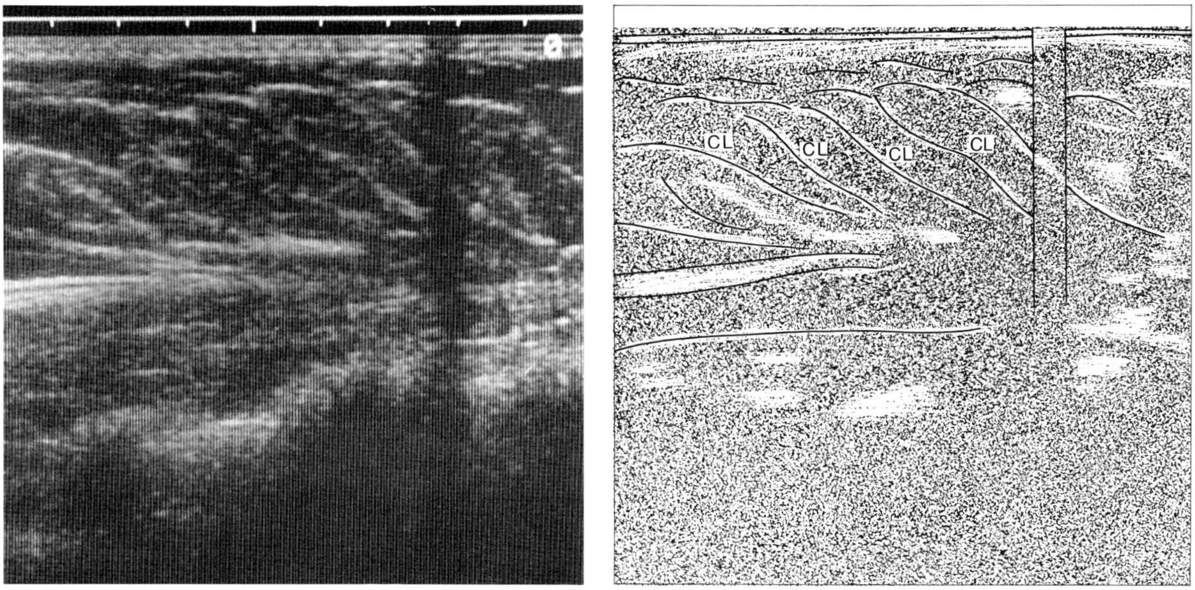 b

Fig. 3.**4** Woman, 55 years of age. The breast parenchyma is largely involuted and is permeated by septumlike Cooper ligaments
a Sonogram. The shadow on the right side of the image is caused by faulty acoustic coupling over the skin
b Schematic drawing (CL = Cooper ligaments)

a
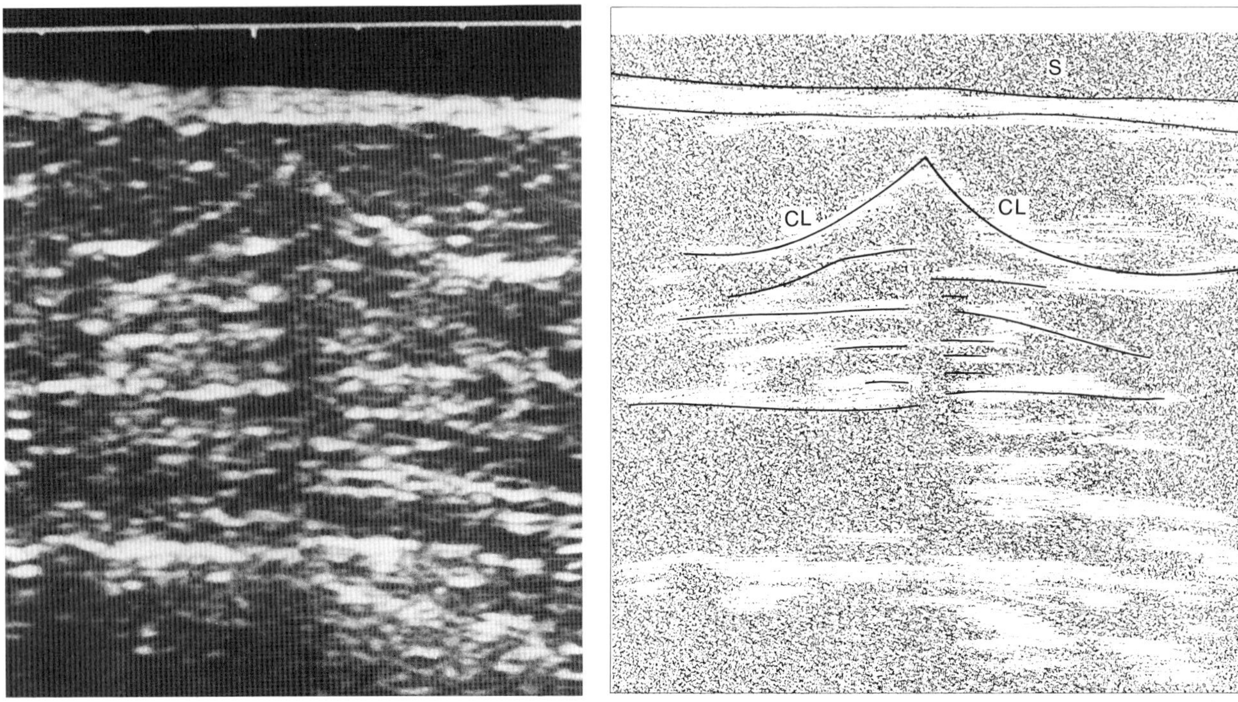

b

Fig. 3.**5** Woman, 29 years of age
a Sonogram with standoff. The tentlike Cooper ligaments attach to the corium. A faint acoustic shadow is seen beneath their point of intersection
b Schematic drawing (CL = Cooper ligaments, S = standoff)

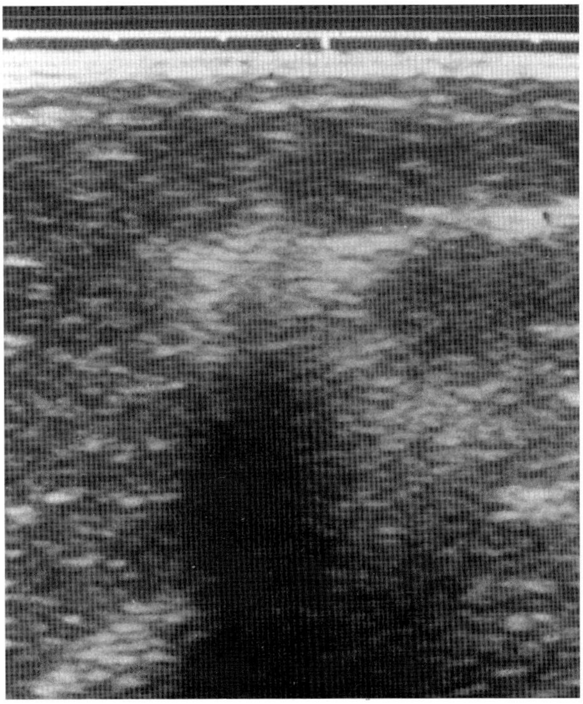

Fig. 3.**6** Woman, 62 years of age, with involuted breast. The intersection of the Cooper ligaments traversing the fat causes marked posterior shadowing (the shadow arises from a hyperechoic area)

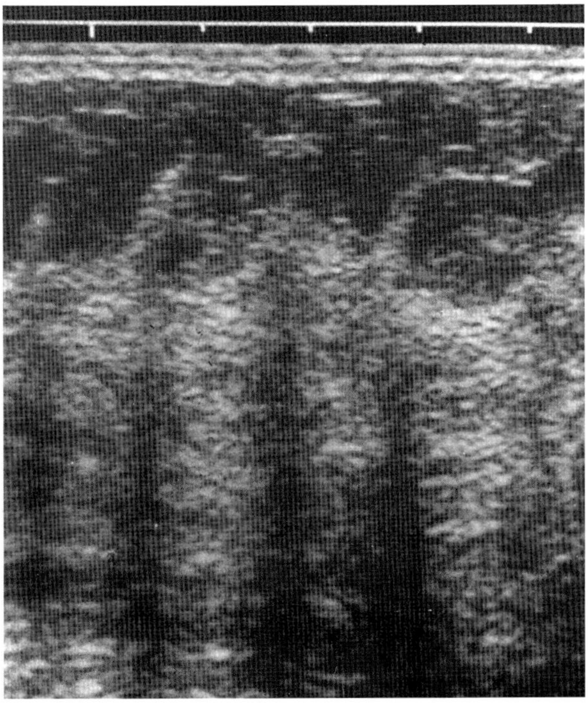

Fig. 3.**7** Woman, 37 years of age. The Cooper ligaments appear as sawtoothlike extensions of the breast parenchyma in the subcutaneous fat. Each casts a shadow

Glandular Region

The glandular region is separated from the subcutaneous fat by the echogenic "superficial fascia". Normally the echogenicity of the glandular region is intermediate between that of the fat and fascial planes. The parenchymal pattern of the breast is an expression of the relative quantities of fibroglandular tissue and fat. This ratio is influenced by age, parity, and hormonal status (pregnancy, lactation, menopausal status). Parenchymal changes relating to the menstrual cycle generally cannot be demonstrated with ultrasound. Four main ultrasound parenchymal patterns are recognized:

1. The juvenile (hyperechoic) breast with little fat (Fig. 3.**8**).
2. The premenopausal, partly involuted breast in which the parenchyma has been partially replaced by fat, and there are increased amounts of subcutaneous and retromammary fat (Fig. 3.**9**).
3. The postmenopausal involuted breast, which has undergone almost complete fatty replacement and is permeated by connective-tissue septa (Fig. 3.**10**).
4. A special pattern is observed during pregnancy and lactation, when the dramatic increase in glandular tissue leads to a finely granular pattern with extreme compression of the subcutaneous and retromammary fat (Fig. 3.**11**).

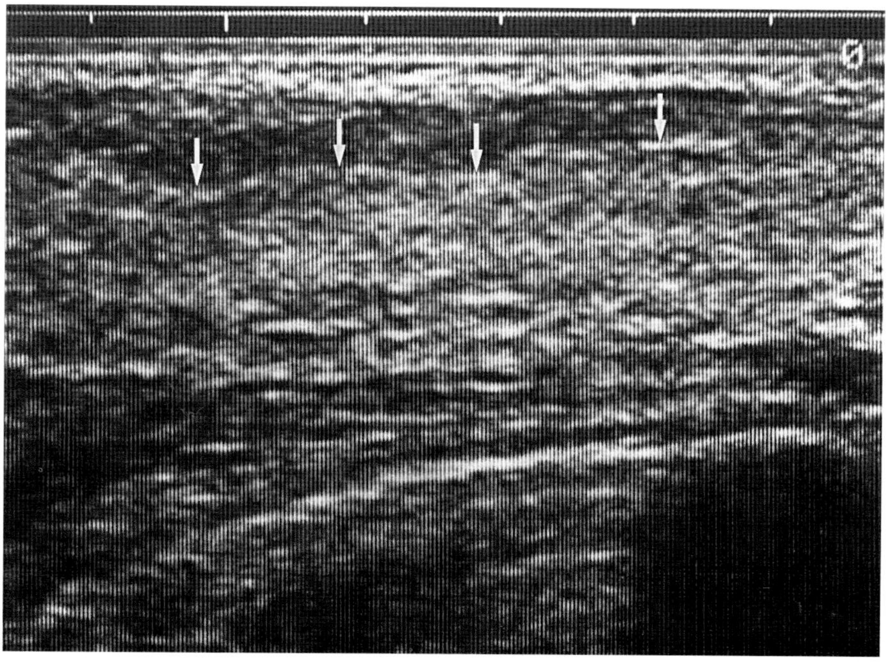

Fig. 3.**8** Juvenile-type parenchymal pattern in a 23-year-old woman with scant subcutaneous fat (arrows: superficial fascia)

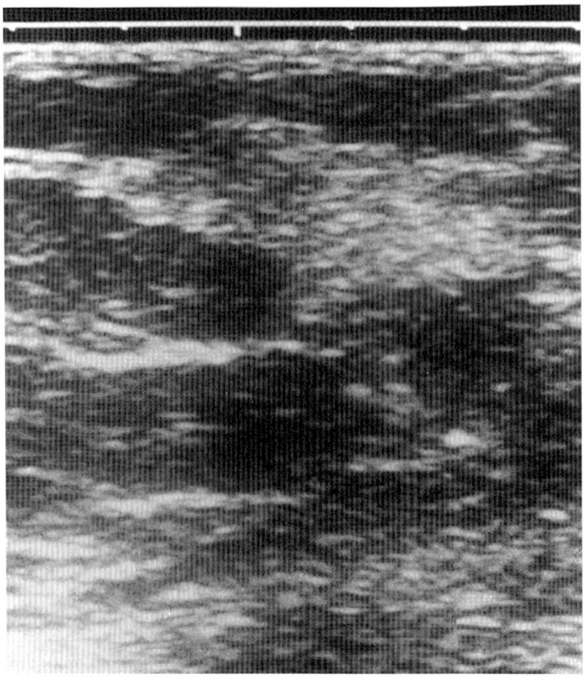

Fig. 3.**9** Breast parenchyma and fat in a 46-year-old premenopausal woman with three children

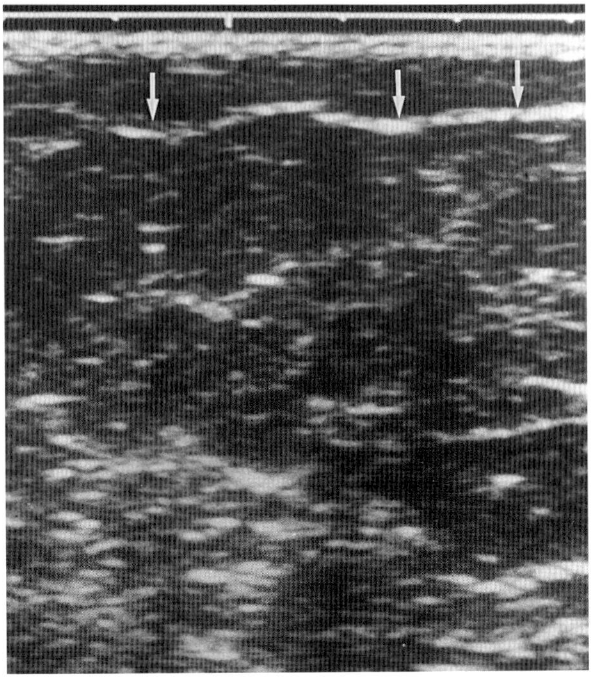

Fig. 3.**10** Involuted fatty breast of a 66-year-old woman. the fat is permeated by connective-tissue septa (arrows: superficial fascia)

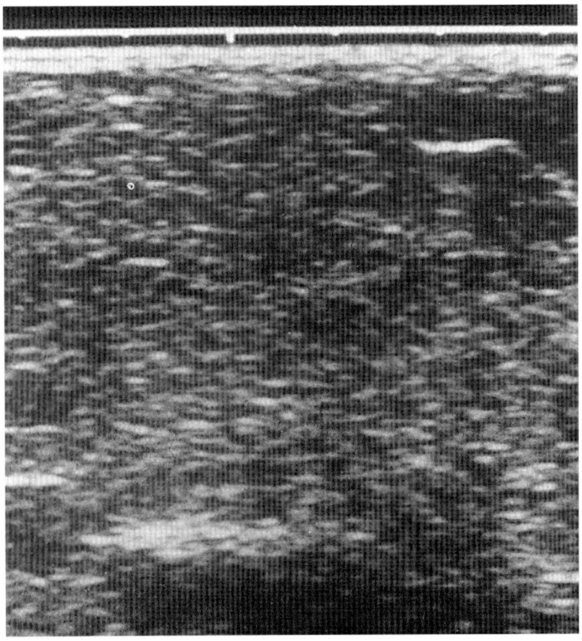

Fig. 3.**11** Lactating breat of a 30-year-old woman, 14 days postpartum

Retromammary Fat

The retromammary fat may appear as a narrow, hypoechoic layer deep to the base of the breast parenchyma, or it may be completely absent. The retromammary fat forms a layer between the deep fascial plane of the breast and the pectoral muscle. It defines the posterior boundary of the glandular tissue.

Pectoral Muscle

The pectoral muscles can be clearly imaged sonographically in the direction of their fibers. They appear as hypoechoic structures above the ribs and parallel to the skin; they are ensheathed by echogenic fascial planes.

Ribs

Sagittal scans through the medial, parasternal, cartilaginous portion of the ribs demonstrate the ribs as oval masses with few internal echoes (Fig. 3.**12**). The round foci produced by the cartilage may be mistaken for benign, solid intramammary lesions. This error can be avoided by giving attention to the deep fascial structures and overlying muscle. The lateral, ossified segments of the ribs appear as hyperechoic crescents with dense posterior shadowing and intervening intercostal muscles (Fig. 3.**13**).

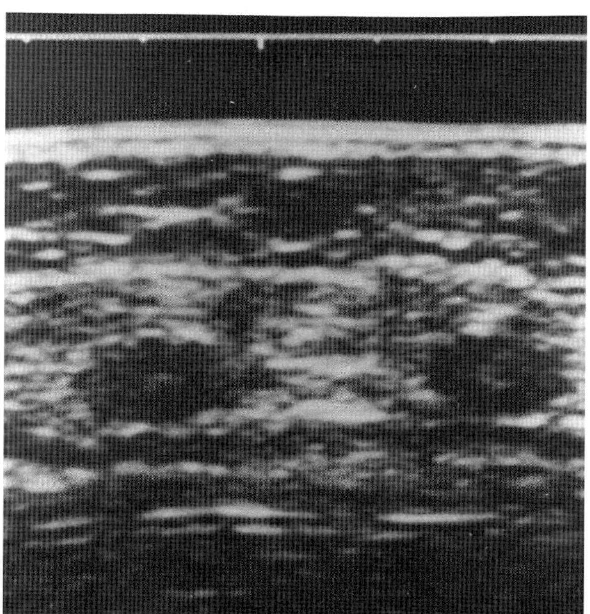

Fig. 3.**12** Parasternal sagittal scan with standoff. The cartilaginous segments of the ribs appear as well-defined oval masses

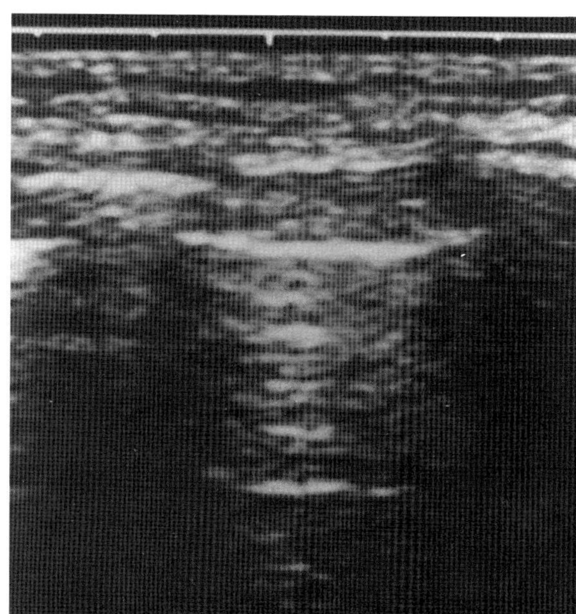

Fig. 3.**13** Sagittal scan at the level of the midclavicular line. The ribs appear as hyperechoic bands with complete posterior shadowing

Nipple Region

An acoustic shadow ("nipple shadow") is commonly seen posterior to the nipple and areola. This shadow is caused largely by the dense connective tissue in the nipple and partly by the connective tissue encasing the lactiferous ducts. The shadowing is most pronounced when the breast is examined without compression (Fig. 3.**14**). Sometimes this shadow can be eliminated by compression or by scanning the subareolar region at a tangential angle (Fig. 3.**15**). The skin of the areola is less echogenic than the rest of the breast skin. The lactiferous ducts are normally collapsed in the nonlactating breast. Dilated lumina are seen only in the region of the lactiferous sinuses just below the nipple (Figs. 3.**16** and 3.**17**).

A knowledge of the structures described in chapter 3 is essential for the interpretation of breast sonograms. Additionally, the examiner must be familiar with limiting acoustic conditions and their interpretation in order to identify focal abnormalities.

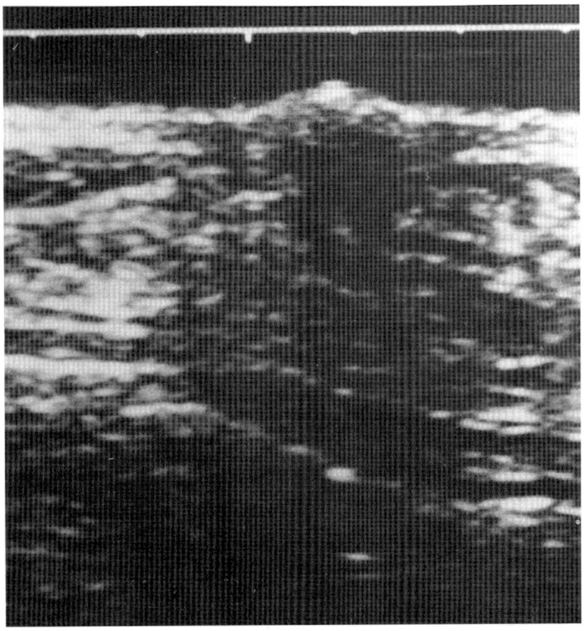

Fig. 3.**14** Sonogram with standoff. Marked nipple shadowing on this plane prevents evaluation of the subareolar region

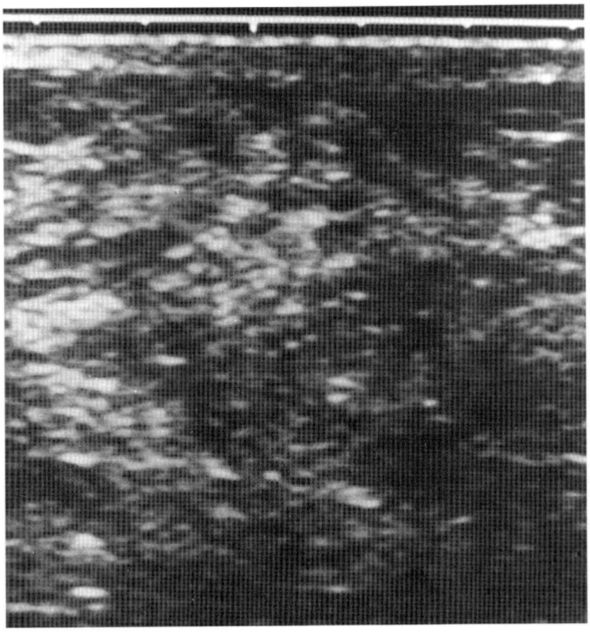

Fig. 3.**15** Tangential scan plane in the nipple region. Here the subareolar tissues can be evaluated

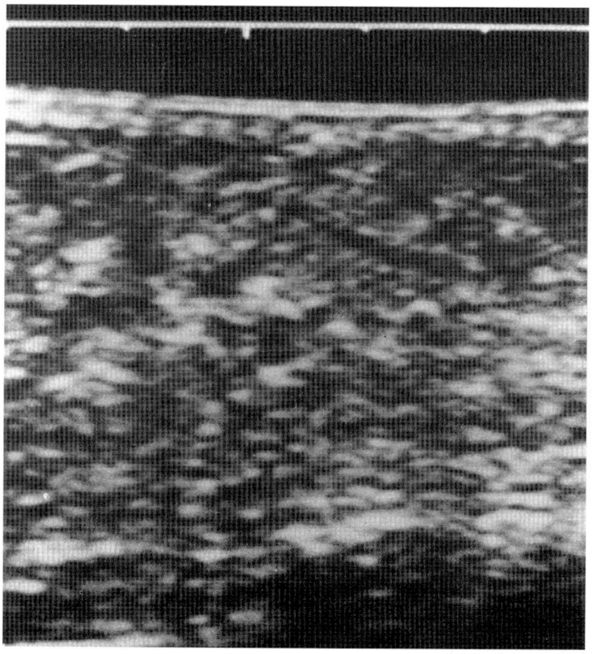

Fig. 3.**16** Good visualization of the subareolar region in a 29-year-old woman. Normal breast skin on the left side of the image contrasts with the adjacent, less echogenic skin of the areola. In the middle third of the image (level of the milk ducts), the dilated ductal lumina are imaged in transverse and longitudinal section (sonogram with standoff)

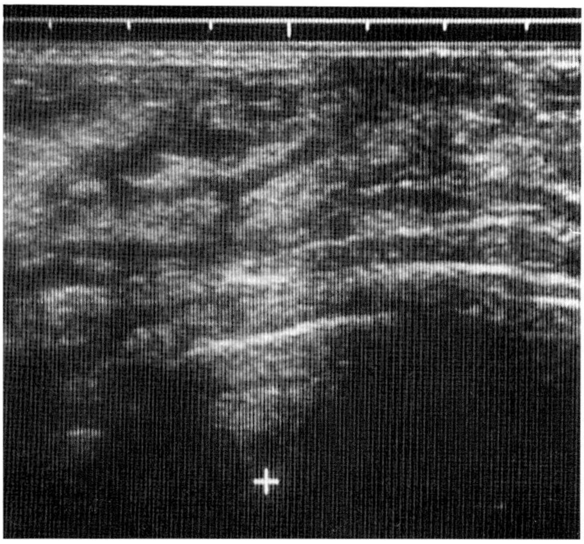

Fig. 3.**17** Subareolar region in a 24-year-old woman. The areola appears less echogenic at skin level. Below it, milk ducts in longitudinal section converge upon the nipple

4 Interpretation of Breast Sonograms

In the interpretation of breast sonograms, we proceed systematically using our standard ultrasound report form (Figs. 4.**10**, 5.**19**). The interpretation stands or falls with the quality of the image (see chapter 2, p. 3f. for more details).

Parenchymal Pattern

The first step in every examination is to identify the breast parenchymal pattern. A glandular region with no interspersed fat lobules is said to be *homogeneously sonodense* (Fig. 4.**1**); this pattern is most commonly seen in young women. Often these breasts lack subcutaneous and even retromammary fat. A homogeneously sonodense breast is easy to evaluate with ultrasound. In particular, focal hypoechoic lesions—a common manifestation of carcinoma—are very clearly portrayed by virtue of their contrast.

The *loosely sonodense* pattern with some interspersed fat lobules is most common in middle-aged women. Again, this type of breast is easy to evaluate with ultrasound (Fig. 4.**2**).

The *partially involuted* pattern in older women can hamper carcinoma detection in areas where involutional processes in the form of fatty degeneration have already taken place (Figs. 4.**3**, 4.**4**).

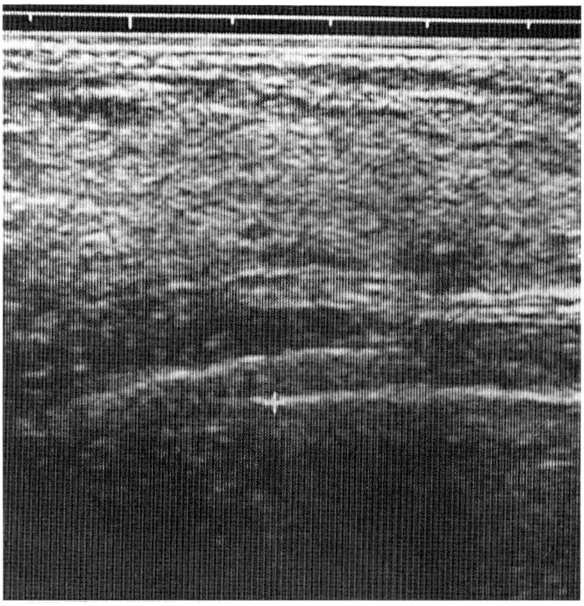

Fig. 4.**1** Homogeneously sonodense breast parenchyma in a 29-year-old woman

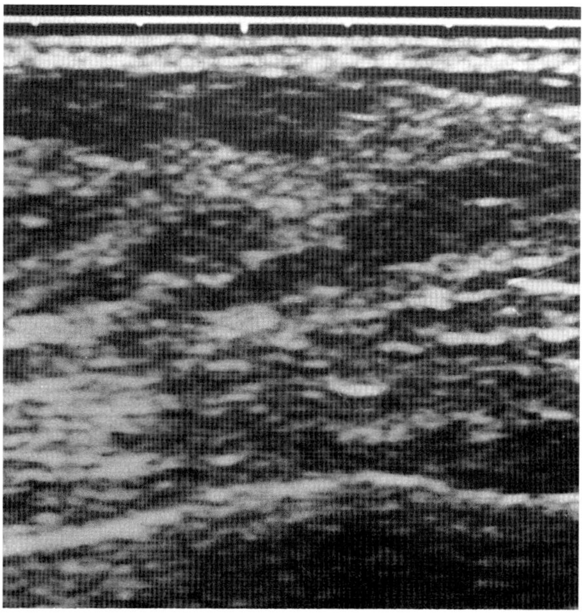

Fig. 4.**2** Loosely sonodense breast parenchyma in a 42-year-old woman

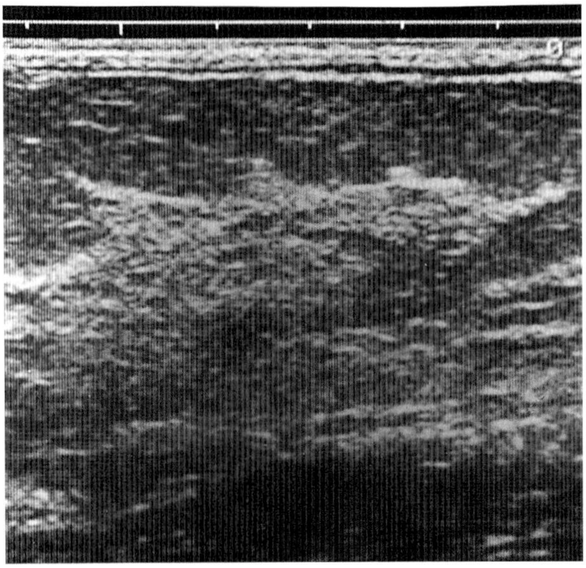

Fig. 4.**3** Partially involuted breast of a 56-year-old woman. The ratio of fat to glandular tissue has shifted in favor of fat

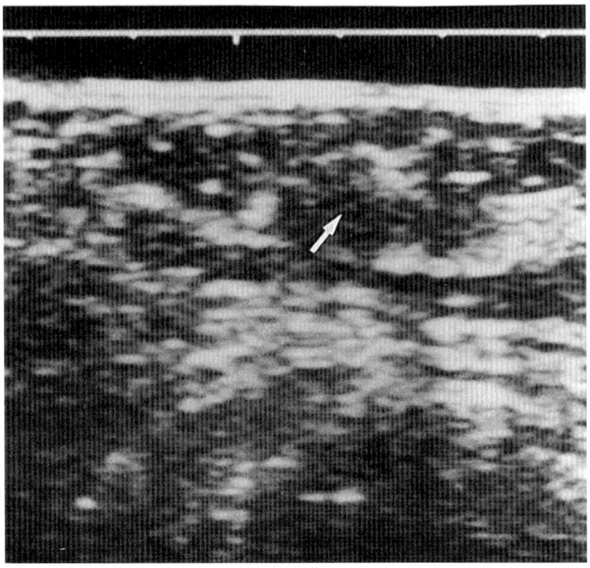

Fig. 4.**4** Involuted breast of a 56-year-old woman. The hypoechoic focal lesion, which is extremely difficult to identify, represents infiltrating ductal carcinoma (arrow; sonogram with standoff)

The *involuted* breast in postmenopausal women is generally hypoechoic and interspersed with connective-tissue septa of high echogenicity. It can create a difficult environment for the detection of sonographically low-echo focal lesions (Fig. 4.**5**).

During pregnancy and lactation, the volume of breast parenchyma increases tremendously (Fig. 3.**11**). As term approaches, the dilated milk ducts become visible as cystic spaces (Fig. 4.**6**). Focal lesions are easily recognized within the lactating breast.

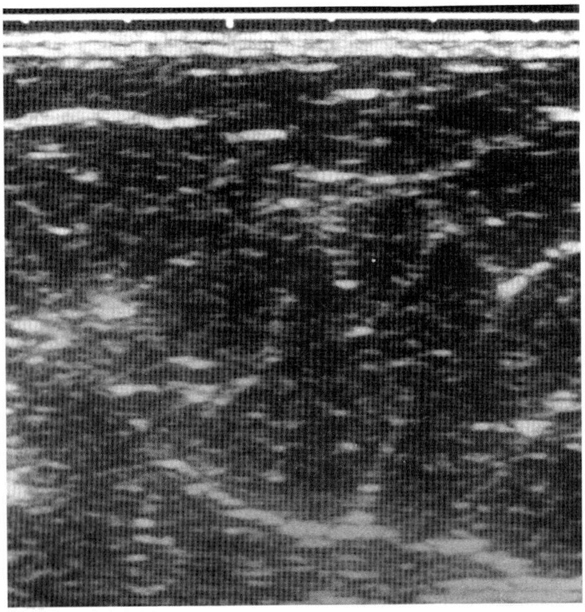

Fig. 4.**5** Involuted breast of a 66-year-old woman. The fat is permeated by connective-tissue septa. Breast parenchyma is no longer visible

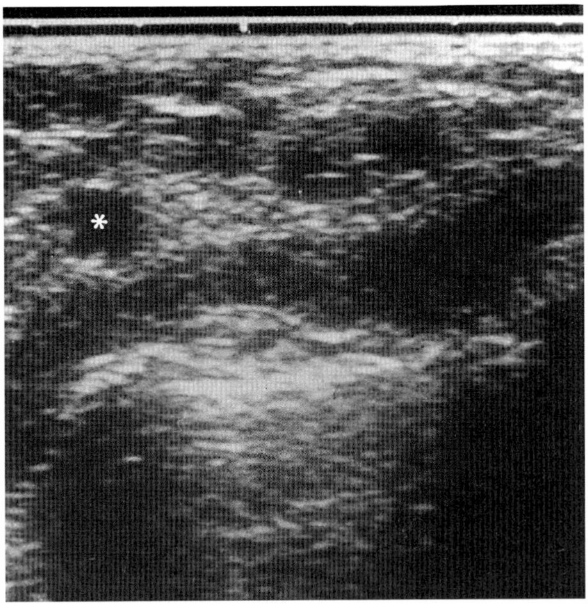

Fig. 4.**6** Congested milk duct (*) in the lactating breast of a 30-year-old woman

Parenchymal pattern identification by ultrasound provides helpful information on the confidence level of the breast evaluation, especially in the absence of a focal sonographic lesion. As a general rule, the higher the ratio of breast parenchyma to fat, the easier it is to detect a focal abnormality.

Readability

Most breast sonograms are easy to read and interpret. Limited or poor readability is most commonly due to acoustic shadowing (Fig. 4.**7**) or local attenuation (Fig. 4.**8**). Either phenomenon can completely obscure a small focal lesion.

Subareolar-Nipple Region

The readability of the region below the nipple and areola should always be noted on the ultrasound report. Frequently this region is obscured by nipple shadowing (Fig. 3.**14**), but this problem can often be eliminated by scanning tangentially (Fig. 3.**15**). Inability to evaluate the subareolar-nipple region should never tempt the examiner to declare an absence of disease.

Focal Sonographic Lesions

The goal of every breast ultrasound examination is to disclose any focal abnormality that is present and, if possible, make an analytic interpretation of the lesion. The hallmark of a focal sonographic lesion is a disruption of normal breast anatomy, known also as an "architectural distortion."

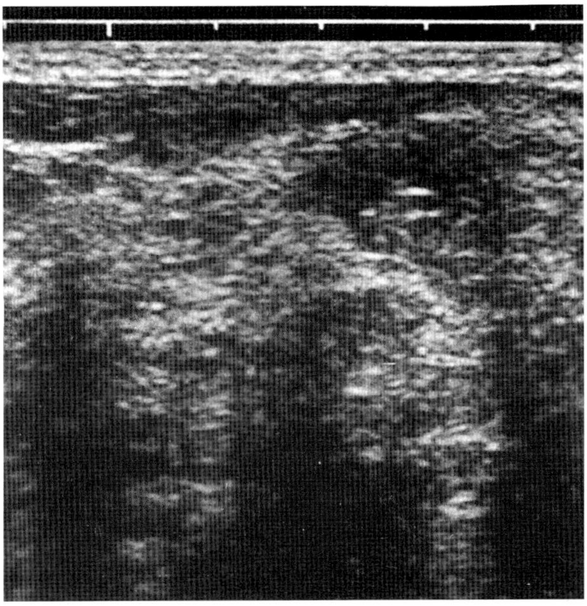

Fig. 4.**7** Acoustic shadowing makes the lower central portion of this sonogram very difficult to read

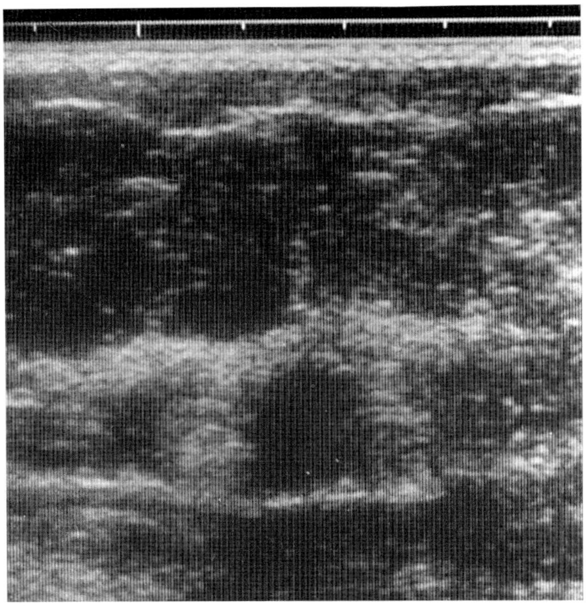

Fig. 4.**8** Readability is seriously limited by strongly attenuating areas

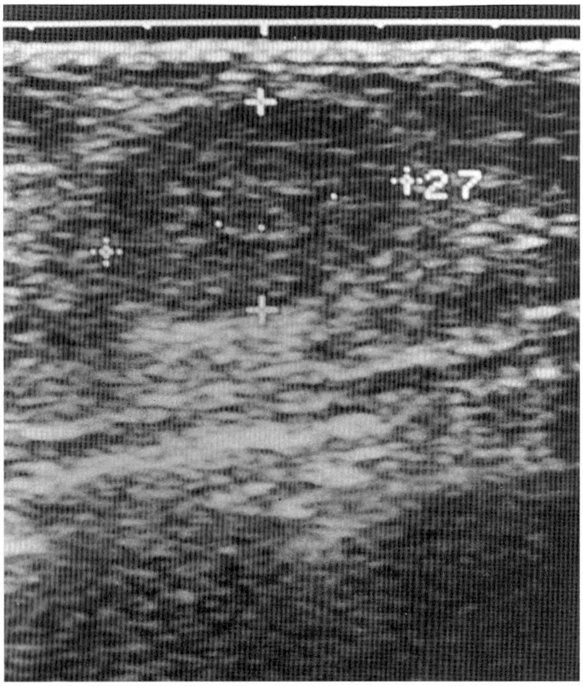

a

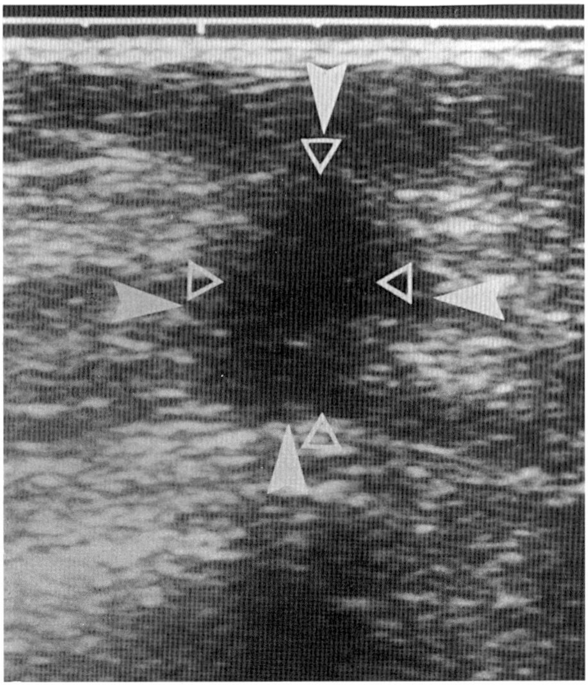

b

Fig. 4.**9** Differences in the margins of breast masses
a Fibroadenoma with sharp, smooth margins. It is easy to position measuring cursors at the periphery of the mass
b Carcinoma with indistinct margins. The boundaries of the mass are difficult to discern (▽ or ▼)

Focal lesions should be measured in three planes whenever possible. Generally this is easily done with benign lesions, which typically have smooth, sharply defined margins (Fig. 4.**9a**). But with carcinoma, it is often difficult to position the measuring cursors accurately, as it may be unclear where the lesion stops and the surrounding tissue response begins (Fig. 4.**9b**). The technique for interpreting and describing the various analytic criteria is discussed in chapter 5.

Infiltration

On detecting a focal sonographic lesion, the examiner should attempt to define its relationship to adjacent structures such as the skin, pectoral muscle, and fascia. Preoperative awareness of infiltrating disease can significantly influence management.

Aspirations

Following the aspirations of a cyst, the volume and color of the aspirate are noted on the report. The aspiration of solid lesions and preoperative needle or wire localization is also indicated.

Calcification Correlates

See chapter 6, p. 184ff.

Lymph Node Status

Ultrasound examination of the lymphatic drainage of the breast is indicated whenever a palpable breast mass has been detected or an intramammary malignancy has been found. The infraclavicular and supraclavicular regions are of particular interest in the search for recurrent or metastatic disease. Scans of these regions will frequently disclose close proximity of the tumor to major blood vessels.

Sonographic Diagnosis

The diagnosis is based on the interpretation of sonographic findings. The implications that may be drawn depend on the experience of the examiner. Highest priority is placed upon the sonographic prediction of whether the lesion is benign or malignant. We have found it useful to categorize this assessment as: no abnormality, benign, indeterminate, or malignant. It is our experience that a detailed verbal narrative is not particularly helpful. We prefer to use a standard breast ultrasound report form (Fig. 4.**10**) that follows the sequence of the examination.

Unfortunately, there is still no international consensus on standard nomenclature for the sonographic appearances of the breast.

Parenchymal pattern

Homogeneously sonodense ☐
Loosely sonodense ☐
Partially involuted ☐
Involuted ☐
Lactating ☐

Readability

Good ☐

Limited ☐
Poor ↓ ↓ ☐

Reason
Marked shadowing ☐
Local attenuation ☐

Readability of subareolar region

Yes ☐
Only on tangential scan ☐
No ☐

Other

Focal sonographic lesion

No ☐
Yes ☐
Size: mm x mm x mm
Margins: m/b
Retrotumoral acoustic effect: i/m/b
Internal echo pattern: m/b
Echogenicity: m/b
Compression (shape): i/b
Compression (internal echoes): i/b

(i=indifferent, m=malignant, b=benign)

Infiltration

Skin ☐
Pectoral fascia ☐
Pectoral muscle ☐

Aspirations

Cyst mL
Color ☐
Solid lesion ☐
Needle localization ☐

Correlation with microcalcifications

Lymph node status

(number and size)
Axillary ☐
Infraclavicular ☐
Supraclavicular ☐

Sonographic diagnosis

No abnormality ☐
Benign ☐
Indeterminate ☐
Malignant ☐

Date ....

Examiner ....

Fig. 4.**10** Breast ultrasound report form used at the Heidelberg University Gynecological Clinic

5 Analytic Criteria for the Interpretation of Focal Sonographic Lesions

(Schematic diagram, Figure 5.**1**)

The sine qua non for an acceptable sonographic breast diagnosis is the detection of focal abnormalities and their analysis. In the past, many groups of workers have attempted to define reliable sonographic criteria for malignancy and benignancy (Gros et al. 1975, Kobayashi 1975, Baum 1977, Kelly-Fry et al. 1977, Pluygers et al. 1977, Kossoff 1977, Rubin et al. 1979, Kasumi et al. 1982). An analytic criterion should satisfy two main requirements:

1. It should describe the finding as accurately as possible.
2. It should differentiate as sharply as possible between benign and malignant processes.

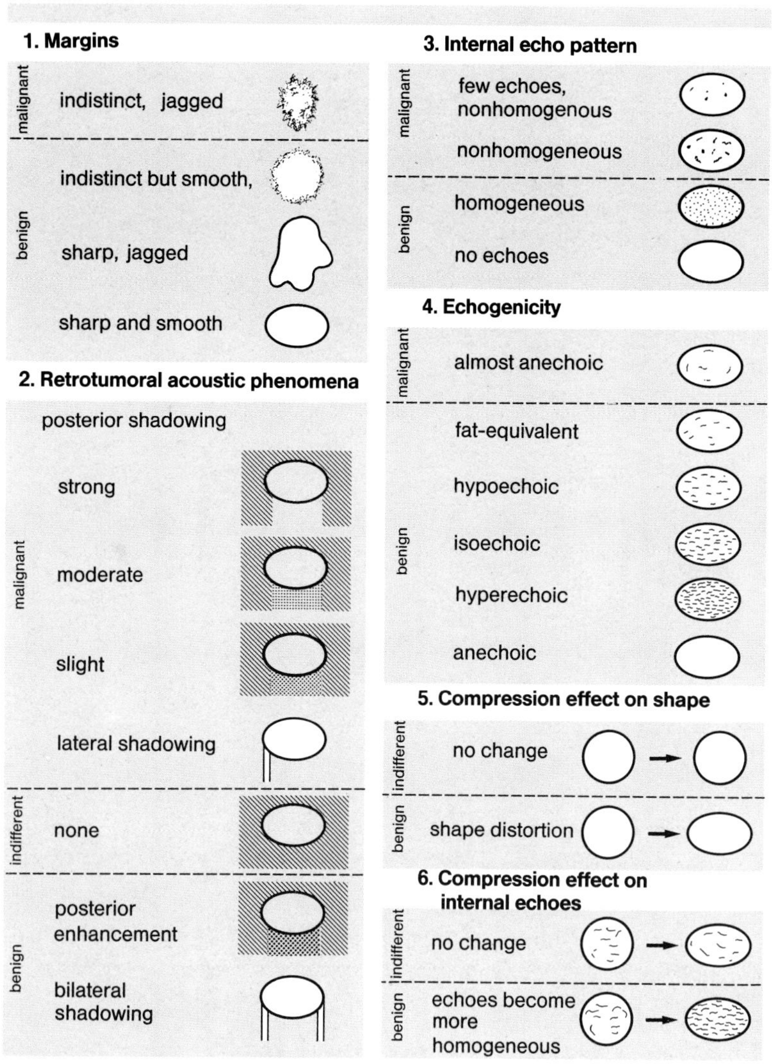

Fig. 5.**1** Schematic representation of our analytic criteria for the interpretation of breast sonograms

Most examiners have based their criteria on histologic diagnoses, assigning acoustic phenomena to different types of carcinoma and to the most commonly encountered benign lesions such as cysts and fibroadenomas. However, we have tailored our analytic criteria toward predicting the benignancy or malignancy of a focal sonographic lesion with the highest possible confidence, regardless of the specific histologic diagnosis (Leucht et al. 1988). The following criteria have proved effective in the analytic interpretation of a focal sonographic abnormality.

Margins

Part of evaluating the margins of a focal lesion is to assess its demarcation with respect to surrounding tissues. In this respect the margins may be described as sharp or indistinct. It is also important to assess the contour of the lesion, which may be smooth or jagged. Thus, the margins of a sonographic lesion can be characterized in any of four ways: 1) indistinct and jagged, 2) indistinct but smooth, 3) sharp and jagged, or 4) sharp and smooth. These patterns are illustrated in Figure 5.**2**. Analysis of our examinations has shown that

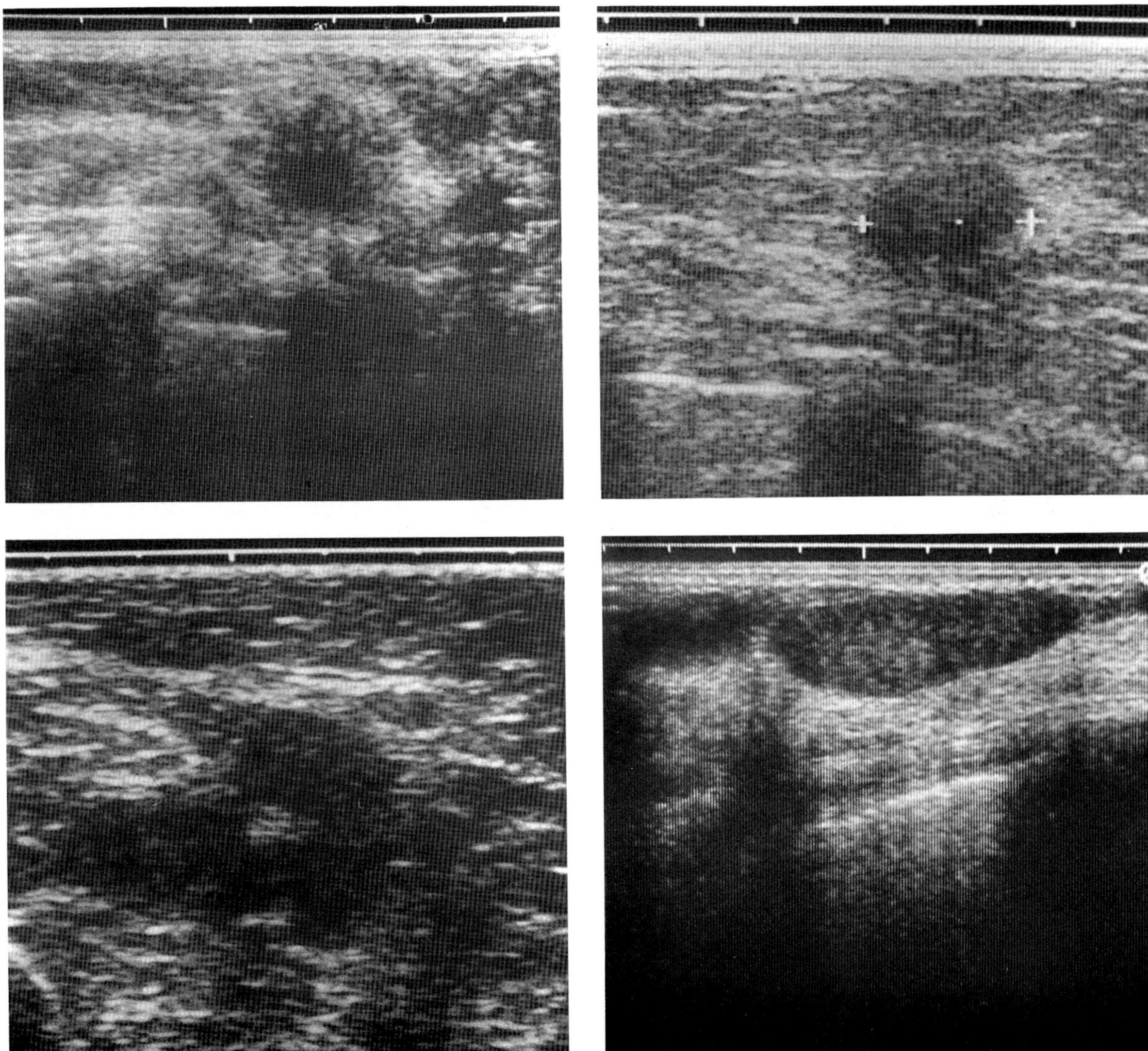

Fig. 5.**2** Margins of breast masses
a Indistinct and jagged; solid carcinoma, 20×15 mm – **b** Indistinct but smooth; solid carcinoma (+...+), 17×15 mm – **c** Sharp and jagged; sudoriparous abscess, 38×28 mm – **d** Sharp and smooth; fibroadenoma, 42×18 mm

only the "indistinct, jagged" pattern signifies a malignant tumor with a reasonably high degree of confidence. the other three patterns are more commonly associated with benign processes.

Retrotumoral Acoustic Phenomena

Any of three acoustic phenomena may be noted deep to a focal sonographic lesion. There can be posterior shadowing, posterior enhancement, or no change in the echoes compared to their surroundings. In our analytic scheme, we have arranged the retrotumoral phenomena in the order of decreasing prognostic importance in terms of malignant potential (see Fig. 5.**1**). Signs suggesting a malignant process are strong, moderate, or slight posterior shadowing or unilateral shadowing phenomena. The degree of shadowing is judged by the "blackness" of the shadow, as sug-

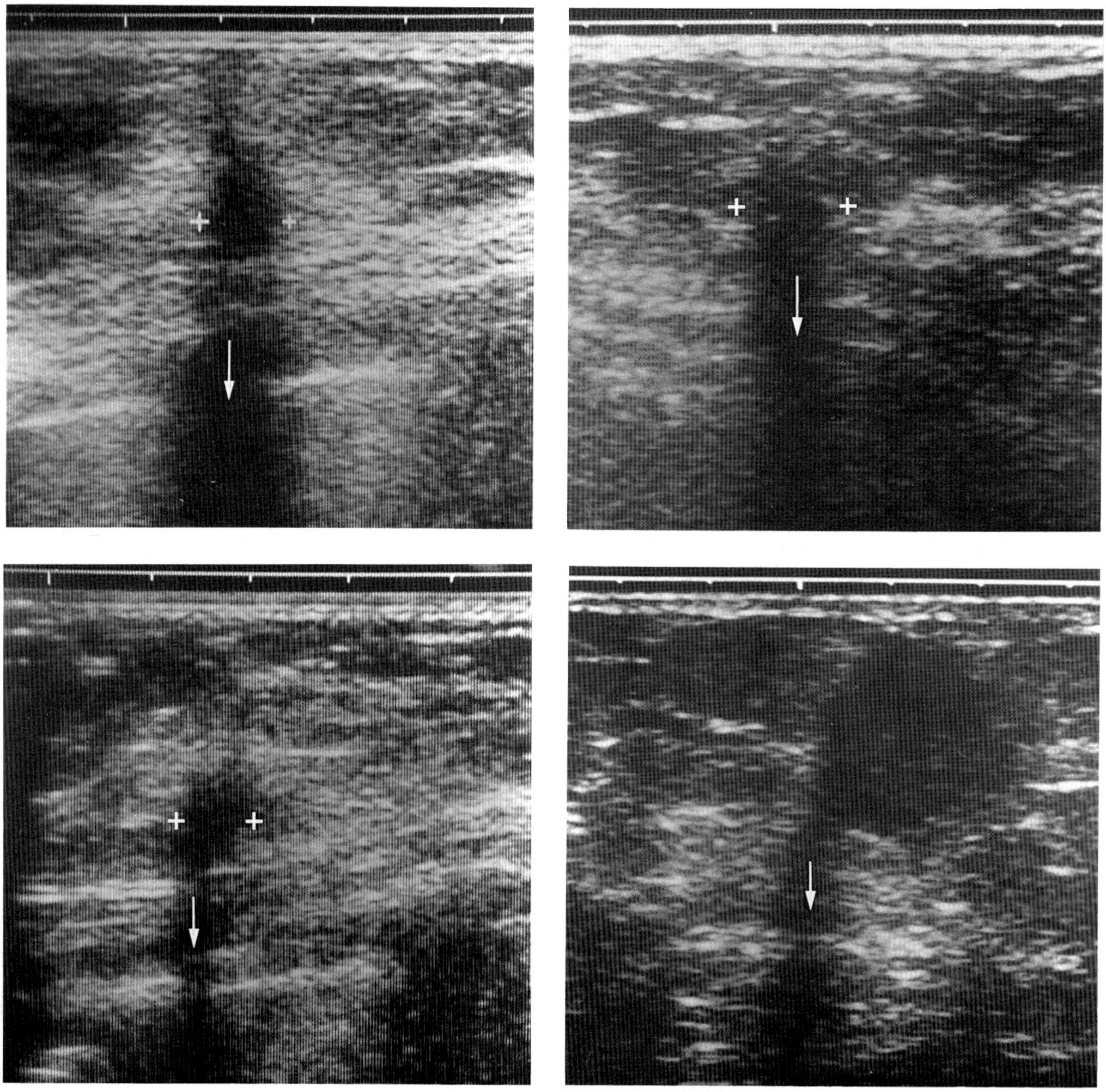

a b c d

gested by Harper et al. (1983), and not by the shadow width. A true posterior shadow can be seen on two different scan planes when tissue compression is applied. Unaltered echoes are not useful for predicting benignancy or malignancy, as they are seen with about equal frequency in both types of lesion. Posterior enhancement and bilateral shadowing phenomena are suggestive of benignancy. Examples are shown in Fig. 5.3.

Areas of acoustic shadowing or enhancement that do not originate from focal sonographic lesions have a different prognostic significance and are discussed in the appendix to this chapter (p. 29).

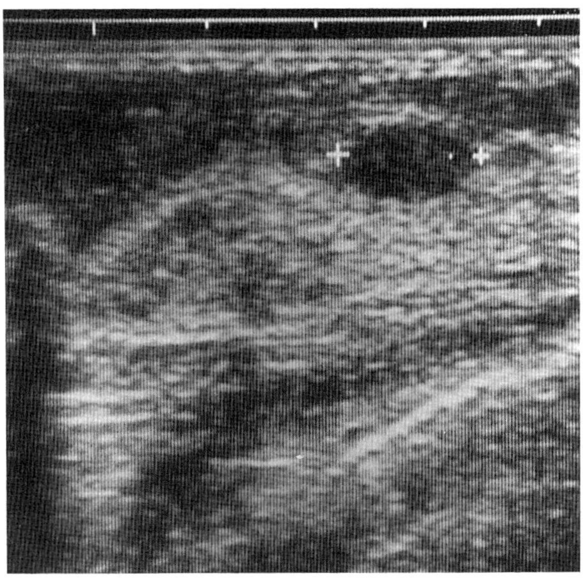
e

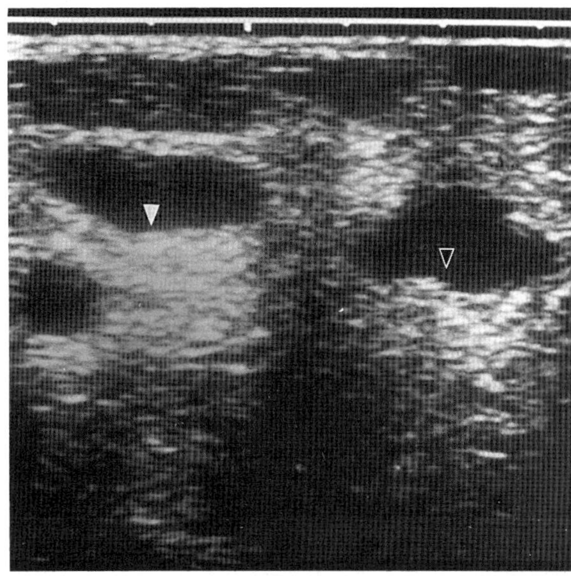
f

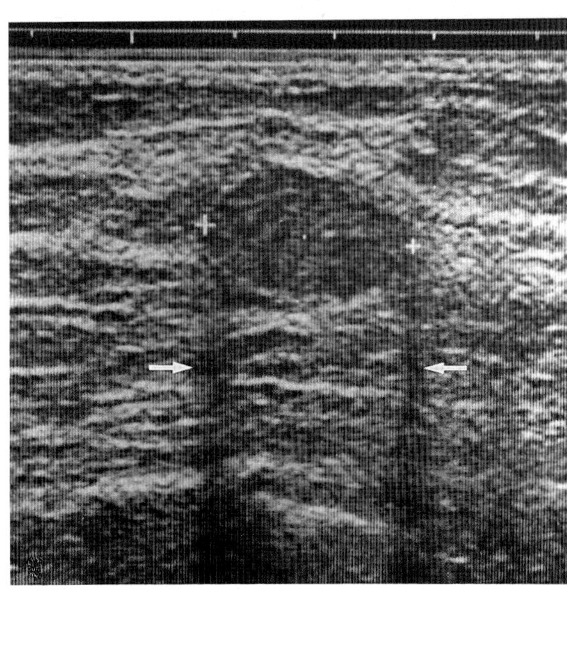
g

△
◁ Fig. 5.**3** Retrotumoral acoustic phenomena
a Strong posterior shadowing (arrow); scirrhous carcinoma (+...+), 10×10 mm
b Moderate posterior shadowing (arrow); infiltrating ductal carcinoma (+...+), 8×8 mm
c Slight posterior shadowing (arrow); adenoid tubular carcinoma (+...+), 8×9 mm
d Unilateral shadowing (arrow); infiltrating ductal carcinoma, 22×20 mm
e Unchanged echoes; pericanalicular fibroadenoma (+...+), 13×19 mm
f Posterior enhancement (▼ strong, ▽ slight); cysts, approx. 20×10 mm
g Bilateral shadowing (arrows); fibroadenoma (+...+), 20×12 mm

Internal Echo Pattern

Internal echo pattern refers to the "texture" or arrangement of echoes within a focal sonographic lesion. A nonhomogeneous arrangement with few echoes, or even more, is suspicious for malignancy. A homogeneous internal echo pattern like that commonly seen in fibroadenoma, or the absence of internal echoes in the case of a cyst, is more characteristic of a benign process (Fig. 5.**4**).

Echogenicity

The echogenicity of a focal lesion is assessed in relation to the echo characteristics of adjacent tissues. The various grades of echogenicity are stated in reference to known structures, i.e., fat and glandular structures.

If a focal lesion appears less echogenic than fat, it is described as "almost anechoic." If it ap-

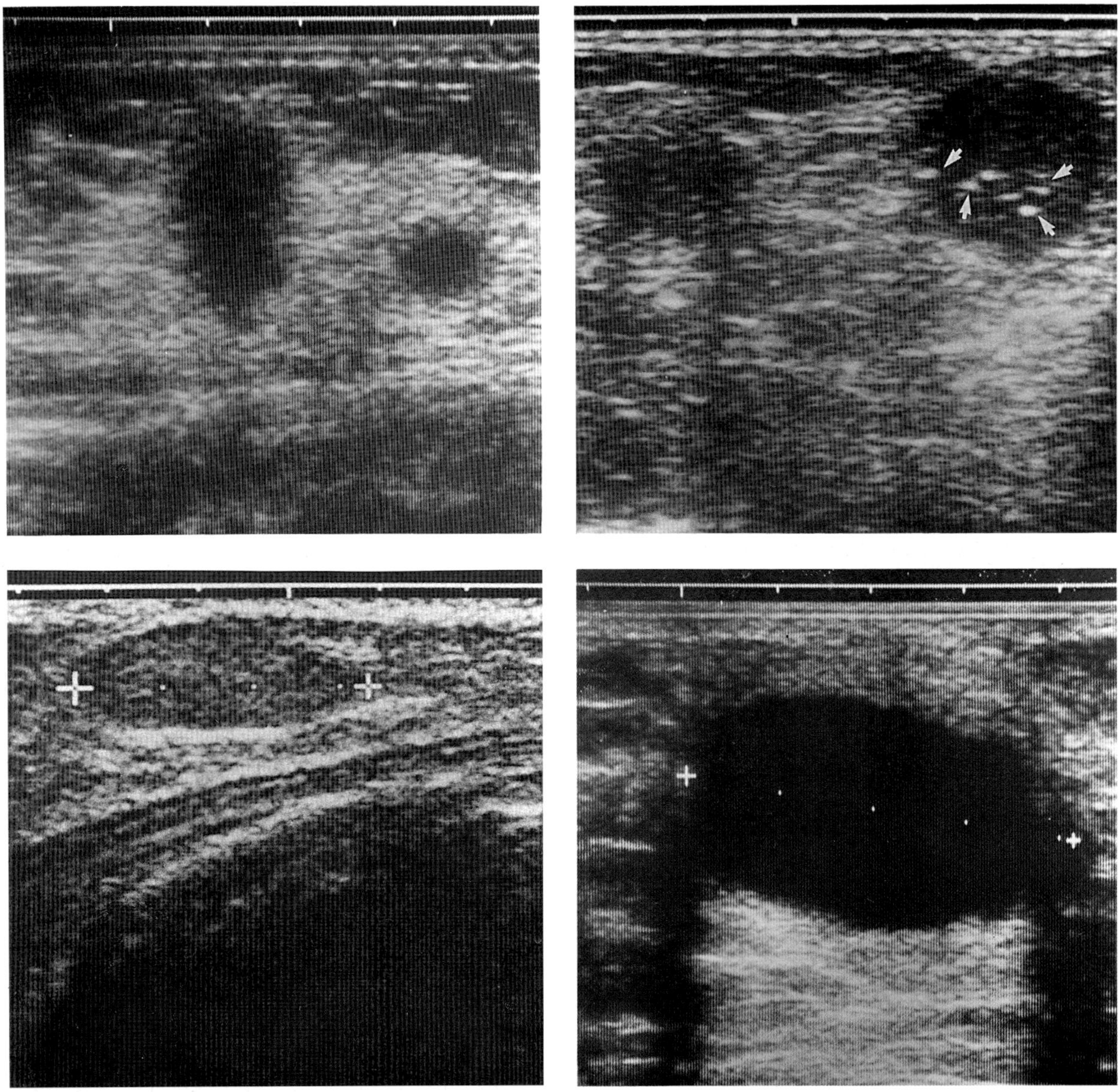

a b c d

Fig. 5.**4** Internal echo pattern
a Few internal echoes, nonhomogeneous; solid multicentric carcinoma
b Nonhomogeneous (echoes more numerous) (arrows); solid carcinoma, 20×20 mm
c Homogeneous; pericanalicular fibroadenoma (+...+), 30×13 mm
d No internal echoes; solitary cyst (+...+), 42×22 mm

pears to have the same echogenicity as fat, it is described as "fat-equivalent." A "hypoechoic" focal lesion is less echogenic than the glandular structures but more echogenic than fat. "Isoechoic" closely approximates the echogenicity of the glandular structures, while "hyperechoic" is used when the focal lesion appears brighter than the surrounding glandular tissue. "Anechoic" is the hallmark of a cystic mass. Several grades of echogenicity are illustrated in Fig. 5.**5**. Malignant tumors usually appear almost anechoic. Fat-equivalent, hypoechoic, isoechoic, or hyperechoic focal lesions are usually benign. Cysts are without echoes.

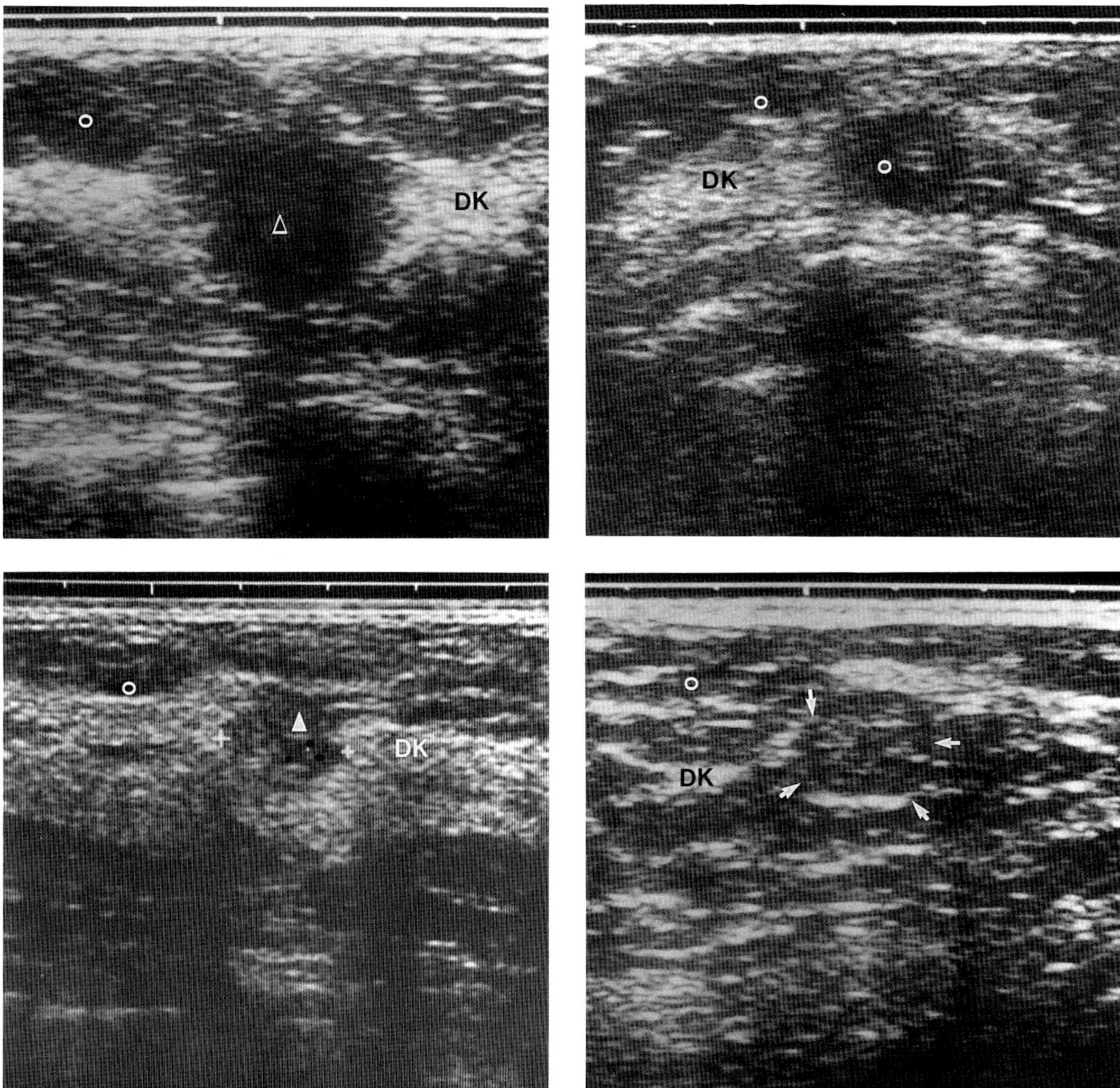

a b c d

Fig. 5.**5** Echogenicity

a Almost anechoic (△); solid carcinoma, 20×20 mm (o = fat, DK = glandular region) – **b** Fat-equivalent (o); intraductal carcinoma with necrotic foci and microcalcifications, 15×14 mm (o = fat, DK = glandular region) – **c** Hypoechoic (▲); fibrocystic disease (+...+), 12×10 mm (o = fat, DK = glandular region) – **d** Isoechoic; adenoma (arrows), 20×15 mm (o = fat, DK = glandular region)

Fig. 5.**5** e u. f ▶

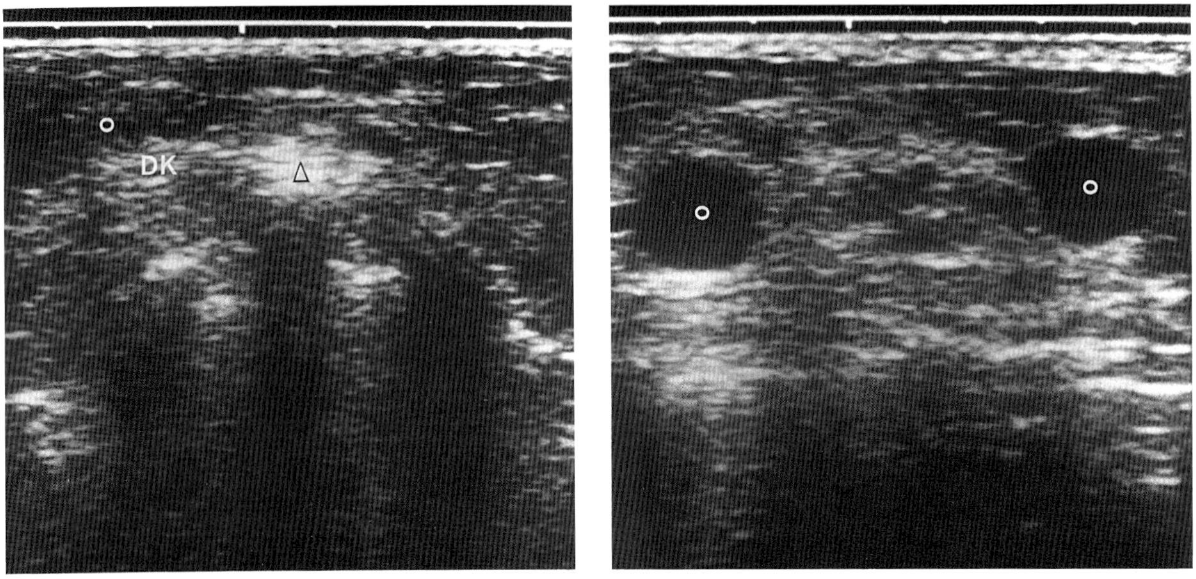

e f

Fig. 5.**5**
e Hyperechoic (△); scar following segmental breast resection (o = fat, DK = glandular region) – **f** Without echoes (anechoic); cysts (o)

Compression Effect on Shape and Internal Echo Pattern

The dynamic phase of the real-time examination is of critical importance. As tissue compression is applied with the transducer or palpating finger, the examiner watches for shape distortion of the focal mass. If shape distortion is noted, the lesion is almost certainly benign (Fig. 5.**6**).

The absence of shape distortion is not a meaningful prognostic criterion, because approximately 50% of all malignant and benign breast lesions are nondeformable. The same applies to the effect of compression on the internal echo pattern. A focal lesion whose internal echoes become more homogeneous under compression is benign in more than 90% of cases (examples in Fig. 5.**7**).

These analytic criteria and their association with benignancy or malignancy are shown schematically in Figure 5.**1**.

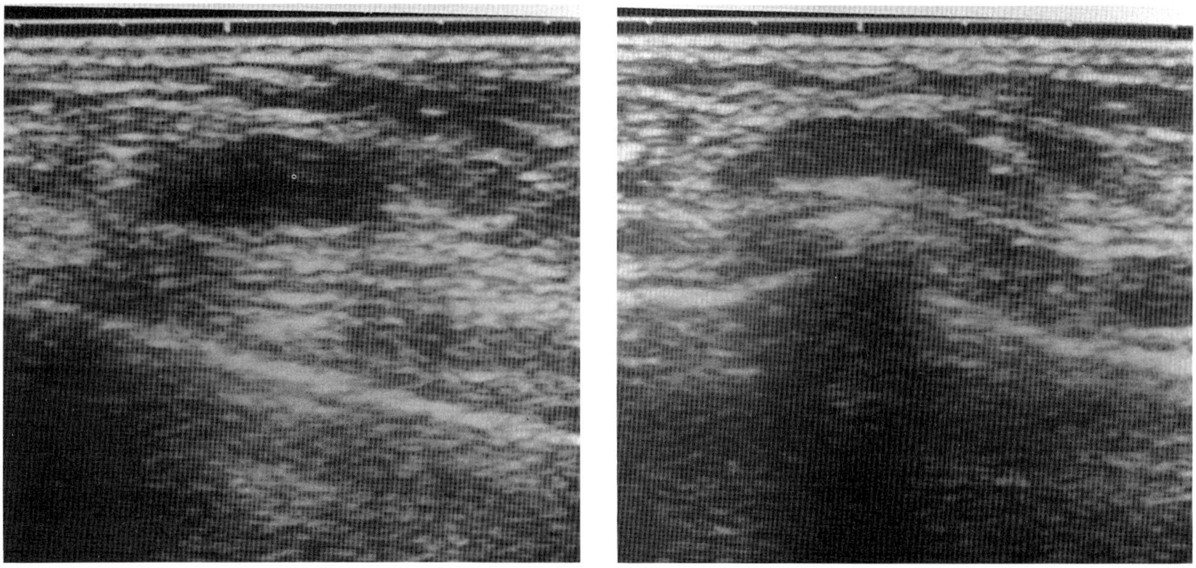

a b

Fig. 5.**6** Effect of compression on shape
a Focal sonographic lesion without significant compression (lipoma)
b Same lesion with compression. There is shape distortion, but the internal echo pattern is unchanged

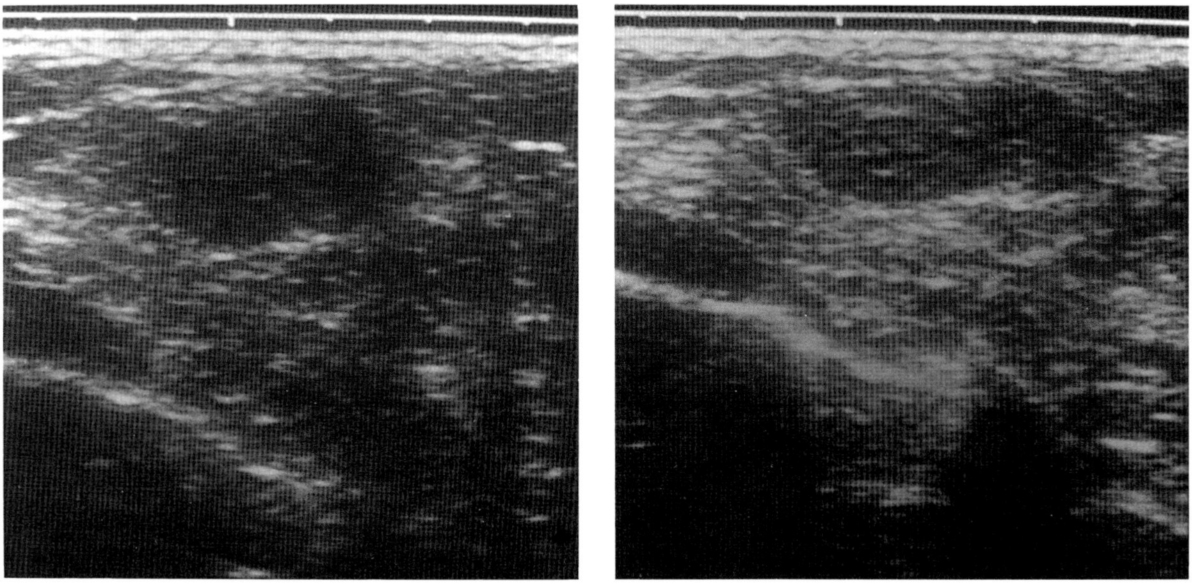

a b

Fig. 5.**7** Effect of compression on internal echo pattern
a Focal sonographic lesion without significant compression (fibroadenoma)
b Same lesion with compression, which produces a more homogeneous internal echo pattern

L/T Ratio

(Ratio of longitudinal to transverse lesion diameter)

The L/T ratio may provide a useful new criterion for evaluating focal breast masses. Preliminary studies indicate that a lesion with a greater longitudinal diameter (L/T ratio > 1) is more likely to be malignant than benign. A greater transverse diameter (L/T ratio < 1) is more characteristic of a benign process (Figs. 5.**8**, 5.**9**).

In making a diagnosis, we do not consider it worthwhile to develop a scoring system from our analytic criteria, or to attempt to add up the criteria on a benignancy–malignancy scale. We believe that the diagnosis must ultimately be based on all of the criteria and on a measure of intuition (Gross 1988). A detailed numerical analysis of our diagnostic criteria has already been published (Leucht et al. 1988).

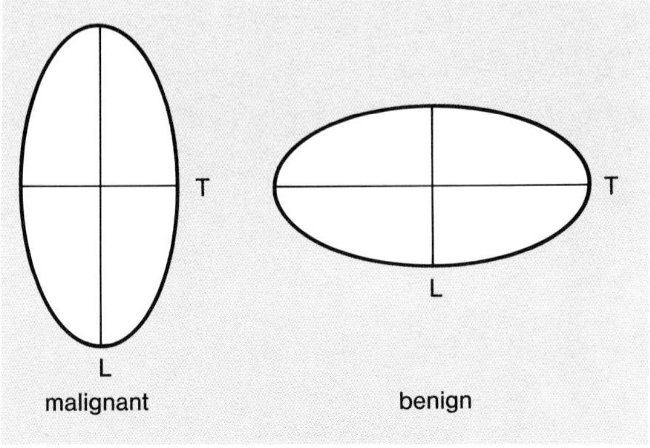

Fig. 5.**8** Schematic representation of the L/T ratio

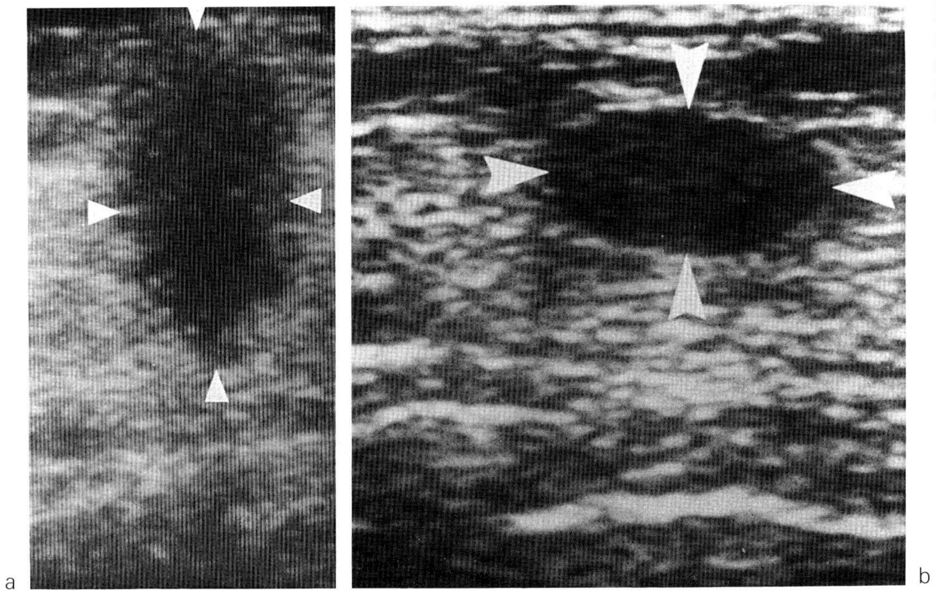

Fig. 5.**9** L/T ratios of different tumors
a L/T ratio > 1 (carcinoma)
b L/T ratio < 1 (fibroadenoma)

Appendix: Shadowing Not Associated with Focal Lesions

Unfortunately, acoustic shadows occur not just "behind" malignant tumors (Fig. 5.**3**), but also in association with other structures such as the Cooper ligaments (Figs. 3.**5–7**), calcifications (Figs. 5.**10**, 5.**11**), scars, fibrosed tissue (Figs. 5.**12**, 5.**13**), and strongly attenuating materials that block sound transmission, such as foreign bodies (p. 173) and air insufflated after cyst aspiration (Fig. 5.**14**). A knowledge of these sources of acoustic shadowing is essential for the interpretation of focal abnormalities. From the standpoint of differential diagnosis, it is important to consider whether an acoustic shadow originates from a focal sonographic lesion or represents an area that cannot be construed as a true focal lesion. An important prognostic consideration, moreover, is whether a shadow originates from a hypoechoic or hyperechoic area. Shadowing behind hypoechoic foci is more likely to signify a malignancy than shadowing behind hyperechoic features such as macrocalcifications or scar fibrosis.

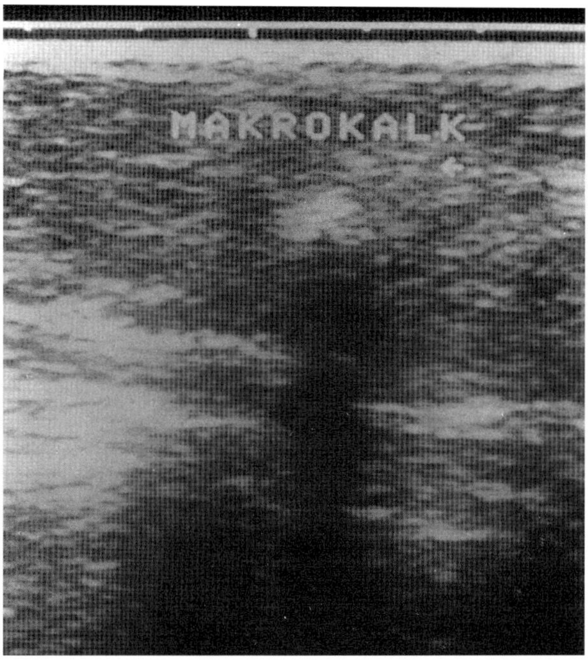

Fig. 5.**10** Hyperechoic area with posterior shadowing. Large calcification

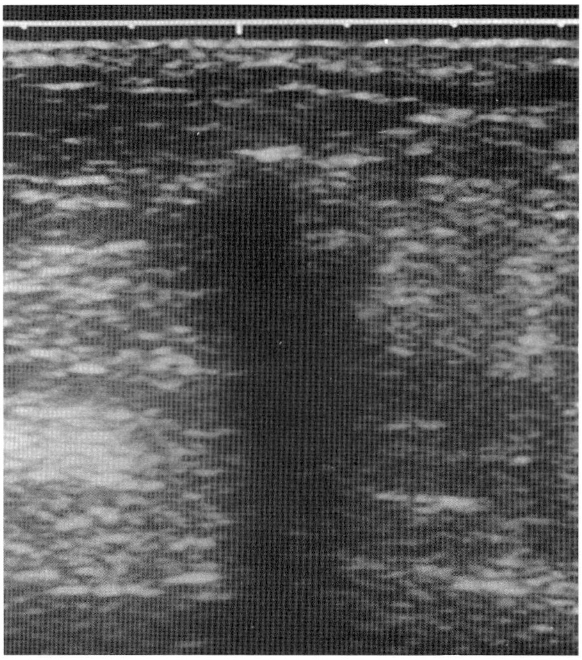

Fig. 5.**11** Marked shadowing not associated with a true focal lesion. Only X-ray mammography, by demonstrating a calcification at this site, can clarify the differential diagnosis

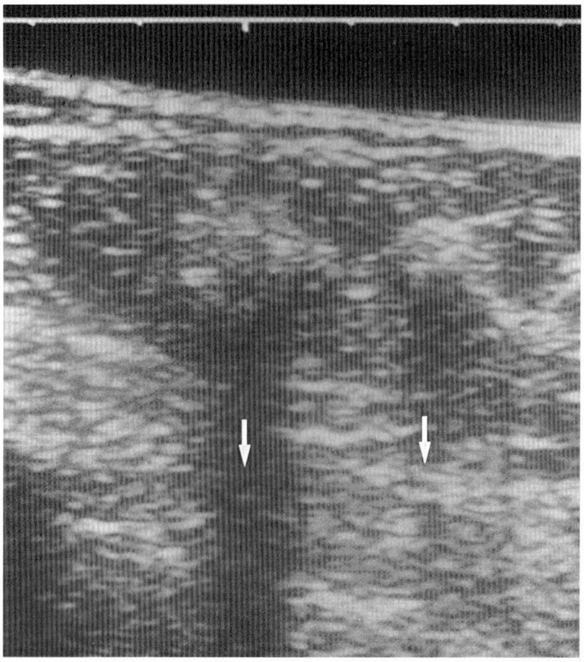

Fig. 5.**12** Center of the image: strong acoustic shadowing (arrow) behind a hyperechoic area (cutaneous and subcutaneous fibrosis). Right side of image: faint shadowing (arrow) below a point of ligament intersection (sonogram with standoff)

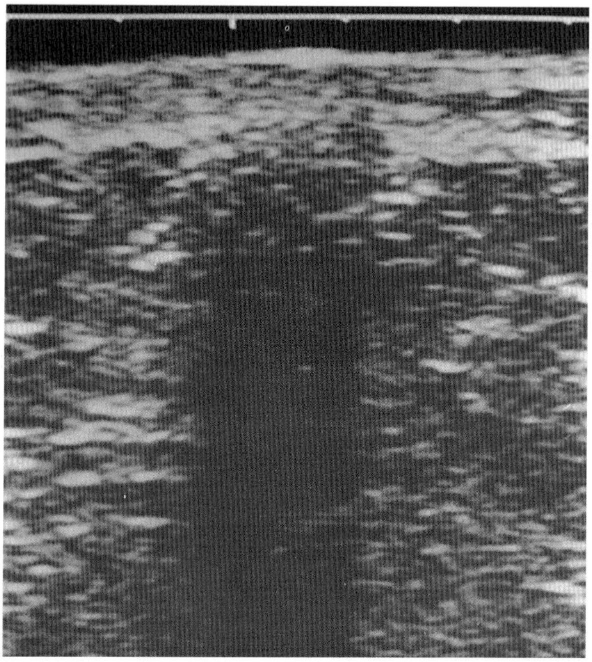

Fig. 5.**13** Sharply marginated shadow not associated with a focal lesion. Older foci of fat necrosis (sonogram with standoff)

a 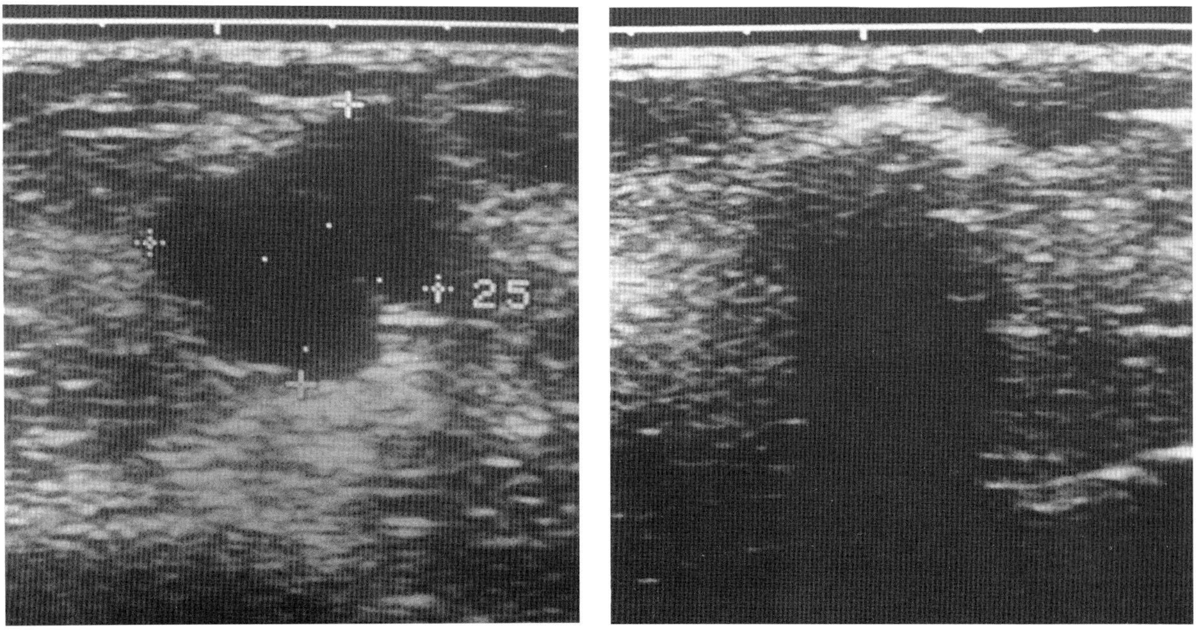 b

Fig. 5.**14** Iatrogenic shadowing
a Cyst with somewhat irregular contour
b Same cyst following aspiration of 4 mL clear fluid and insufflation of 4 mL air. Complete shadowing is seen deep to the hyperechoic air crescent

References

Baum, G.: Ultrasound mammography. Radiology 122 (1977) 199

Bloomberg, T. J., R. C. Chivers, J. L. Price: Real-time ultrasonic characteristics of the breast. Clin. Radiol. 35 (1984) 21

Cole-Beuglet, C. M., R. A. Beique: Continuous ultrasound B-scanning of palpable breast masses. Radiology 117 (1975) 123

Cole-Beuglet, C., G. Schneck, A. B. Kurtz, A. S. Patchefsky, B. B. Goldberg: Ultrasound mammography for the augmented breast. Radiology 146 (1983) 737

Dodd, G. D.: Present status of thermography, ultrasound and mammography in breast cancer detection. Cancer (Philad.) 39 (1977) 2796

Fields, S. I.: Ultrasound mammographic-histopathologic correlation. Ultrason. Imag. 2 (1980) 150

Friedrich, M.: Ultraschalluntersuchung der Brust – Erfahrungen mit einem hochauflösenden „Real-time"-Gerät. Radiologe 20 (1980) 209

Gros, Ch., G. Dale, B. Gairard, P. Hachnel: Échographie des épithéliomas mammaires avant et après traitement. J. Radiol. Électrol. 56, Suppl. 1 (1975) 318

Gross, R.: Intuition. Dtsch. Ärztebl. 85 (1988) 22

Guyer, P. B., K. C. Dewburry: Ultrasound of the breast in the symptomatic and x-ray dense breast. Clin. Radiol. 36 (1985) 69

Hackelöer, B. J., V. Duda, G. Lauth: Ultraschall-Mammographie: Methoden, Ergebnisse, diagnostische Strategien. Springer, Berlin 1986

Harper, P. A., E. Kelly-Fry, J. S. Noe, J. R. Bies, V. P. Jackson: Ultrasound in the evaluation of solid breast masses. Radiology 146 (1983) 731

Hayashi, N., N. Tamaki, Y. Yonekura, M. Senda, K. Yamamoto, K. Torizuka: Real-time sonography of palpable breast masses. Brit. J. Radiol. 58 (1985) 611

Jackson, V. P., P. A. Rothschild, D. L. Kreipke, J. T. Mail, R. W. Holden: The spectrum of sonographic findings of fibroadenoma of the breast. Invest. Radiol. 21 (1986) 34

Jellins, J., G. Kossoff, T. S. Reeve, B. B. Barraclough: Ultrasonic gray-scale visualization of breast disease. Ultrasound Med. Biol. 1 (1975) 393

Jellins, J., T. S. Reeve, J. Croll, G. Kossoff: Results of breast echographic examination in Sydney, Australia, 1972–1979. Semin. Ultrasound 3 (1982) 58

Kasumi, F., A. Fukami, K. Kuno, T. Kajitani: Characteristic echographic features of circumscribed cancer. Ultrasound Med. Biol. 8 (1982) 369

Kelly-Fry, E., F. J. Fry, G. W. Gardner: Recommendations for widespread application of examination of the female breast. Ultrasound Med. Biol. 3 (1977) 1085

Kelly-Fry, E.: Breast cancer screening for younger United States women. In Jellins, J., T. Kobayashi: Ultrasonic Examinations of the Breast. Wiley, New York 1983

Kobayashi, T., T. Takatani, N. Hattori, K. Kimura: Differential diagnosis of breast tumors. The sensitivity grades method of ultrasonotomography and clinical evaluation of its diagnostic accuracy. Cancer (Philad.) 33 (1974) 940

Kobayashi, T.: Review – ultrasonic diagnosis of breast cancer. Ultrasound Med. Biol. 1 (1975) 383

Kobayashi, T.: Gray scale echography for breast cancer. Radiology 122 (1977) 207

Kossoff, G.: Improved techniques in ultrasound cross sectional echography. Ultrasonics 10 (1972) 221

Kossoff, G.: Classification of soft tissues by grey-scale echography. Ultrasound Med. Biol. 3 (1977) 1869

Leucht, W. D. Rabe, R. Boos, D. von Fournier, W. Schmidt: Stellenwert der Real-time-Echomammographie bei röntgenmammographisch unklaren Befunden. In Judmaier, G., H. Frommhold, A. Kratochwil: Ultraschalldiagnostik 84. Thieme, Stuttgart 1985

Leucht, W., D. von Fournier, D. Rabe, K. D. Humbert, W. Kühn, W. Schmidt: Mikrokalk in der Mammasonographie – Darstellung und Bewertung. Ultraschall Klin. Prax. 2 (1987) 195

Leucht, W., D. Rabe: Sonographic findings following conservative surgery and irradiation for breast carcinoma. Ultrasound Med. Biol. 14, Suppl. 1, (1988) 27

Leucht, W., D. Rabe, W. Schmidt: Beurteilungskriterien für die Mammasonographie. Geburtsh. u. Frauenheilk. 48 (1988) 78

Pluygers, E., M. Rombaut, M. Beauduin, B. Hendrickx, F. Devergnies, A. Picron, G. Tomignaux: Possibilities, results and indications of breast echography. J. belge Radiol. 60 (1977) 181

Rabe, D., W. Leucht, H. Schmid, W. Schmidt: Sonographische Diagnostik von Lokalrezidiven nach operativer Therapie eines Mammacarcinoms. Arch. Gynecol. 242 (1987) 342

Rubin, C., A. B. Kurtz, B. B. Goldberg, S. A. Feig, C. Cole-Beuglet: Ultrasonic mammographic parenchymal patterns. A preliminary report. Radiology 130 (1979) 515

Schneck, C. D., D. A. Lehman: Sonographic anatomy of the breast. Semin. Ultrasound 3 (1982) 13

Smallwood, J. A., P. Guyer, K. Dewburry, S. Mengatti, A. Herbert, G. T. Royle, J. Taylor: The accuracy of ultrasound in the diagnosis of breast disease. Ann. roy. Coll. Surg. Engl. 68 (1986) 19

Teubner, J., A. Müller, G. van Kaick; Echomorphologie der Brustdrüse. Radiologe 23 (1983) 97

Wagai, T., M. Tsutsumi: Mass screening of breast cancer by grey-scale serial echography. Ultrasound Med. Biol. 3 (1977) 1147

Wagai, T., M. Tsutsumi, A. Ishihara: Detection of breast cancer by grey-scale serial echography. Ultrasound Med. Biol. 3 (1977) 1143

Wild, J. J., J. M. Reid: Further pilot echographic studies on the histologic structure of tumors of the living intact human breast. Amer. J. Path. 28 (1952) 839

(This reference list includes all publications cited in the text as well as a selection of publications for further reading.)

6 Indications for Breast Ultrasound

The currently recognized indications for breast sonography are listed in Table 6.**1**. Although most examiners stress that the essential role of breast ultrasound is in the differentiation of cystic and solid masses, it is our experience that the range of indications extends well beyond this capacity. In the sections that follow, we shall present illustrative cases arranged according to the indications that prompted breast sonography.

Table 6.**1** Indications for breast ultrasound

Palpable breast mass
Radiographically dense breast   Fibrocystic disease
Mammographically indeterminate lesion
Pregnancy and lactation

Oncologic follow-up
  After mastectomy (chest wall)
  After breast-conserving surgery (residual breast)

Postoperative follow-up   Hematomas, seromas, prostheses

Ultrasound-guided aspirations
  Cyst aspiration
  Aspiration of solid lesions
  Preoperative needle localization

Axillary lymph nodes
Microcalcifications (relative indication)

Palpable Breast Mass

Ultrasound should always be the first study in the diagnostic workup of a palpable breast mass. If a cyst is found, it can be aspirated directly under sonographic vision, and further diagnostic measures such as a cytologic analysis or pneumocystogram can follow. Solid masses necessitate further investigation in accordance with prevailing expert opinion. Guidelines for these investigations can be found in all textbooks dealing with the breast and its disorders.

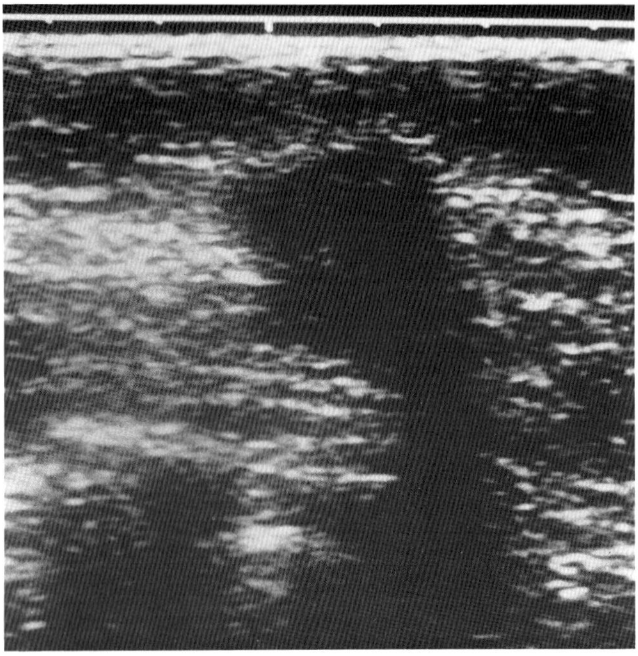

Analysis

1. **Margins**	indistinct, jagged
2. **Retrotumoral acoustic phenomena**	unilateral shadowing phenomena
3. **Internal echo pattern**	few echoes, nonhomogeneous
4. **Echogenicity**	almost anechoic
5. **Compression effect** on **shape**	no deformation
6. **Compression effect** on **internal echoes**	no change

History

The 59-year-old woman had noticed a lump in the upper outer quadrant of her right breast 1 month before. She had a known history of chronic fibrocystic breast disease with a marked proliferative tendency.

Palpable Findings

Firm, mobile, subareolar mass extending into the upper outer quadrant of the right breast, with slight overlying skin retraction.

Sonography

Figure: sagittal scan over the palpable mass.

Readability: good.

Focal sonographic lesion, 20×25 mm, with no apparent infiltration of the skin or the pectoralis major muscle.

Interpretation

All the sonographic criteria suggest a malignant tumor.

Histology

Infiltrating ductal carcinoma of the right breast (pT2 pN1 MX).

History

The 61-year-old woman complained of pain in her right breast. A lump, present for 3 years, had begun to enlarge.

Palpable Findings

Firm, mass, approximately 5×6 cm, with orange-peel dimpling of the skin in the upper outer quadrant of the right breast. Two suspicious, firm lymph nodes in the right axilla.

Sonography

Figure: sagittal scan over the mass.

Readability: good.

Focal lesion, 28×22 mm, with infiltration of the skin (obvious disruption of skin line, *arrows*).

Interpretation

All sonographic criteria suggest a malignant process.

The bright central echoes are clustered microcalcifications by X-ray mammography; they are responsible for the well-defined, columnar posterior shadow. The shadowing obscures possible infiltration of the pectoral muscle.

Histology

Poorly differentiated, predominantly solid infiltrating ductal carcinoma with infiltration of the skin and extensive infiltration of the pectoral muscle. Tumor approximately 30 mm in diameter.

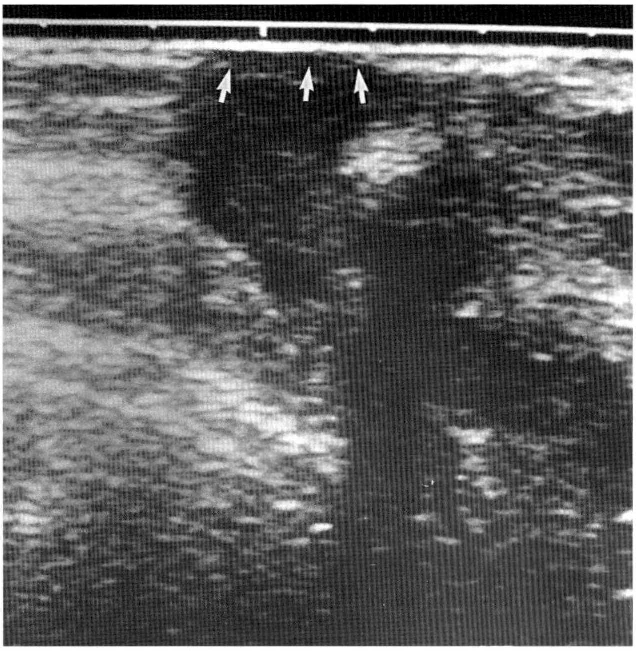

Analysis

1. **Margins**	indistinct, jagged
2. **Retrotumoral acoustic phenomena**	strong posterior shadowing
3. **Internal echo pattern**	nonhomogeneous
4. **Echogenicity**	almost anechoic
5. **Compression effect** on **shape**	no deformation
6. **Compression effect** on **internal echoes**	no change

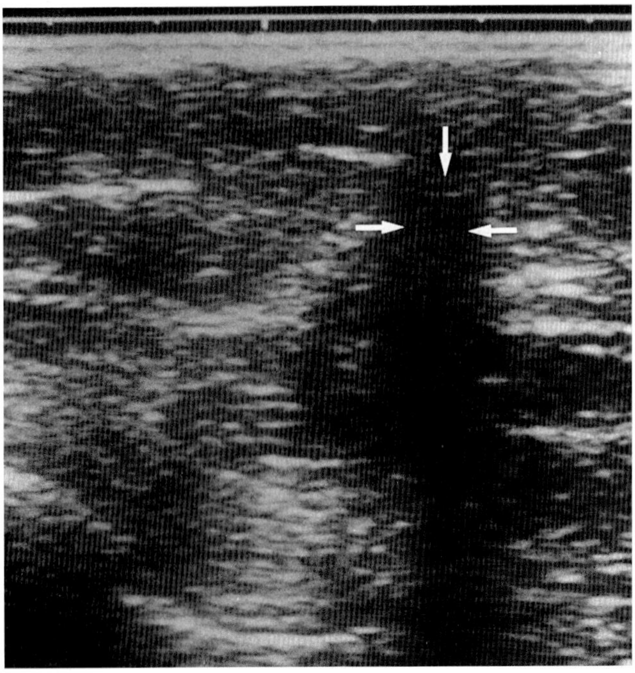

a

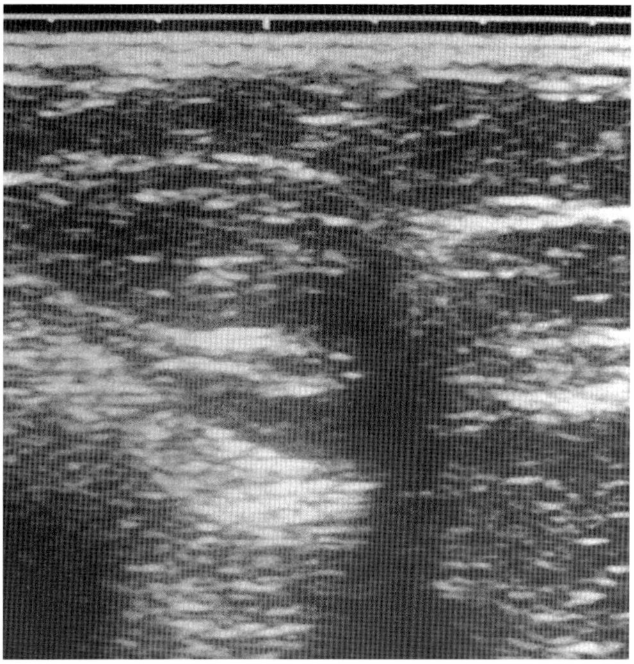

b

History

The 45-year-old woman had noted a lump in the upper outer quadrant of her right breast 1 month before.

Palpable Findings

Approximately 4 cm, firm, suspicious mass in the upper outer quadrant of the right breast with overlying skin retraction. A 2 cm mass was also palpated in the upper inner quadrant of the left breast.

Sonography

Figure **a**: right breast. Sagittal scan over the palpable mass.
Readability: good despite pronounced involution.
Focal lesion approx. 1 cm in size *(arrows)* with posterior shadowing.

Figure **b**: left breast. Sagittal scan over the palpable mass.
Readability: good despite pronounced involution.
Focal lesion, approximately 10×14 mm, with posterior shadowing.

Interpretation

Right side (**a**): Criteria 2, 3, 4, 5 and 6 are suggestive of malignancy. It is noteworthy that the roentgen and histologic tumor dimensions were greater than the sonographic dimensions. The boundaries depicted by ultrasound are probably limited to the tumor core, which casts a very dense acoustic shadow.
Left side (**b**): All analytic criteria suggest a malignant process. The sonographic picture closely resembles that on the right side.

Histology

Right side: infiltrating ductal carcinoma with some tubular elements.
Size: 25×20 mm.
Left side: infiltrating ductal carcinoma with mixed solid and tubular elements.
Size: 15×10 mm.

History

The 55 year-old woman had previously undergone a left mastectomy for breast cancer and had had several subsequent local–regional recurrences.

Palpable Findings

Follow-up disclosed a poorly circumscribed mass in the upper outer quadrant of the contralateral breast with overlying skin fixation.

Sonography

Figure: sagittal scan over the mass.

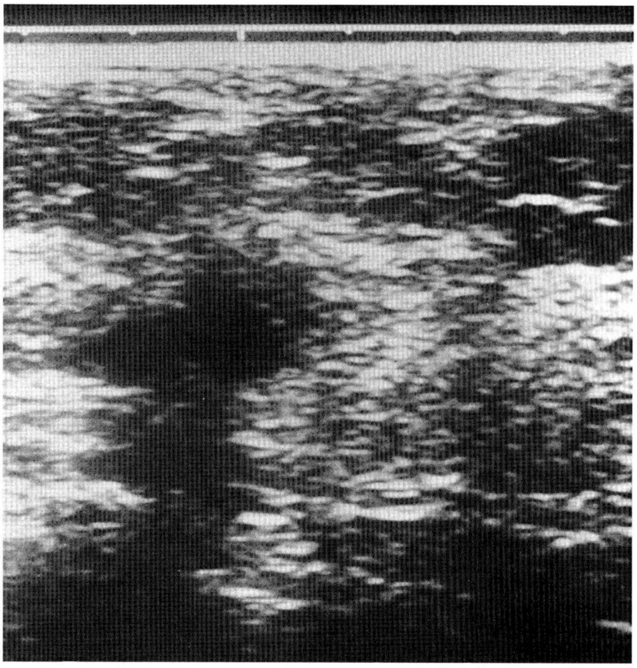

Readability: good

Focal lesion, 25×12 mm, with shadowing, near the chest wall.

Interpretation

All sonographic criteria are consistent with malignancy. The lesion is near the chest wall. The marked posterior shadowing obscures possible involvement of the pectoral fascia or muscle. Despite clinical skin fixation, there is no sonographic evidence that the subcutaneous fat or skin have been infiltrated.

Histology

Infiltrating ductal carcinoma, 30 mm, with mucinous elements and lymphatic invasion; no infiltration of the pectoral fascia or skin.

Analysis

1. **Margins**	indistinct, jagged
2. **Retrotumoral acoustic phenomena**	strong posterior shadowing
3. **Internal echo pattern**	few echoes, nonhomogeneous
4. **Echogenicity**	almost anechoic
5. **Compression effect** on **shape**	no deformation
6. **Compression effect** on **internal echoes**	no change

◁

Analysis

	a	b
1. **Margins**	indistinct but smooth	indistinct, jagged
2. **Retrotumoral acoustic phenomena**	strong posterior shadowing	strong posterior shadowing
3. **Internal echo pattern**	few echoes, nonhomogeneous	few echoes, nonhomogeneous
4. **Echogenicity**	almost anechoic	almost anechoic
5. **Compression effect** on **shape**	no deformation	no deformation
6. **Compression effect** on **echoes**	no change	no change

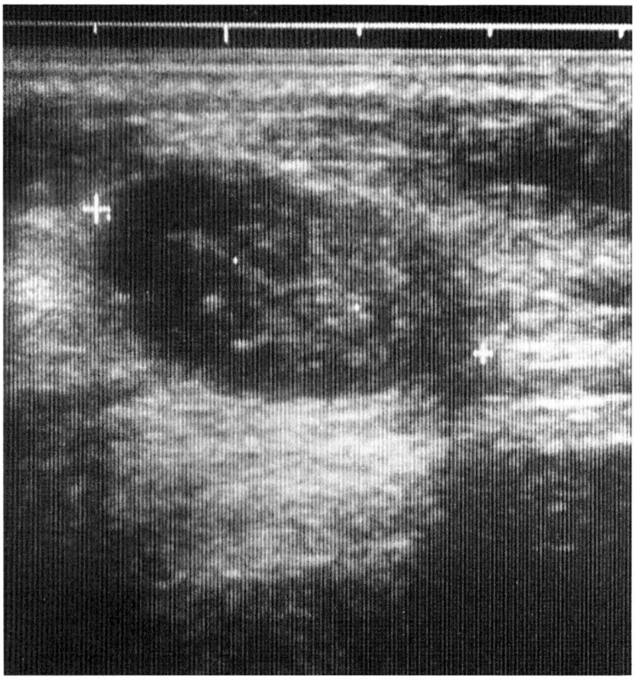

Analysis

1. Margins	indistinct but smooth
2. Retrotumoral acoustic phenomena	slight posterior shadowing
3. Internal echo pattern	nonhomogeneous
3. Echogenicity	mixed, almost anechoic to hypoechoic
5. Compression effect no **shape**	(slight) distortion
6. Compression effect on **internal echoes**	no change

History

The 79-year-old woman had noticed a lump in her right breast 3 weeks before.

Palpable Findings

Prominent, relatively soft, fixed, walnut-sized mass in the lower inner quadrant of the right breast.

Sonography

Figure: transverse scan over the palpable mass.

The palpable mass appears sonographically as a focal lesion. Acoustic coupling on the left side the image is poor because the whole transducer could not be applied flush to the breast surface.

Size: 29×18 mm.

Interpretation

Criteria 3 and 4 are consistent with a malignant lesion, while the others are more suggestive of benignancy. Closer scrutiny reveals extremely pronounced differences in tumor echogenicity. The almost anechoic crescent-shaped area in the left half of the mass contrasts sharply with the more echogenic texture of the right half. This may result from areas of tumor necrosis.

Histology

Undifferentiated breast carcinoma, 25×22 mm, with medullary structure and central necrosis.

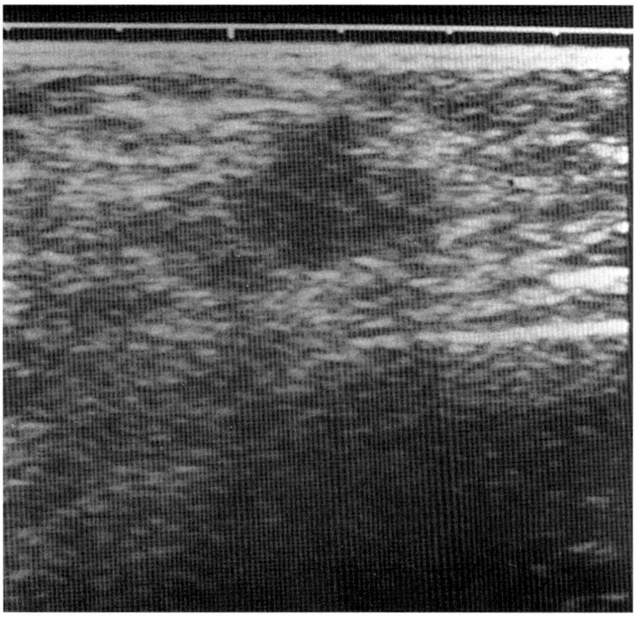

History

The 42-year-old woman noticed a lump in the left breast during her last menstruation.

Palpable Findings

Firm, hazelnut-sized mass in the lower outer quadrant of the left breast at 3 o'clock.

Sonography

Figure: transverse scan over the palpable mass.

Readability: good.

Focal sonographic lesion, 20×13 mm.

Interpretation

All sonographic criteria suggest a malignant process.

Histology

Infiltrating ductal adenocarcinoma with mixed solid and cribriform elements.
Size: 22×13 mm.

Analysis

1. **Margins**	indistinct, jagged
2. **Retrotumoral acoustic phenomena**	nonmodified echoes
3. **Internal echo pattern**	nonhomogeneous
4. **Echogenicity**	almost anechoic
5. **Compression effect** on **shape**	no deformation
6. **Compression effect** on **internal echoes**	no change

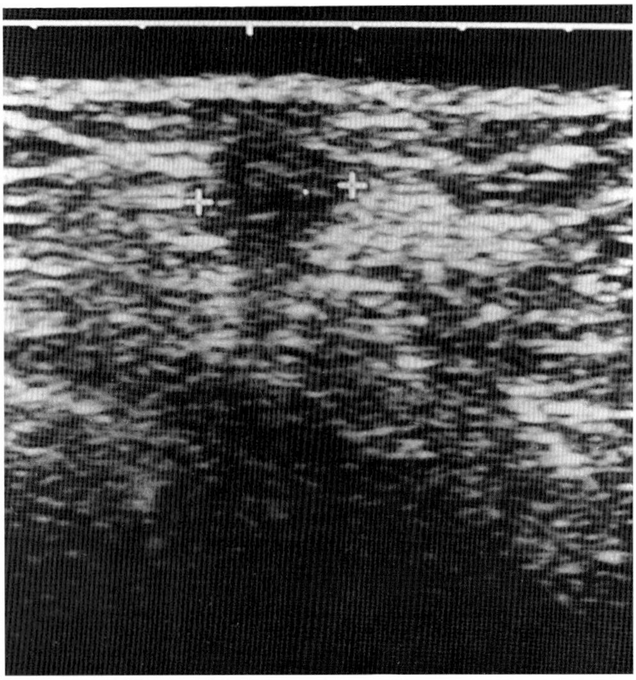

Analysis

1. Margins	indistinct, jagged
2. Retrotumoral acoustic phenomena	unchanged echoes
3. Internal echo pattern	nonhomogeneous
4. Echogenicity	fat-equivalent
5. Compression effect on **shape**	no deformation
6. Compression effect on **internal echoes**	no change

History

The 60-year-old woman had felt a lump in her left breast 1 week before.

Palpable Findings

Firm, mobile, approximately 1.5 cm mass in the lower outer quadrant of the left breast.

Sonography

(with standoff)

Figure: transverse scan over the palpable mass.

Readability: good.

Focal sonographic lesion, 14×21 mm.

Interpretation

Criteria 1, 2 and 3 imply malignancy. The deep, nodular tumor extension is noteworthy. The pectoral fasciae are not visualized, so it cannot be determined whether muscle infiltration has occurred.

Histology

Moderately differentiated infiltrating ductal carcinoma with tubular elements (pT1).

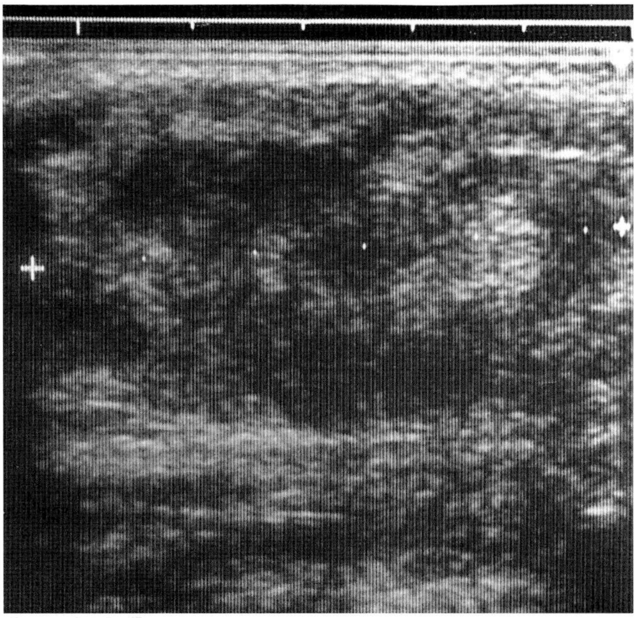

History

The 34-year-old woman noticed a rapidly enlarging lump in her right breast during pregnancy. She did not seek medical attention until after the lactation period, approximately 6 months after the lesion first appeared.

Palpable Findings

Large, firm, very suspicious mass involving both outer quadrants of the right breast, with livid discoloration of the overlying skin.

Sonography

Figure: sagittal scan over the mass.

The entire field is occupied by a tumor that has destroyed the normal glandular architecture and cannot be encompassed in one image. Analysis is not feasible.

Interpretation

The extensive architectural disarray is striking. The change cannot be described as a true focal lesion since there is no intact glandular tissue for comparison. This type of pattern is sometimes seen in severe fibrocystic disease or diffuse mastitides. When the physical findings are considered, a malignant tumor is the most likely diagnosis.

Histology

Solid medullary carcinoma!
Size: 70×90×40 mm.

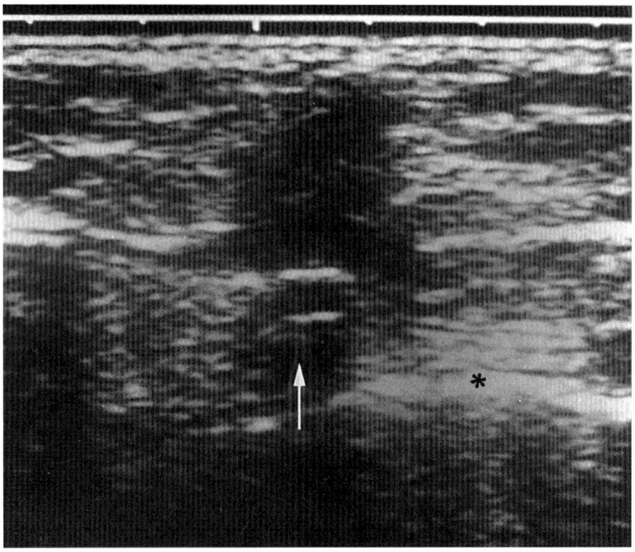

a

Analysis

1. Margins	indistinct, jagged
2. Retrotumoral acoustic phenomena	unchanged echoes
3. Internal echo pattern	few echoes, nonhomogeneous
4. Echogenicity	almost anechoic
5. Compression effect on **shape**	no deformation
6. Compression effect on **internal echoes**	no change

History

The 46-year-old woman had noticed a lump in her right breast 3 weeks before.

Palpable Findings

Firm, nodular density with skin protrusion directly adjacent to the sternum, in the lower inner quadrant of the large, ptotic right breast.

Sonography

Figure **a**: sagittal scan over the palpable mass.

Readability: good.

Focal lesion over a rib suspicious for carcinoma.

Interpretation

All sonographic criteria suggest a malignant process. The tumor lies directly over a rib *(arrow)*. Deeper infiltration is apparent on the right side of the image next ro the rib. There is infiltration of the pectoralis, but the pleura (*) is not involved.

Note: The preoperative assessment of the extent of a carcinoma in relation to adjacent structures is important for treatment planning. However, breast-conserving therapy is contraindicated from the outset in such cases regardless of the tumor size.

X-ray Mammography

Figure **b**: The mediolateral projection following three cyst aspirations with air insufflation (pneumocystography) showing no correlate to the focal sonographic lesion because the tumor is near the chest wall. The craniocaudal projection likewise fails to demonstrate the mass.

Histology

Infiltrating ductal carcinoma with predominantly solid and tubular components. Invasion of adjacent pectoral muscle.
Size: 45 mm in diameter.

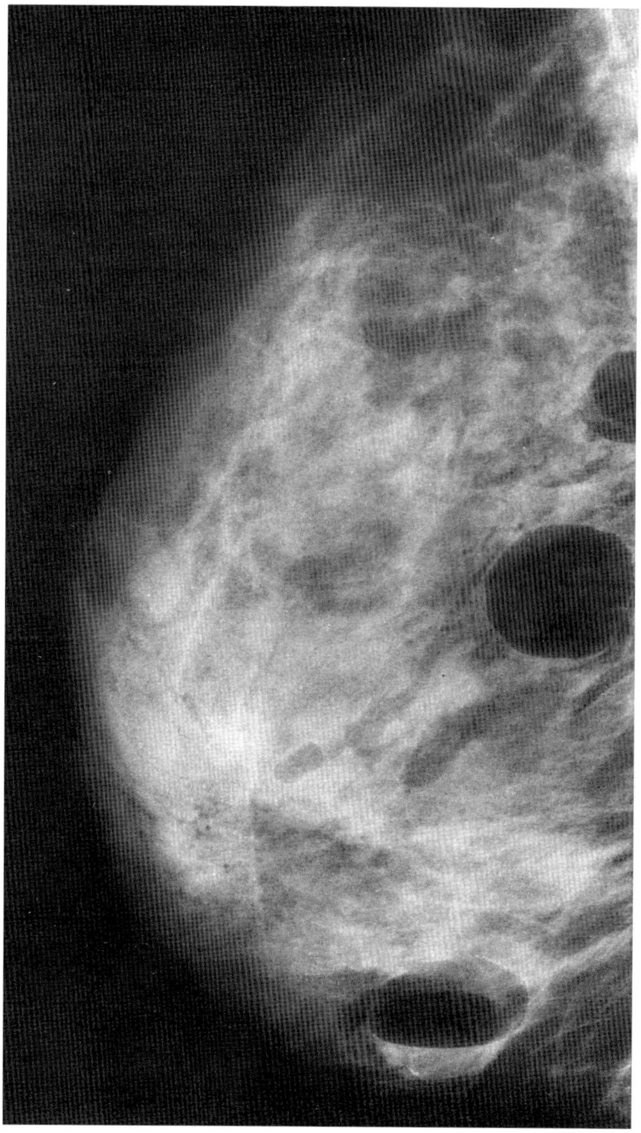

b

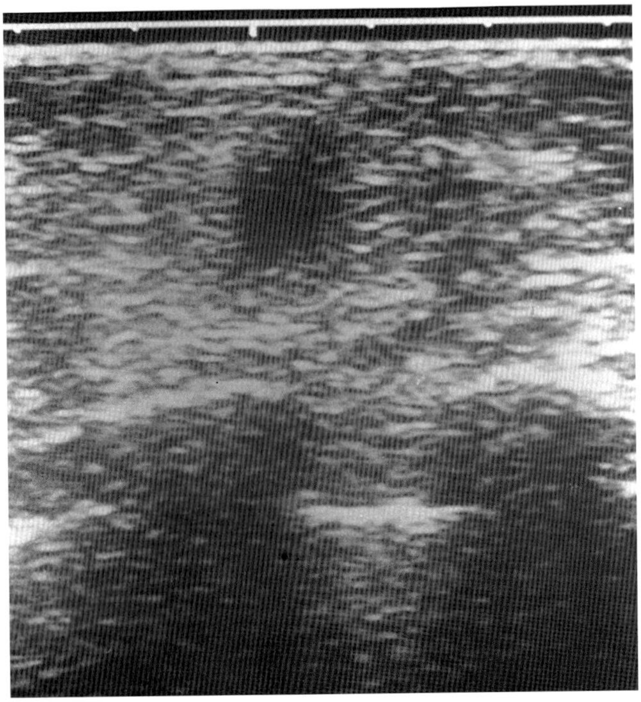

Analysis

1. Margins	indistinct, jagged
2. Retrotumoral acoustic phenomena	unchanged echoes
3. Internal echo pattern	few echoes, non-homogeneous
4. Echogenicity	almost anechoic
5. Compression effect on **shape**	no deformation
6. Compression effect on **internal echoes**	no change

History

The 59-year-old woman had a palpable mass in the lower outer quadrant of the right breast detected on routine examination.

Palpable Findings

Firm, fixed, approximately 1-cm mass in the lower outer quadrant of the right breast.

Sonography

Figure: sagittal scan over the palpable mass.

Readability: good.

Focal sonographic lesion, 16×10 mm, occurring within an area altered by fibrocystic disease.

Interpretation

All sonographic criteria are consistent with malignancy.

The contrast between the almost anechoic focal mass and its relatively hyperechoic (fibrocystic) surroundings is impressive.

Histology

Infiltrating lobular carcinoma with subtle tubular components and associated microcalcifications. Fibrocystic disease.

History

The 36-year-old woman had noticed a lump in her left breast about 2 weeks before.

Palpable Findings

Suspicious mass approximately 2×3 cm in size palpated deep to the nipple in the left breast.

Sonography

Figure: sagittal scan over the palpable mass.

Readability: good.

Focal lesion, 24×21 mm.

Interpretation

All sonographic criteria suggest a malignant process.

Histology

Moderately differentiated infiltrating ductal carcinoma with a predominantly solid, clear-cell composition.

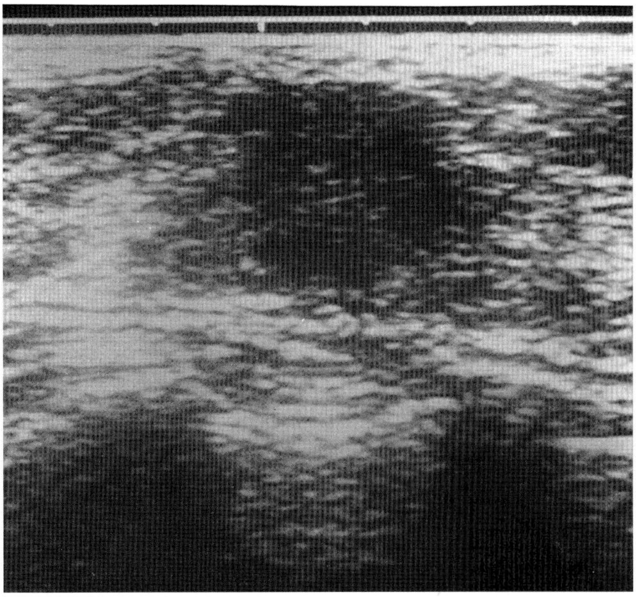

Analysis

1. **Margins**	indistinct, jagged
2. **Retrotumoral acoustic phenomena**	unchanged echoes
3. **Internal echo pattern**	nonhomogeneous
4. **Echogenicity**	almost anechoic
5. **Compression effect** on **shape**	no deformation
6. **Compression effect** on **internal echoes**	no change

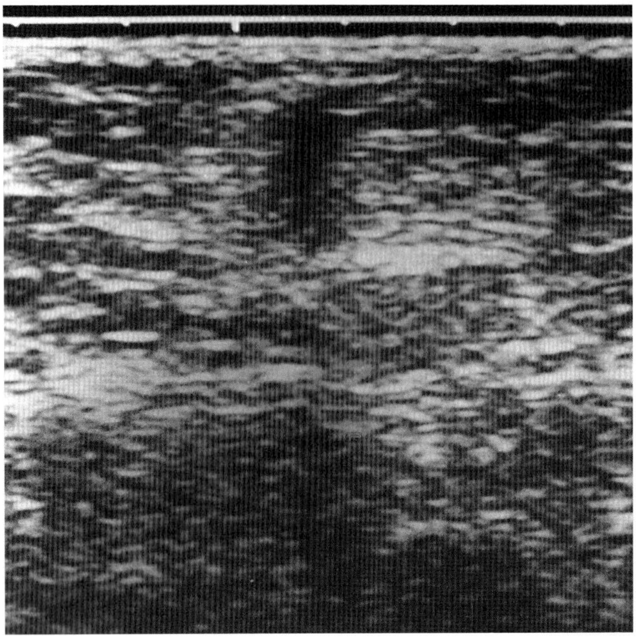

Analysis

1. Margins	indistinct, jagged
2. Retrotumoral acoustic phenomena	unchanged echoes
3. Internal echo pattern	few echoes, nonhomogeneous
4. Echogenicity	almost anechoic
5. Compression effect on **shape**	no deformation
6. Compression effect on **internal echoes**	no change

Note: The L/T ratio of this mass (> 2) is impressive (see chapter 5, p. 28).

History

This woman, 74 years of age, had been aware of a lump in her right breast for 3 weeks.

Palpable Findings

Approximately 15-mm, firm mass in the upper outer quadrant of the right breast. A freely mobile lymphoma was detected in the right axilla.

Sonography

Figure: sagittal scan over the palpable mass.

Readability: good.

Focal sonographic lesion, 12×15×7 mm.

Interpretation

All sonographic criteria, including the L/T ratio, are consistent with malignancy.

Histology

Moderately differentiated, predominantly solid infiltrating ductal carcinoma.
Size: 15 mm in diameter.

History

The 64-year-old woman had a lump in the right breast, first noticed by her daughter.

Palpable Findings

Relatively large, ptotic right breast with flattening and retraction of the areola. A relatively soft, poorly demarcated mass about as large as the ball of the thumb was palpable in the subareolar region.

Sonography

Figure: sagittal scan over the palpable mass.

Readability: good.

Suspicious focal sonographic lesion, 20×20 mm.

Interpretation

Typical sonographic presentation of carcinoma.

Histology

Poorly differentiated infiltrating lobular breast carcinoma (25 mm) with extensive lymphatic invasion.

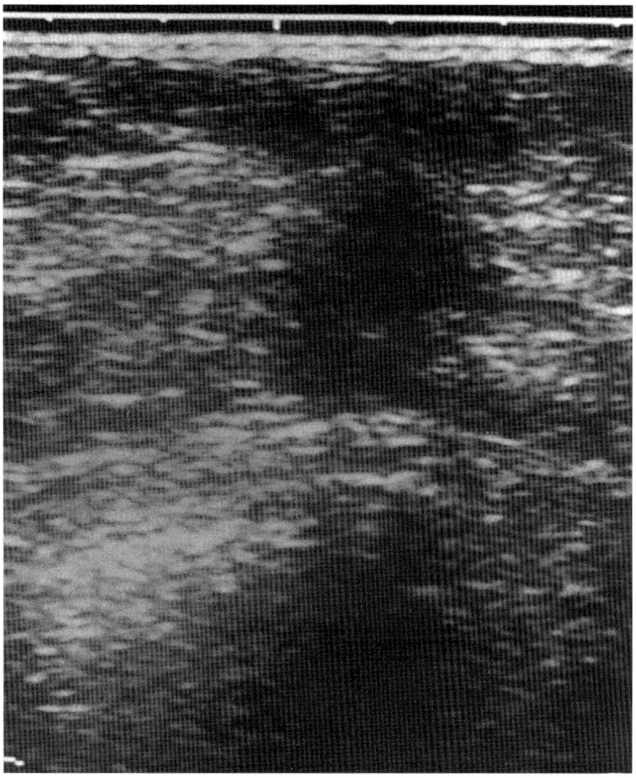

Analysis

1. Margins	indistinct, jagged
2. Retrotumoral acoustic phenomena	unchanged echoes
3. Internal echo pattern	few echoes, nonhomogeneous
4. Echogenicity	almost anechoic
5. Compression effect on **shape**	no deformation
6. Compression effect on **internal echoes**	no change

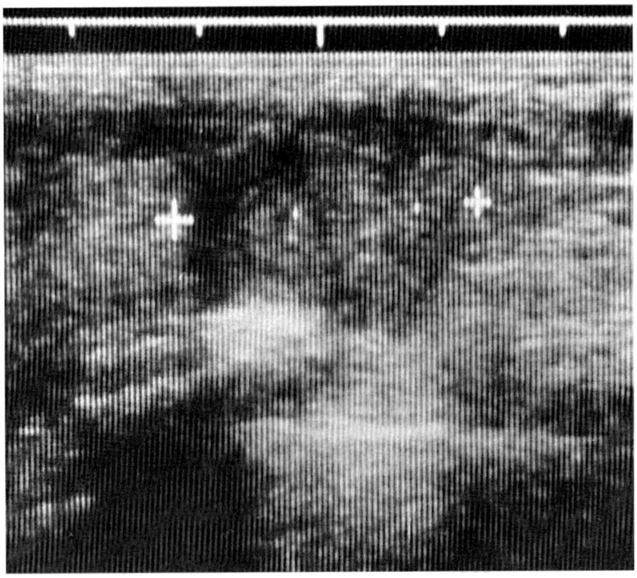

Analysis

1. Margins	indistinct, jagged
2. Retrotumoral acoustic phenomena	posterior enhancement
3. Internal echo pattern	mixed homogeneous and nonhomogeneous
4. Echogenicity	hypoechoic, with an almost anechoic border beneath the skin
5. Compression effect on **shape**	no deformation
6. Compression effect on **internal echoes**	no change

History

The 83-year-old woman had fallen onto her right breast 14 days before and later noticed a painful lump within the breast.

Palpable Findings

Firm, painful, approximately chestnut-sized, polygonal mass above the nipple of the right breast, associated with slight brownish skin discoloration. Clinical differential diagnosis included carcinoma and hematoma.

Sonography

Figure: transverse scan over the palpable mass.

Readability: good.

Focal lesion, 30×20 mm.

Interpretation

The sonographic criteria initially imply a benign lesion; both the history and sonographic findings are consistent with an organizing hematoma. But posterior enhancement is also seen with colloid carcinoma (see the case on p. 204). Hematoma and colloid carcinoma are indistinguishable by ultrasound in this case.

X-ray Mammography

An elliptical density, approximately 25×30 mm, with suspicious microcalcifications is seen in the subareolar region of the right breast. Roentgen findings are strongly suggestive of malignancy.

Histology

Colloid carcinoma.

History

The 49-year-old woman had felt a lump in her left breast 3 weeks before.

Palpable Findings

Firm, extensive mass with nipple retraction in the upper inner quadrant of the left breast.

Sonography

Figure: transverse scan over the mass.

Readability: good.

Focal lesion, 34×26 mm, with partial posterior shadowing. Involuted parenchyma.

Interpretation

All sonographic criteria are characteristic of malignancy. It is noteworthy that the shadowing does not appear behind the entire tumor. In the left part of the image the pectoral fascia appears intact *(arrow)*, but in the shadowed portion on the right, fascial integrity cannot be assessed.

X-ray Mammography

Stellate density in the left breast, suspicious for malignancy.

Histology

Predominantly small-cell infiltrating lobular carcinoma with lymphatic invasion (pT2).

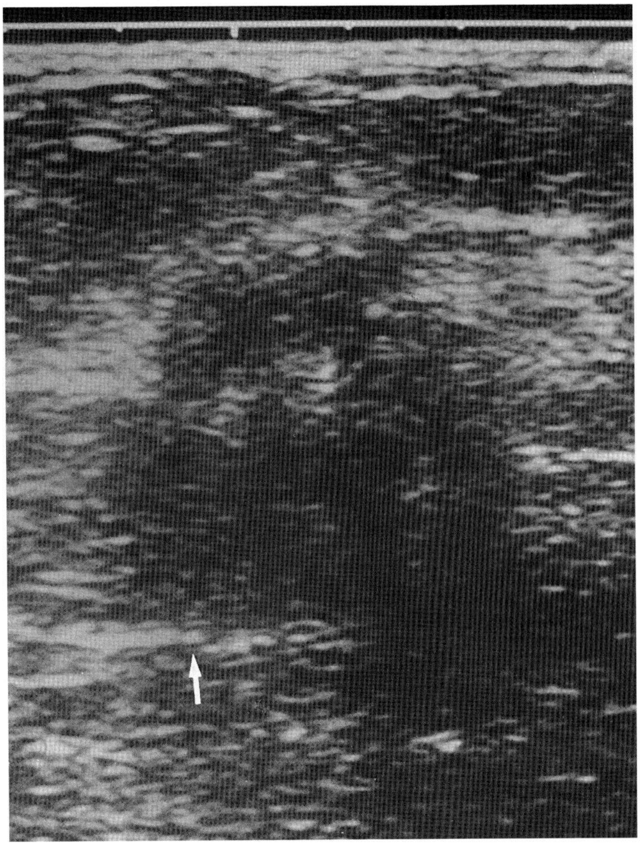

Analysis

1. **Margins**	indistinct, jagged
2. **Retrotumoral acoustic phenomena**	strong posterior shadowing (not behind the entire tumor)
3. **Internal echo pattern**	nonhomogeneous
4. **Echogenicity**	almost anechoic to fat-equivalent
5. **Compression effect** on **shape**	no deformation
6. **Compression effect** on **internal echoes**	no change

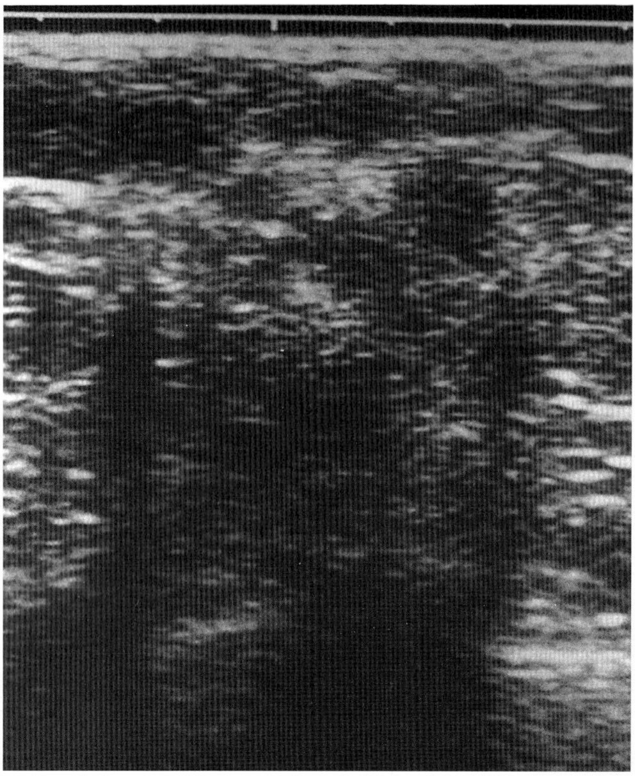

Analysis

1. Margins	indistinct, jagged
2. Retrotumoral acoustic phenomena	strong posterior shadowing
3. Internal echo pattern	nonhomogeneous
4. Echogenicity	almost anechoic to isoechoic
5. Compression effect on **shape**	no deformation
6. Compression effect on **internal echoes**	no change

Note: Posterior shadowing in this case is caused by the multiple interfaces of the infiltrating cancer.

History

The 37-year-old woman was hospitalized elsewhere for thrombosis and subsequently referred for evaluation of a right breast mass.

Palpable Findings

Firm, apple-sized mass with marked plateau sign in both lateral quadrants of the right breast.

Sonography

Figure: sagittal scan over the mass.

Readability: good.

Approximately 40 mm area with strong posterior shadowing, which appears to originate from several smaller focal lesions.

Interpretation

All sonographic criteria support a diagnosis of malignancy, the leading criterion being the dense, distinct posterior shadowing. It is noteworthy that the shadow originates from sites with different echogenicities.

Histology

Infiltrating ductal carcinoma, with predominantly solid extensions into the adjacent fat and connective tissue (60×40 mm).

History

The 53-year-old woman noticed a lump in her left breast. She had a family history of breast cancer.

Palpable Findings

Approximately 2-cm, fixed subareolar mass with skin retraction and incipient ulceration.

Sonography

Figure **a**: sagittal scan over the palpable mass (direct contact).

Readability: good.

Suspicious focal lesion, 18×23 mm, with posterior shadowing.

Figure **b**: same plane as in Figure **a** (with water path).

Suspicious focal abnormality with no posterior shadowing.

Interpretation

In Figure **a** (no water path), all sonographic criteria suggest a malignant process. In Figure **b**, most of the criteria are likewise consistent with malignancy. However, skin infiltration is depicted much more clearly *(arrows)*.

Histology

Infiltrating ductal carcinoma with tubular elements and dermal involvement. Maximum tumor diameter 25 mm.

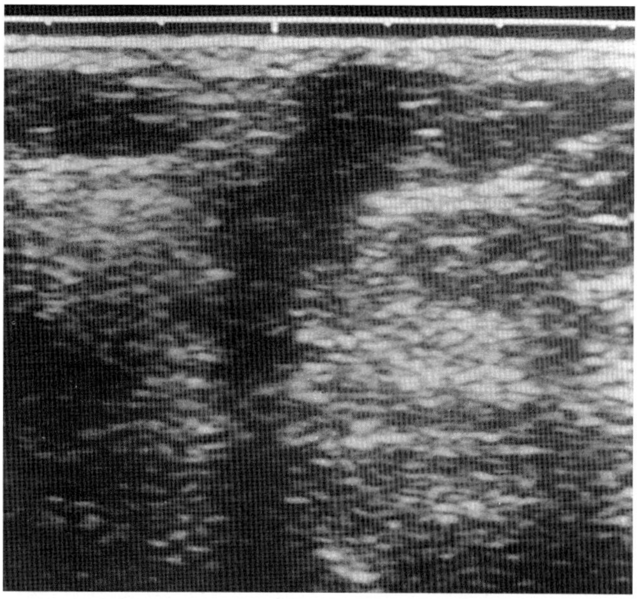

a

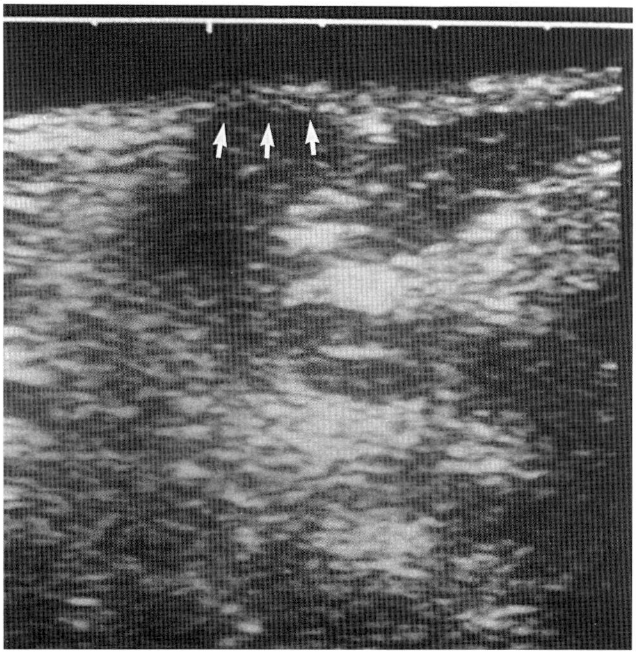

b

Analysis

	a	b
1. **Margins**	indistinct, jagged	indistinct, jagged
2. **Retrotumoral acoustic phenomena**	strong posterior shadowing	unchanged echoes
3. **Internal echo pattern**	few echoes, nonhomogeneous	nonhomogeneous
4. **Echogenicity**	almost anechoic	fat-equivalent
5. **Compression effect** on **shape**	no deformation	cannot be tested!
6. **Compression effect** on **internal echoes**	no change	cannot be tested!

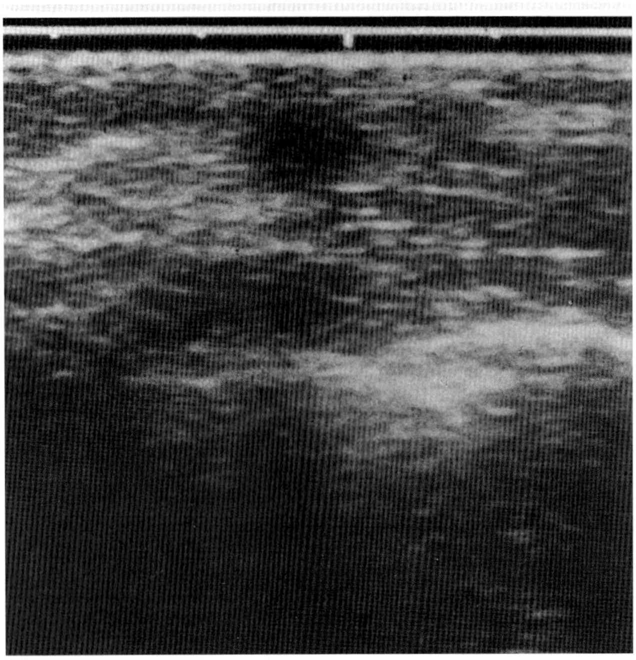

Analysis

1. **Margins**	indistinct, jagged
2. **Retrotumoral acoustic phenomena**	unchanged echoes
3. **Internal echo pattern**	few echoes, nonhomogeneous
4. **Echogenicity**	almost anechoic
5. **Compression effect** on **shape**	no deformation
6. **Compression effect** on **internal echoes**	no change

History

The 42-year-old woman noticed a small, painful lump in the upper outer quadrant of her left breast.

Palpable Findings

Firm, fixed, approximately 1-cm mass in the axillary tail of the left breast.

Sonography

Figure: transverse scan over the palpable mass.

Readability: good.

Focal sonographic lesion, 8×6 mm.

Interpretation

Despite the small size of the lesion, all sonographic criteria support the diagnosis of a malignant process.

Histology

Infiltrating ductal carcinoma with predominantly solid tumor proliferating within the ducts.

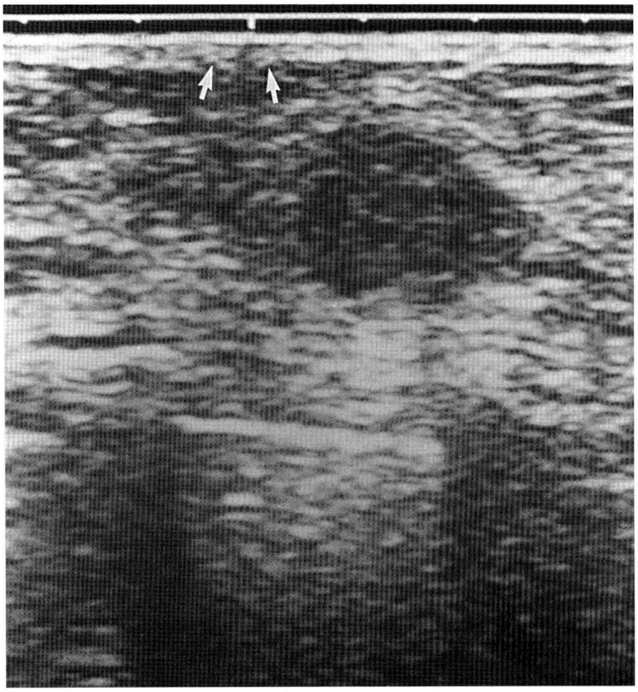

History

The 47-year-old woman with a family history of breast cancer had undergone two mammographic examinations in the past 2 years. She presented now with a right breast lump that she detected herself.

Palpable Findings

Firm, relatively fixed mass, 3×3 cm, in the upper outer quadrant of the right breast.

Sonography

Figure: sagittal scan over the mass.

Readability: good.

Conspicuous focal sonographic lesion beneath the areola (*arrows* indicate nipple).

Size: 19×15 mm.

Interpretation

All ultrasound criteria imply a benign tumor. However, when the clinical findings are taken into account, breast carcinoma must be suspected despite the sonographic analysis.

X-ray Mammography

Previous mammograms had demonstrated a smoothly marginated focal lesion in the right breast that was interpreted as a cyst. It was not until the patient herself reported a palpable mass that carcinoma was suspected.

Histology

Moderately differentiated infiltrating lobular carcinoma with lymphatic invasion.
Size: 20×25 mm.

Analysis

1. Margins	indistinct, jagged
2. Retrotumoral acoustic phenomena	unchanged echoes
3. Internal echo pattern	homogeneous
4. Echogenicity	hypoechoic
5. Compression effect on **shape**	no deformation
6. Compression effect on **internal echoes**	no change

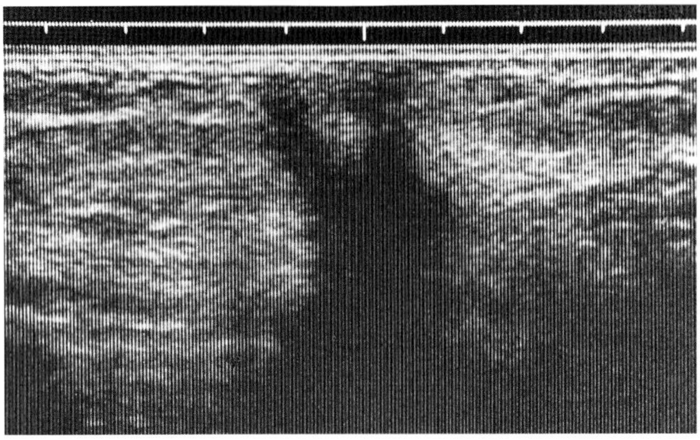

Analysis

1. Margins	indistinct, jagged
2. Retrotumoral acoustic phenomena	strong posterior shadowing
3. Internal echo pattern	few echoes, nonhomogeneous
4. Echogenicity	almost anechoic
5. Compression effect on **shape**	no deformation
6. Compression effect on **internal echoes**	no change

History

The 83-year-old woman, who had never had a screening examination, presented with a lump an skin retraction in the left breast.

Palpable Findings

Firm, fixed, approximately walnut-sized mass with skin fixation and orange-peel dimpling in the upper outer quadrant of the left breast.

Sonography

Figure: sagittal scan over the mass.

Readability: good.

Scan demonstrates an almost anechoic, focal lesion, 27×23 mm. Two fingerlike tumor projections with skin invasion are particularly striking.

Interpretation

All sonographic criteria are suggestive of breast carcinoma infiltrating the skin. The posterior boundary of the tumor (pectoral muscle) is not defined by ultrasound.

Histology

Infiltrating ductal carcinoma with skin infiltration and lymphatic invasion.
Size: 23×21 mm.

History

The 63-year-old woman had a mass in the left breast discovered on routine examination.

Palpable Findings

Soft, freely mobile, approximately 1.5 cm mass in the upper inner quadrant of the left breast.

Sonography

Figure: transverse scan over the mass.

Readability: good.

Focal lesion *(arrows)*, 10×10 mm, with posterior shadowing.

Interpretation

All sonographic criteria are suggestive of a malignant tumor.

Clinical and X-ray mammographic findings were more consistent with a benign tumor (e.g., adenolipoma). Ultrasound furnished a compelling indication for breast biopsy.

X-ray Mammography

Subtle density of indeterminate nature visible in both projections.

Histology

Infiltrating ductal carcinoma, approximately 30 mm in diameter, with predominantly intraductal spread; lymphatic invasion.

Note: The discrepancy between sonographic and histologic tumor size results from the fact that ultrasound did not demonstrate the intraductal tumor component.

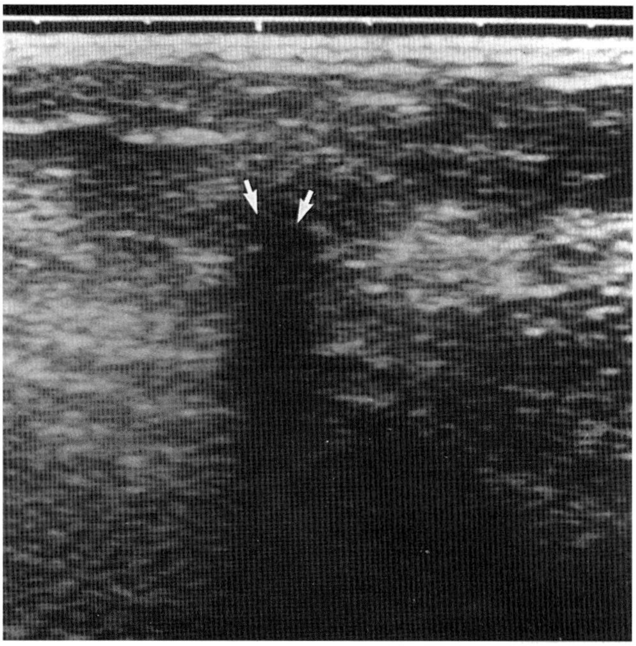

Analysis

1. **Margins**	indistinct, jagged
2. **Retrotumoral acoustic phenomena**	strong posterior shadowing
3. **Internal echo pattern**	few echoes, nonhomogeneous
4. **Echogenicity**	almost anechoic
5. **Compression effect** on **shape**	no deformation
6. **Compression effect** on **internal echoes**	no change

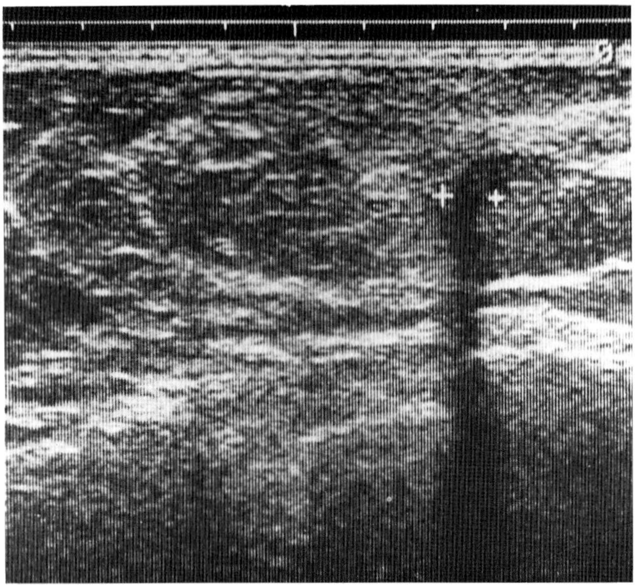

a

Analysis

1. **Margins**	sharp, jagged
2. **Retrotumoral acoustic phenomena**	strong posterior shadowing
3. **Internal echo pattern**	few echoes, nonhomogeneous
4. **Echogenicity**	almost anechoic
5. **Compression effect** on **shape**	no deformation
6. **Compression effect** on **internal echoes**	no change

History

The 62-year-old woman underwent screening mammography, which showed a stellate mass with microcalcifications in the left breast.

Palpable Findings

Both breasts were relatively firm. An indeterminate mass was palpated in the upper outer quadrant of the left breast. A small, mobile lymphoma was found in the axilla.

Sonography

Figure **a**: transverse scan through the left upper outer quadrant.

Readability in involuted parenchyma: good.

Conspicuous focal lesion, 8×7 mm, with posterior shadowing.

Interpretation

Sonographic criteria 2, 3, 4, 5 and 6 suggest a malignant process. The very dense shadow despite the small size of the lesion is impressive.

X-ray Mammography

Figure **b**: craniocaudal projection showing a lateral stellate density with clustered microcalcifications.

Histology

Infiltrating carcinoma with mixed lobular and scirrhous components; maximum diameter 8 mm.

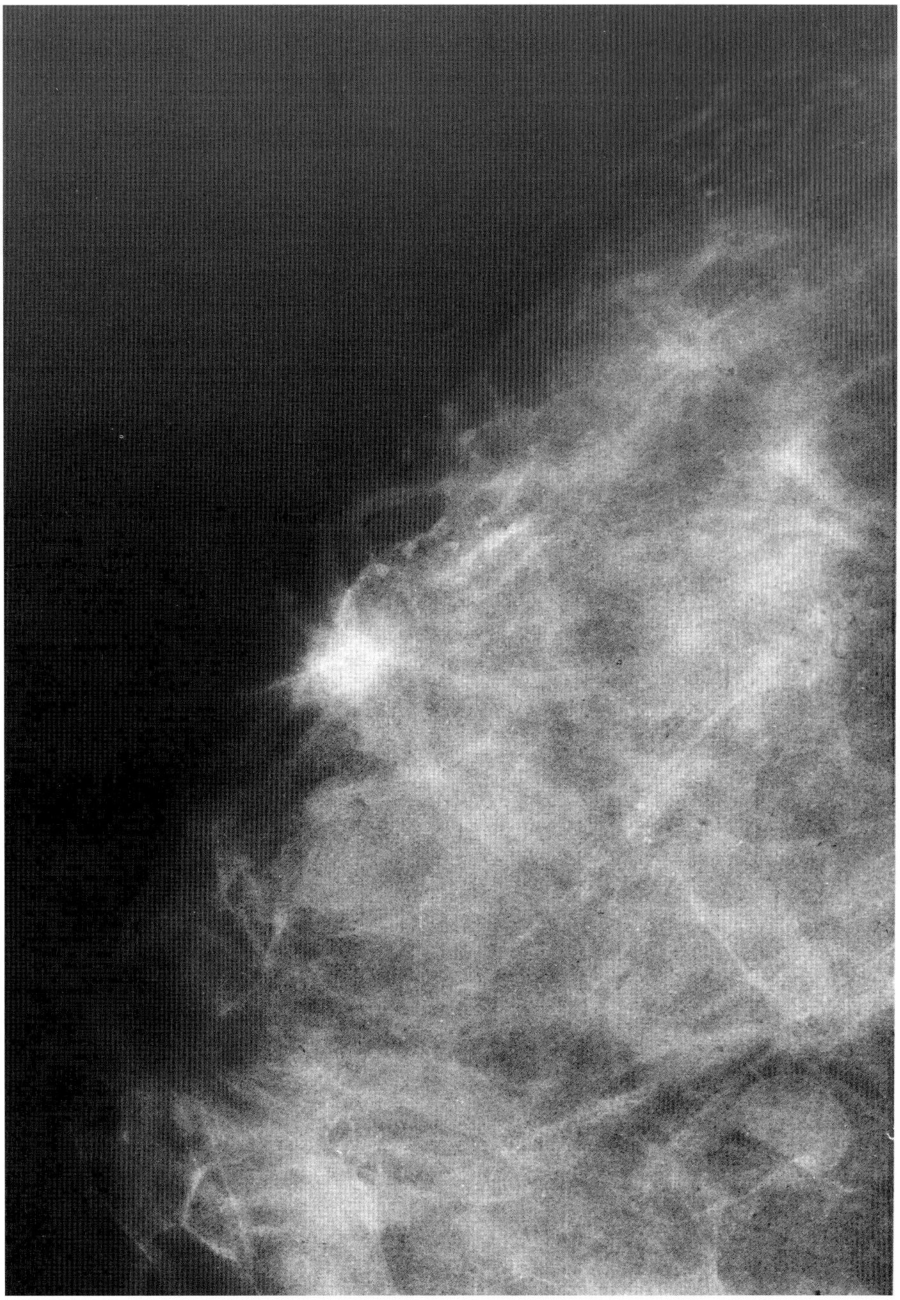

b

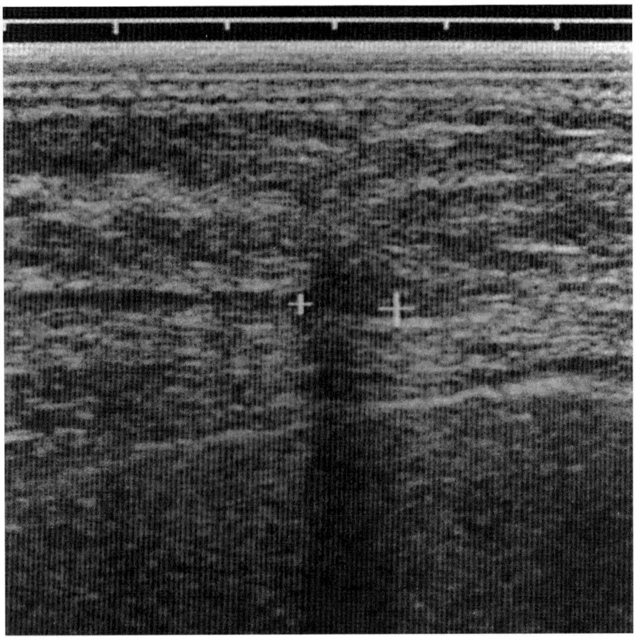

Analysis

1. Margins	indistinct, jagged
2. Retrotumoral acoustic phenomena	moderate posterior shadowing
3. Internal echo pattern	few echoes, nonhomogeneous
4. Echogenicity	almost anechoic
5. Compression effect on **shape**	no deformation
6. Compression effect on **internal echoes**	no change

History

The 78-year-old woman had undergone left breast biopsy elsewhere 6 weeks before. Histologic diagnosis: fibrocystic disease.

Patient again noticed the nodule that had been present before biopsy.

Palpable Findings

Freely mobile, bean-sized mass in the left breast at 12 o'clock, approximately 5 cm from the nipple.

Sonography

Figure: transverse scan over the palpable mass.

Readability: good.

Focal lesion, 9×4×5 mm, near the chest wall; posterior shadowing.

Interpretation

All analytic criteria suggest a malignant process.

X-ray Mammography

The mass is located relatively high in the breast, so it is not seen on the mediolateral projection and is only partly imaged on the craniocaudal view. Consequently, mammograms are not useful for benign/malignant differentiation.

Histology

Scirrhous-type infiltrating ductal carcinoma. Histologic size: 10 mm in diameter.

History

The 69-year-old woman, who had never had a screening examination, was referred for gynecologic consultation during a hospital stay.

Palpable Findings

Firm, mobile, approximately 5-cm mass in the upper outer quadrant of the right breast, which otherwise appeared normal.

Sonography

Figure: sagittal scan over the mass.

Readability: good.

Lobulated mass, 25×16 mm.

Interpretation

Except for tumor margins, all the sonographic criteria are suggestive of malignancy.

Histology

Infiltrating ductal carcinoma, 25 mm in diameter, with lymphatic invasion.

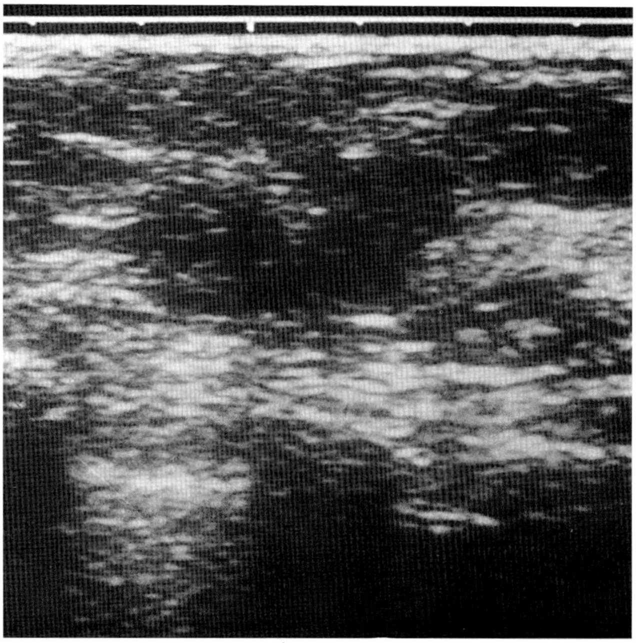

Analysis

1. **Margins**	sharp, jagged
2. **Retrotumoral acoustic phenomena**	unchanged echoes
3. **Internal echo pattern**	few echoes, nonhomogeneous
4. **Echogenicity**	almost anechoic
5. **Compression effect** on **shape**	no deformation
6. **Compression effect** on **internal echoes**	no change

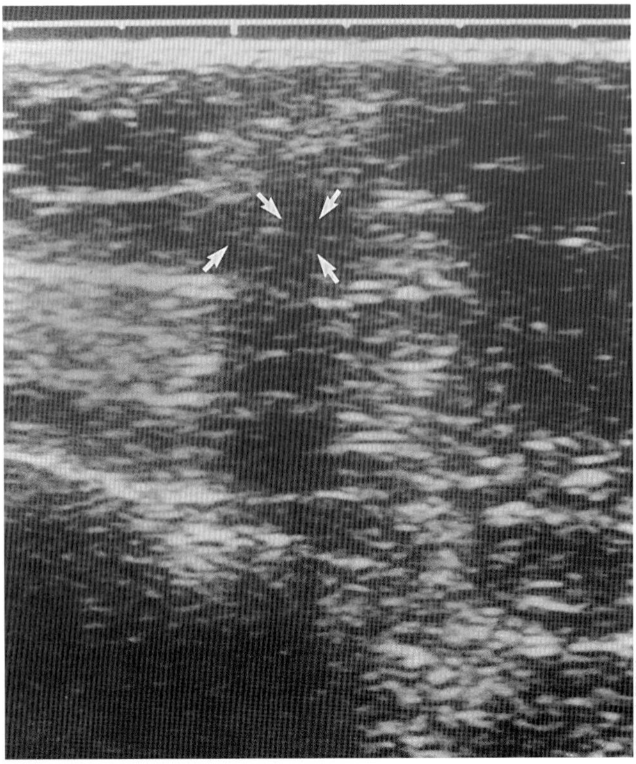

Analysis

1. **Margins**	indistinct, jagged
2. **Retrotumoral acoustic phenomena**	moderate posterior shadowing
3. **Internal echo pattern**	few echoes, nonhomogeneous
4. **Echogenicity**	fat-equivalent
5. **Compression effect** on **shape**	no deformation
6. **Compression effect** on **internal echoes**	no change

History

The 57-year-old woman had undergone mastectomy for carcinoma of the left breast 1 year before. She had also a right breast biopsy (elsewhere) 2 months earlier for a mass she detected herself.

Histologic diagnosis: carcinoma in situ.

Induration was later noted above the nipple during a routine follow-up examination.

Palpaple findings

Firm mass, approximately 1×2 cm, located about 10 cm above the right nipple on the midclavicular line. Lesion was not seen on mammograms due to its peripheral location.

Sonography

Figure: transverse scan over the palpable mass.

Readability: good.

Focal lesion, 14×12 mm *(arrows)*, with posterior shadowing.

Interpretation

All the sonographic criteria except echogenicity suggest a malignant process.

Histology

Scirrhous-solid ductal carcinoma with large-cell elements, 25×20 mm.

History

The 31-year-old woman had noticed a lump in her right breast 1 year before. Aspiration cytology (elsewhere) at that time was negative.

The mass had been enlarging for 6 months when the patient presented for examination.

Palpable Findings

Firm, mobile, poorly circumscribed, walnut-sized mass in the upper outer quadrant of the right breast. Repeat aspiration cytology: Papanicolaou grade V.

Sonography

Figure: transverse scan in the upper outer quadrant over the mass.

Readability: good.

Focal lesion, 25×20 mm.

Interpretation

Despite some nonmalignant sonographic criteria, the nonhomogeneous internal echo pattern with scattered high-level echoes (microcalcifications) creates a very high index of suspicion for malignancy. The posterior enhancement is caused by necrotic foci within the mass.

Histology

Highly cellular infiltrating ductal carcinoma, 25×20 mm, with little stroma (solid).

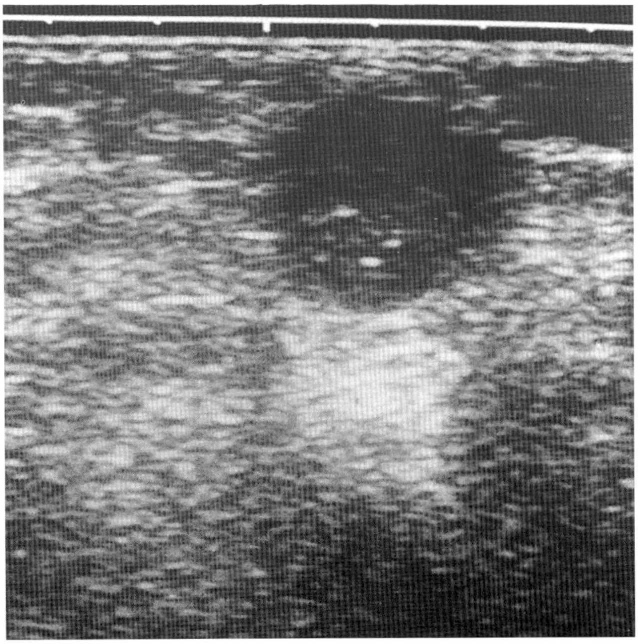

Analysis

1. **Margins**	indistinct but smooth
2. **Retrotumoral acoustic phenomena**	posterior enhancement
3. **Internal echo pattern**	nonhomogeneous
4. **Echogenicity**	almost anechoic
5. **Compression effect** on **shape**	no deformation
6. **Compression effect** on **internal echoes**	no change

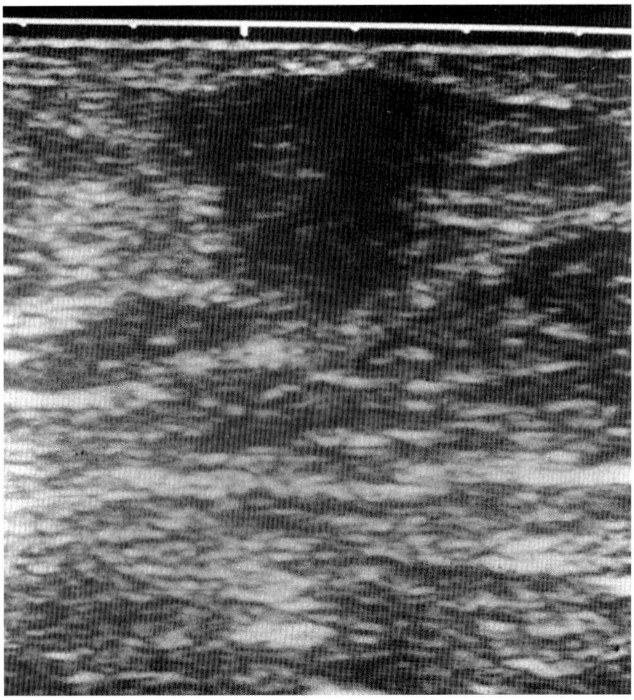

a

Analysis

1. Margins	indistinct, jagged
2. Retrotumoral acoustic phenomena	unmodified echoes
3. Internal echo pattern	few echoes, non-homogeneous
4. Echogenicity	almost anechoic
5. Compression effect on **shape**	no deformation
6. Compression effect on **internal echoes**	no change

History

The 69-year-old woman presented with right nipple retraction noted by her family doctor 2 weeks before.

Palpable Findings

Poorly demarcated mass at the lower inner border of the right areola.

Sonography

Figure **a**: sagittal scan over the mass. Involuted breast parenchyma.

Readability: good.

Focal lesion, 27×24 mm, with no evidence of skin or pectoralis infiltration.

Interpretation

All sonographic criteria suggest a malignant process.

X-ray Mammography

Figure **b**: mediolateral projection of the right breast.

Figure **c**: mediolateral projection of the left breast.

Asymmetric retroareolar density increase with no circumscribed focal lesion.

Histology

Ductolobular carcinoma (maximum extent, 32 mm).

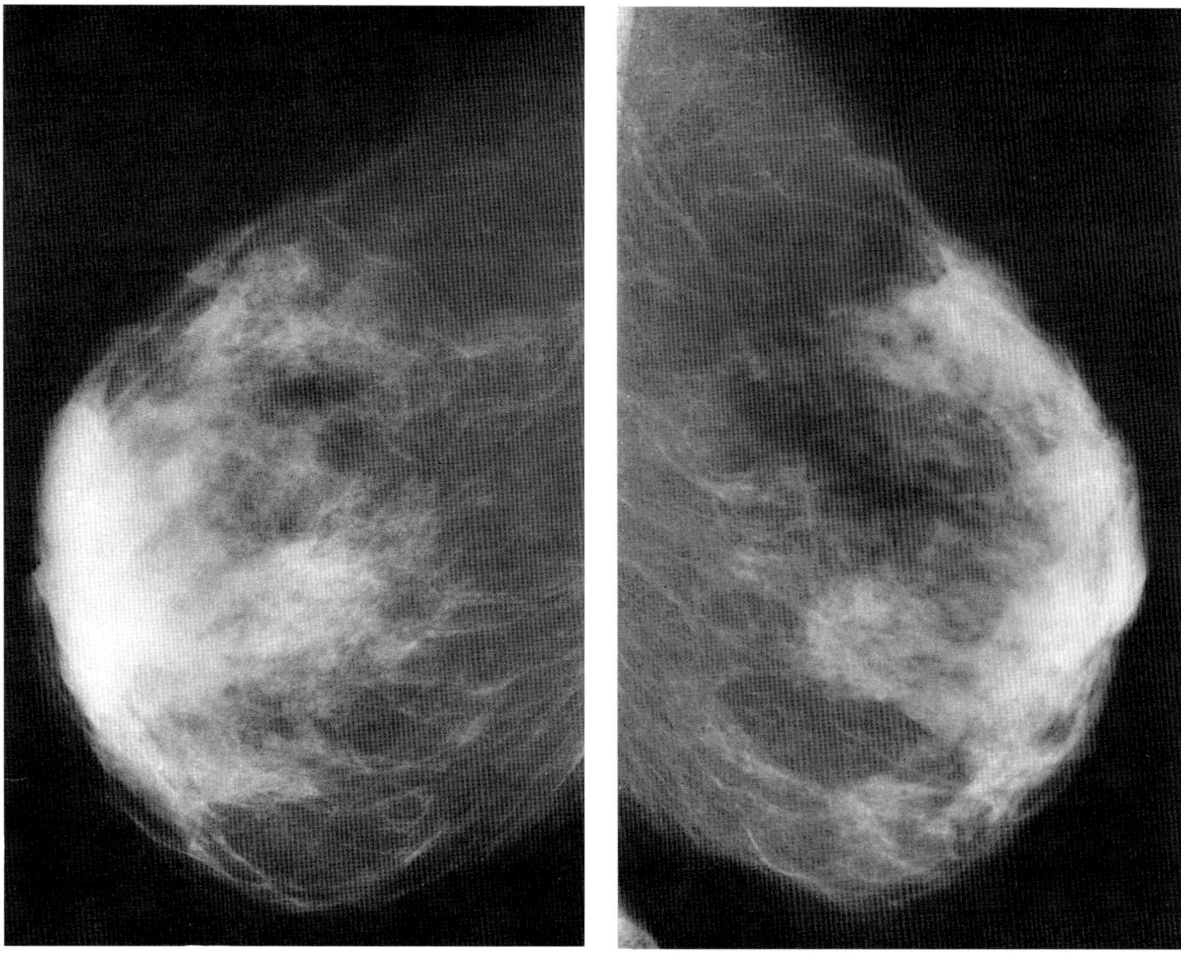

b c

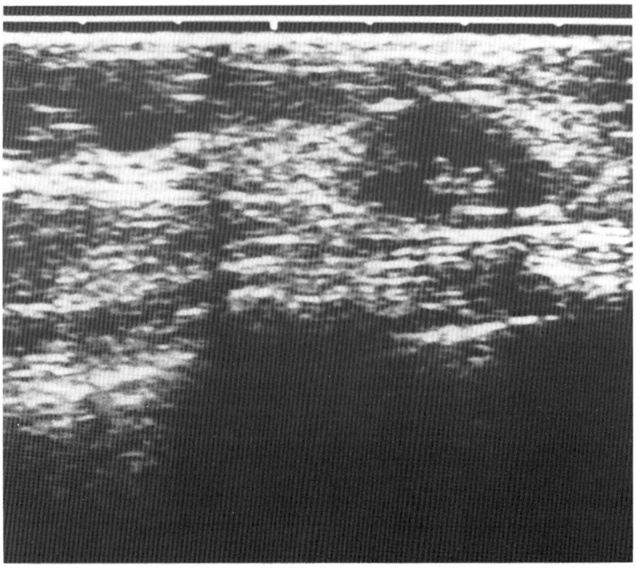

a

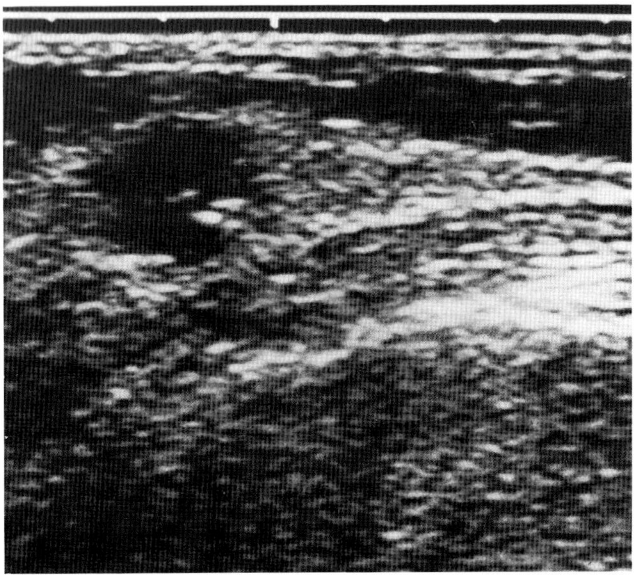

b

History

The 61-year-old woman noticed a lump in her right breast.

Palpable Findings

Mobile, smoothly marginated mass, 2×2 cm, at 12 o'clock in the right breast.

Sonography

Figure **a**: sagittal scan over the palpable mass (7.5 MHz).

Readability: good.

Focal lesion, 20×13 mm.

Figure **b**: transverse scan over the palpable mass (5 MHz).

Interpretation

All sonographic criteria are suggestive of a malignancy. The major difference between the two ultrasound frequencies is that scanning at 7.5 MHz demonstrates more microcalcification equivalents.

Aspiration Cytology

Scant suspicious cellular material (Papanicolaou grade III).

Analysis

1. **Margins** (5 MHz)	indistinct, jagged
2. **Retrotumoral acoustic phenomena**	unmodified echoes
3. **Internal echo pattern**	few echoes, nonhomogeneous
4. **Echogenicity**	almost anechoic
5. **Compression effect** on **shape**	no deformation
6. **Compression effect** on **internal echoes**	no change

Note: The subtle echo clusters are the ultrasound correlates of the roentgen microcalcifications.

X-ray Mammography

Figure **c**: mediolateral projection shows a poorly circumscribed density with centrally clustered microcalcifications suspicious for carcinoma.

Histology

Cut surface shows a grossly nondemarcated tumor mass (tumor size also could not be determined histologically). Moderately differentiated infiltrating ductal carcinoma.

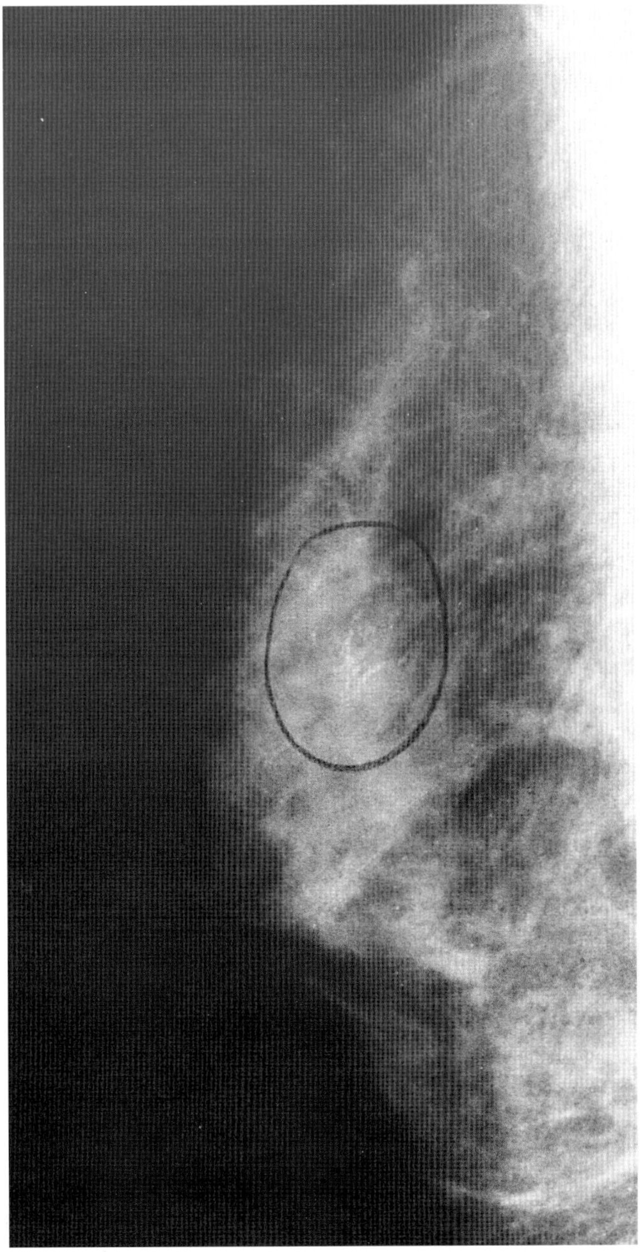

c

History

The 29-year-old woman noticed a lump in her right breast. She had a several-year history of premenstrual syndrome.

Palpable Findings

Coarsely nodular breasts. Mass, approximately 1×1 cm, in the upper inner quadrant of the right breast.

Sonography

Figure: sagittal scan over the palpable mass (with water path).

Readability: good.

Superficial focal lesion, 7×10 mm, with no evidence of skin infiltration.

Interpretation

The sonographic criteria are somewhat equivocal in terms of predicting benignancy or malignancy. However, the overall impression of "architectural distortion" produced by the mass creates a very high index of suspicion for malignancy.

X-ray Mammography

Dysplastic breast parenchyma with disseminated microcalcifications covering an area of 50×30 mm.

Suspicion of extensive carcinoma in situ.

Aspiration Cytology

(from palpable lesion)

Abundant lipid-containing cells suspicious for tumor (Papanicolaou grade IV).

Histology

Infiltrating ductal carcinoma with a predominantly intraductal tumor component (probably only a small, invasive component was visible on sonograms).

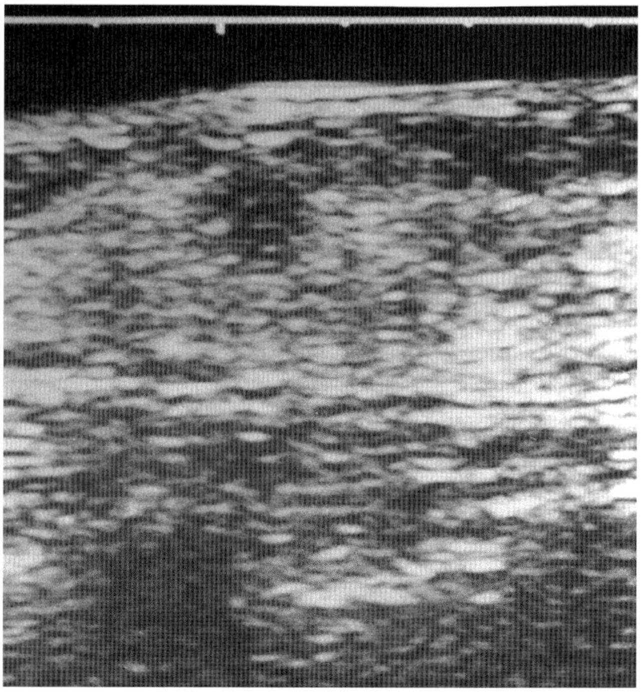

Analysis

1. **Margins**	indistinct but smooth
2. **Retrotumoral acoustic phenomena**	unmodified echoes
3. **Internal echo pattern**	nonhomogeneous
4. **Echogenicity**	fat-equivalent
5. **Compression effect** on **shape**	no deformation
6. **Compression effect** on **internal echoes**	no change

Note: The sonographic lesion contains foci with very different echogenicities; these may be interpreted as microcalcifications.

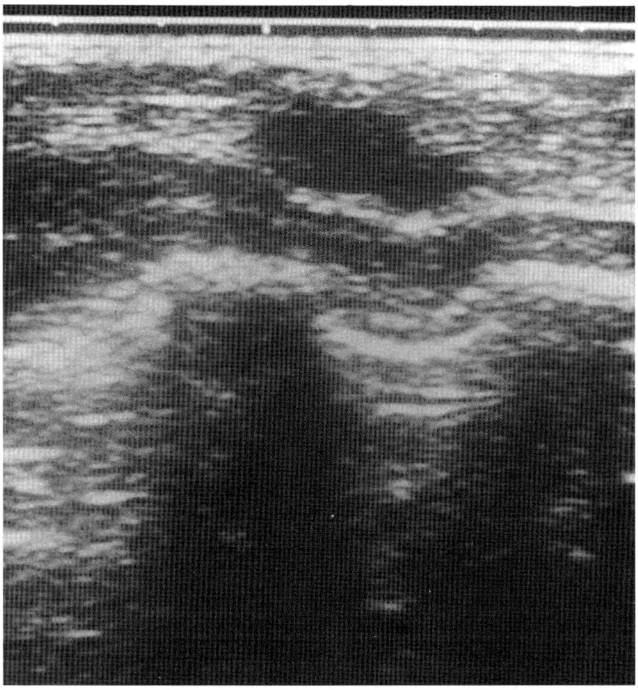

Analysis

1. **Margins**	sharp, jagged
2. **Retrotumoral acoustic phenomena**	unmodified echoes
3. **Internal echo pattern**	few echoes, nonhomogeneous
4. **Echogenicity**	almost anechoic
5. **Compression effect** on **shape**	no deformation
6. **Compression effect** on **internal echoes**	no change

Note: L/T ratio < 0.5 implies a benign lesion.

History

The 27-year-old woman had noticed a lump in her right breast 8 weeks before.

Palpable Findings

Dense breasts. Approximately 3-cm, mobile mass in the upper outer quadrant of the right breast. Also a small mobile lymphoma in the right axilla.

Sonography

Figure: sagittal scan over the mass in the upper outer quadrant of the right breast.

Readability: good.

Focal lesion, 22×10 mm.

Interpretation

The sonographic criteria do not permit a confident prediction of benignancy for malignancy. Differential diagnosis must include lobulated fibroadenoma as well as medullary carcinoma.

X-ray Mammography

Dysplastic breast type with no apparent focal abnormality.

Histology

Cherry-sized pericanalicular fibroadenoma.

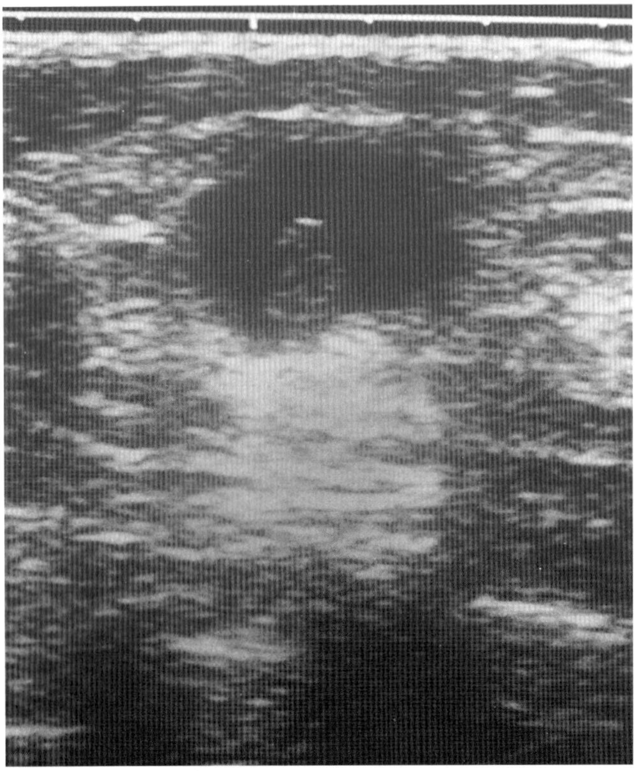

Analysis

1. Margins	sharp, jagged
2. Retrotumoral acoustic phenomena	posterior enhancement, bilateral shadowing phenomena
3. Internal echo pattern	no echoes (intracystic structure arising from the posterior wall)
4. Echogenicity	anechoic
5. Compression effect on **shape**	no deformation
6. Compression effect on **internal echoes**	no change

History

The 49-year-old woman was referred for evaluation of a palpable left breast mass with suspicious cystic aspirate.

Palpable Findings

Smoothly marginated, slightly mobile mass about as large as the ball of the thumb located in the left breast at 3 o'clock.

Sonography

Figure: sagittal scan over the palpable mass.

Readability: good.

Focal sonographic lesion (24×20 mm) with cystic appearance.

Interpretation

The sonographic criteria are characteristic of a benign cystic lesion.

A conspicuous finding is the sonographically indeterminate structure projecting into the cyst from its posterior wall. This feature may represent an intracystic carcinoma or papilloma. Intracystic vegetations of this kind always warrant biopsy!

X-ray Mammography

Round lesion in the left breast with predominantly smooth margins but an indistinct posterior wall, where extensions project into surrounding tissues.

Histology

Proliferative cystic mastopathy presenting with intraductal papillomatosis of large and intermediate glandular ducts. Sclerosing adenosis. No evidence of malignant growth.

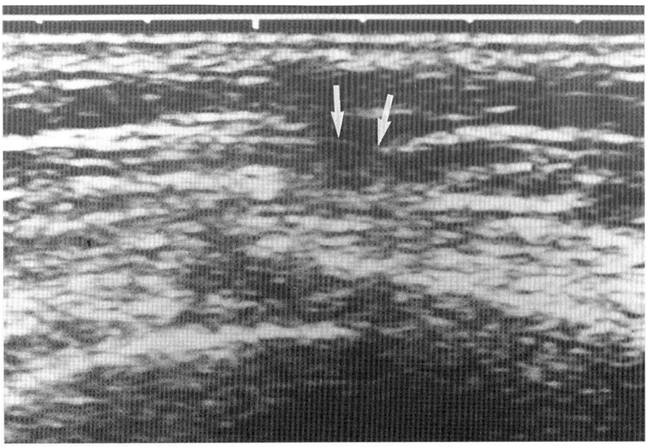

History

The 74-year-old woman, who had undergone an extensive right breast biopsy 5 years before, presented for an ultrasound examination of the scar region.

Palpable Findings

No palpable intramammary masses. The scar region was indurated for its entire length.

Sonography

Figure: transverse scan perpendicular to the scar.

Readability: good.

A true focal sonographic lesion is not demonstrated. The only remarkable finding is the disruption of a connective tissue septum *(arrows)*. There ist apparent fat replacement in the gap.

Analysis

There is no focal lesion, so the usual analytic criteria cannot be applied.

Interpretation

Typical appearance of a scar, which does not necessarily cast an acoustic shadow. A focal lesion is not defined. The absence of skin changes is noteworthy.

The sonographic picture remained unchanged in several follow-ups over a 2-year period.

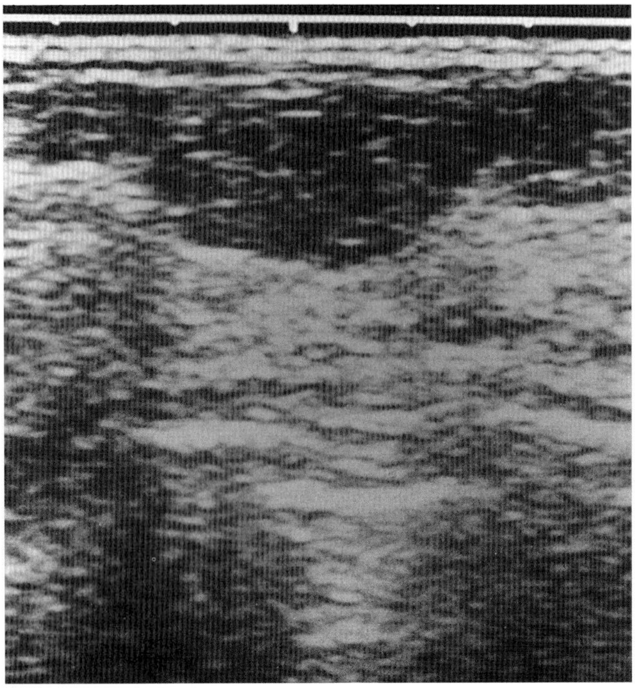

Analysis

1. Margins	sharp and smooth
2. Retrotumoral acoustic phenomena	posterior enhancement
3. Internal echo pattern	homogeneous
4. Echogenicity	fat-equivalent
5. Compression effect on **shape**	shape distortion
6. Compression effect on **internal echoes**	become more homogeneous

History

The 54-year-old woman was noted to have a palpable breast mass during a hospital stay.

Palpable Findings

Soft, mobile mass in the upper outer quadrant of the left breast.

Sonography

Figure: sagittal scan over the palpable mass.

Readability: good.

Focal lesion, 35×14 mm, with little echo contrast.

Interpretation

All the analytic criteria suggest a benign lesion. The lesion is relatively difficult to separate from the skin on sonographic image analysis and tends to blend with the layer of subcutaneous fat.

Presumptive sonographic diagnosis: lipoma.

X-ray Mammography

Onionskin-like density, 2×4×4 cm, in the left breast. Radiographic features consistent with adenolipoma.

Histology

Excised fatty specimen shows extensive lipomatous permeation of the glandular tissue with no evidence of atypia. The glandular tissue simply exhibits fibrocystic change.

History

The 16-year-old girl had noticed a lump in her right breast 2 weeks before.

Palpable Findings

Firm, approximately cherry-sized, clinically innocent-appearing retroareolar mass in the right breast.

Sonography

(with water path)

Figure: transverse scan over the palpable mass.

Readability: good.

Subcutaneous focal sonographic lesion, 23×17 mm.

Interpretation

The quality and degree of all sonographic criteria are consistent with fibroadenoma.

X-ray Mammography

Radiography was withheld in consideration of the young age of the patient.

Histology

Intracanicular fibroadenoma.

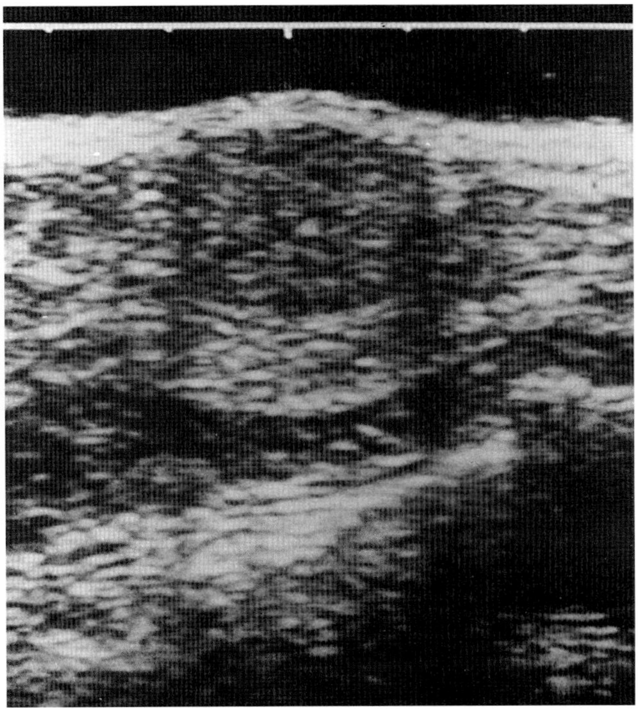

Analysis

1. **Margins**	sharp and smooth
2. **Retrotumoral acoustic phenomena**	bilateral shadowing phenomena
3. **Internal echo pattern**	homogeneous
4. **Echogenicity**	hypoechoic
5. **Compression effect** on **shape**	no deformation
6. **Compression effect** on **internal echoes**	no change

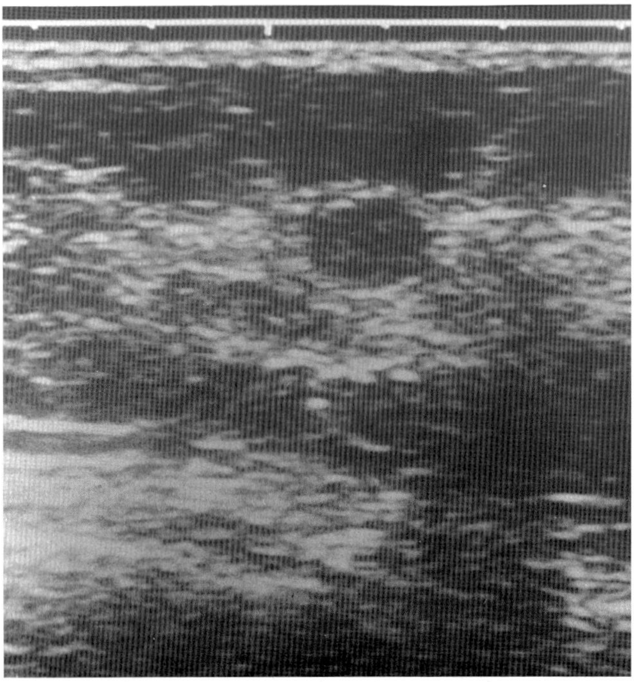
a

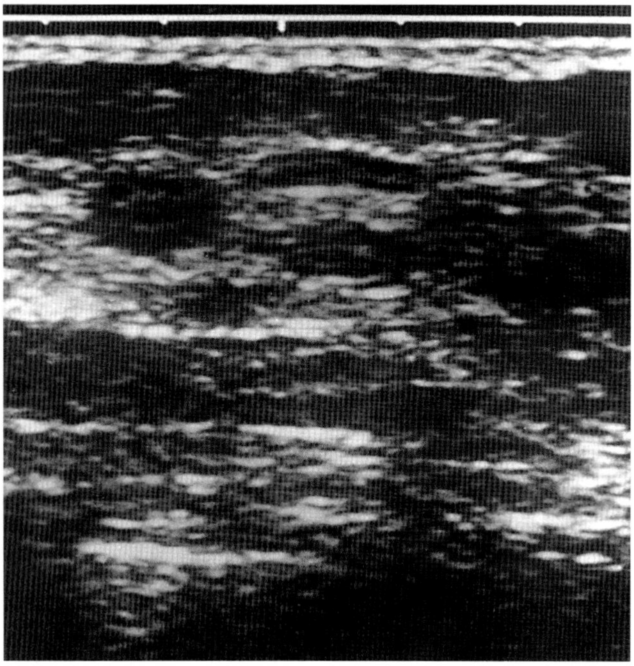
b

History

The 32-year-old woman had felt two painful nodules in her left breast 4 weeks before.

Palpable Findings

Both breast were very nodular. The examining physician was unable to detect any definite lesions.

Sonography

Figure **a**: transverse scan through the upper outer quadrant of the left breast over the site indicated by the patient.

Focal sonographic lesion (10×7 mm).

Figure **b**: transverse scan through the lower outer quadrant of the left breast.

Focal sonographic lesion (10×7 mm).

Readability: good.

Interpretation

The sonographic criteria suggest that both lesions are benign. The quality and degree of the criteria raise a very strong suspicion of fibroadenomas.

X-ray Mammography

Two smoothly marginated, innocent-appearing round lesions.

Histology

Two pericanalicular fibroadenomas.

Analysis

	a	b
1. **Margins**	sharp and smooth	sharp and smooth
2. **Retrotumoral acoustic phenomena**	unmodified echoes	unmodified echoes
3. **Internal echo pattern**	homogeneous	nonhomogeneous
4. **Echogenicity**	almost anechoic	fat-equivalent
5. **Compression effect** on **shape**	no deformation	no deformation
6. **Compression effect** on **internal echoes**	no change	no change

History

The 32-year-old woman felt a small lump in her left breast. Aspiration cytology (elsewhere) indicated Papanicolaou grade III pathology.

Palpable Findings

Firm, mobile, 1 cm mass with predominantly smooth margins in the upper inner quadrant of the left breast.

Sonography

Figure: oblique scan over the palpable mass (with water path).

Readability: good.

Well-demarcated focal sonographic lesion, 12×7 mm.

Interpretation

All sonographic criteria are suggestive of a benign process.

The quality and degree of the criteria are consistent with fibroadenoma. The ovoid contour of the lesion shows slight extension toward the left side of the image, but even there the margins are smooth.

Histology

Intracanalicular fibroadenoma.

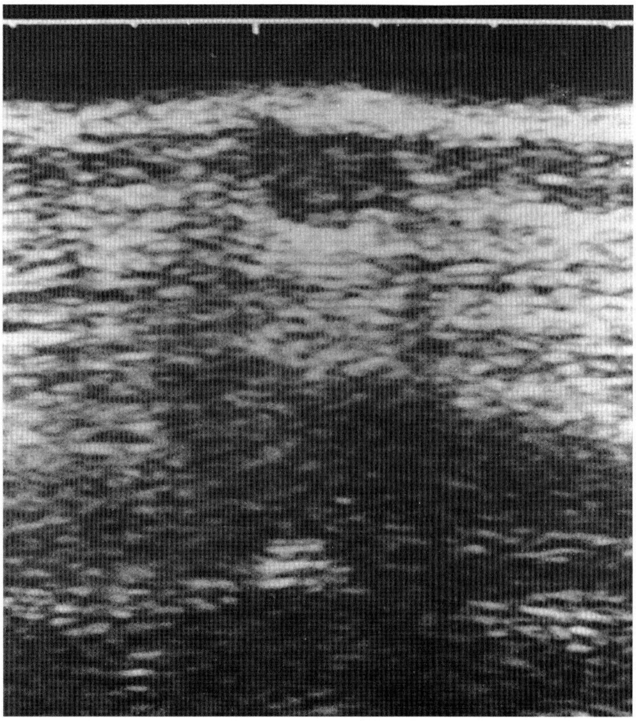

Analysis

1. **Margins**	sharp and smooth
2. **Retrotumoral acoustic phenomena**	very slight posterior enhancement and faint bilateral shadowing phenomena
3. **Internal echo pattern**	homogeneous
4. **Echogenicity**	fat equivalent
5. **Compression effect** on **shape**	no deformation
6. **Compression effect** on **internal echoes**	no change

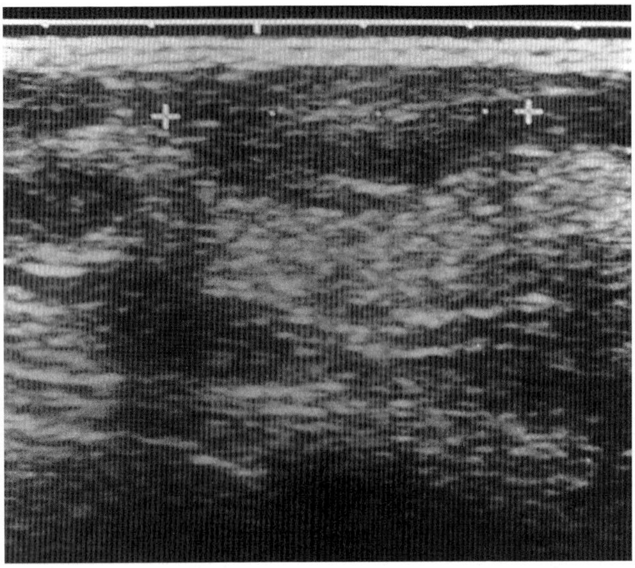
a

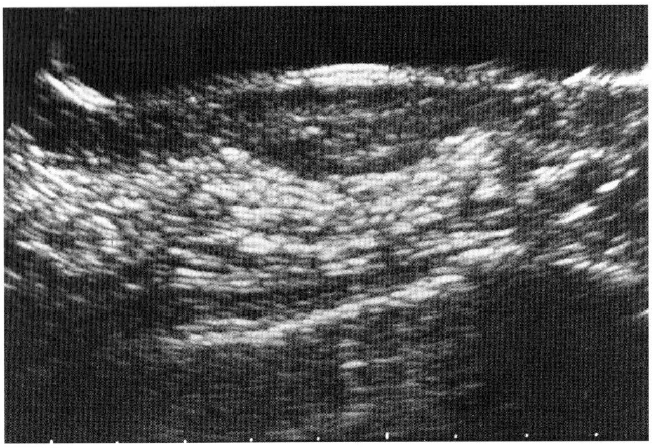
b

Analysis

1. Margins	sharp and smooth
2. Retrotumoral acoustic phenomena	subtle posterior enhancement
3. Internal echo pattern	homogeneous
4. Echogenicity	fat-equivalent
5. Compression effect on **shape**	deformed
6. Compression effect on **internal echoes**	echoes become more homogeneous

History

The 43-year-old woman was known for some years to have lipomas at multiple sites throughout the body.

Palpable Findings

Soft, cylindrical mass palpable 3 cm above the nipple of the left breast.

Sonography

Figure **a** (linear scan): transverse scan over the mass.

Readability: good.

Focal sonographic lesion, 34×13 mm.

Figure **b** (sector scan with standoff): same findings as in Figure **a**.

Interpretation

The analytic criteria point to a benign lesion. Figure **b** clearly localizes the mass to the level of the subcutaneous fat, with which it is continuous on both sides. A standoff is advantageous for imaging subcutaneous lesions.

Histology

Lipoma.

History

The 34-year-old woman had been aware of a steadily enlarging lump beneath the nipple of her right breast for 1 year. Recurrent nipple discharge had also been present for a short time.

Palpable Findings

Firm, mobile, walnut-sized mass deep to the nipple of the right breast.

Sonography

(sector scan with standoff)

Figure: transverse scan over the palpable mass.

Readability: good.

Sharply demarcated focal sonographic lesion, 31×15 mm.

Interpretation

The sonographic criteria suggest a benign lesion. Although the mass has contrasting central and peripheral echogenicities, it is very likely a fibroadenoma by ultrasound. The differential diagnosis must also include colloid carcinoma (see the cases on pp. 48 and 204).

X-ray Mammography

Smoothly marginated subareolar round lesion in the right breast. Galactography showed no abnormalities.

Histology

Fibroadenoma with regressive change.

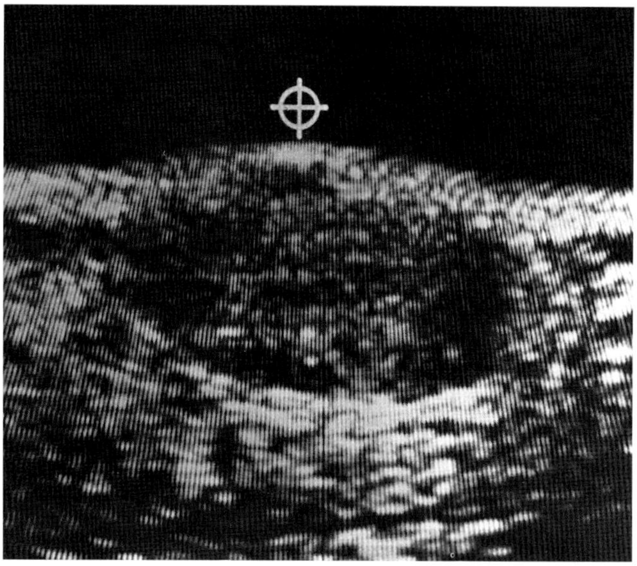

Analysis

1. **Margins**	sharp and smooth
2. **Retrotumoral acoustic phenomena**	slight posterior enhancement
3. **Internal echo pattern**	homogeneous (except for lesion periphery)
4. **Echogenicity**	hypoechoic
5. **Compression effect** on **shape**	no deformation
6. **Compression effect** on **internal echoes**	no change

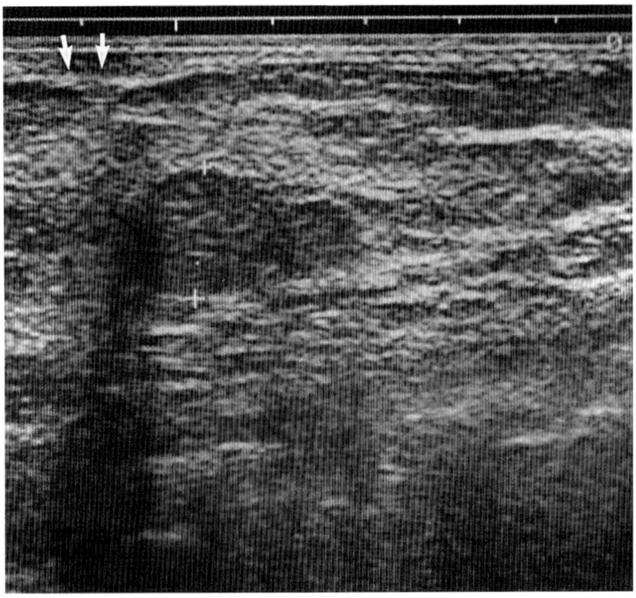

Analysis

1. Margins	sharp and smooth
2. Retrotumoral acoustic phenomena	nonmodified echoes
3. Internal echo pattern	homogeneous
4. Echogenicity	hypoechoic
5. Compression effect on **shape**	no deformation
6. Compression effect on **internal echoes**	no change

History

The 49-year-old woman with a family history of breast cancer had undergone right breast biopsy 4 years before. She recently underwent unsuccessful excision of a mammographically indeterminate focal lesion.

Palpable Findings

Mammographic lesion was located approximately 3 cm beneath the nipple of the right breast; difficult to palpate.

Sonography

Figure: sagittal scan over the barely palpable mass.

Readability: good.

Lobulated focal lesion, 27×15×18 mm, partly beneath the earlier biopsy scar.

Interpretation

The sonographic criteria imply a benign mass. A smaller focal lesion is seen directly adjacent to the larger mass, but both lesions are well demarcated with respect to their surroundings. The analytic criteria are consistent with a lobulated fibroadenoma. The left border of the lesion is obscured by an acoustic shadow from the earlier biopsy scar. This interpretation is made possible by a knowledge of the clinical presentation, although a discontinuity in the skin line *(arrows)* can be seen above the shadow.

X-ray Mammography

Lobulated round lesion, 25×20 mm, with predominantly sharp margins.

Histology

Intracanalicular fibroadenoma.

History

The 48-year-old woman had noticed marked enlargement of a left breast mass in previous weeks.

Palpable Findings

Tense, smoothly marginated, slightly mobile, approximately egg-sized mass involving both upper quadrants of the left breast.

Sonography

Figure: transverse scan over the mass.

Readability: good.

Sharply marginated focal lesion, 45×27 mm.

Interpretation

The criteria are suggestive of a benign lesion and show all the typical features of a tense, solitary breast cyst.

Aspiration Cytology

Aspiration yielded 10.5 mL of al clear, serous fluid; Papanicolaou grades I/II.

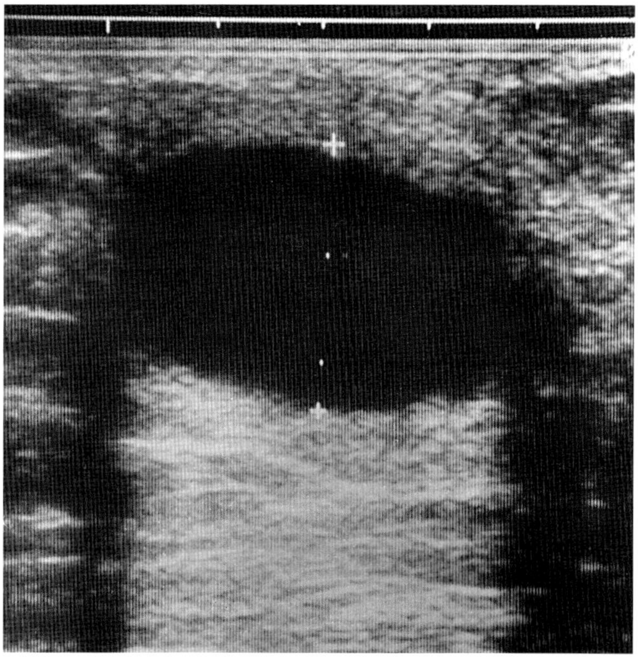

Analysis

1. **Margins**	sharp and smooth
2. **Retrotumoral acoustic phenomena**	posterior enhancement and bilateral shadowing phenomena
3. **Internal echo pattern**	no echoes
4. **Echogenicity**	no echoes
5. **Compression effect** on **shape**	deformed
6. **Compression effect** on **internal echoes**	no change

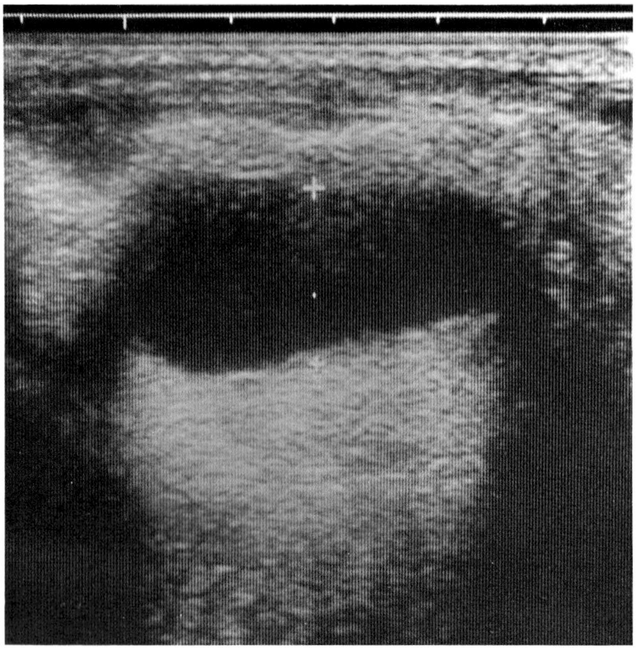

Analysis

1. **Margins**	sharp and smooth
2. **Retrotumoral acoustic phenomena**	posterior enhancement and bilateral shadowing phenomena
3. **Internal echo pattern**	no echoes
4. **Echogenicity**	no echoes
5. **Compression effect** on **shape**	deformed
6. **Compression effect** on **internal echoes**	no change

Note: The multiple low-level echoes issuing from the center of the anterior wall and projecting into the echo-free space are reverberations.

History

This woman, 44 years of age, had known fibrocystic breast disease.

Palpable Findings

Typical nodular breast. A soft, mobile, but well-demarcated, plum-sized mass was palpated in both upper quadrants of the right breast.

Sonography

Figure: transverse scan over the palpable mass.

Readability: good.

Well-demarcated focal lesion, 40×18 mm.

Interpretation

All the criteria suggest a benign cystic lesion. Unlike the lesion in the previous figure, this cyst is not distended with fluid. The reverberations at the anterior wall can be confusing. If a similar structure occurs at the posterior wall, ist should be interpreted as an intracystic growth until proved otherwise.

Note: If the characteristics of a cystic mass are somewhat unclear (as the margins are here), at the least aspiration cytology and pneumocystography should be performed to clarify the situation.

Aspiration Cytology

Aspiration yielded 8.4 mL of a clear, amber-colored fluid; Papanicolaou grades I/II.

History

The 42-year-old woman noticed recent enlargement of a right breast mass that had been present for at least 6 months.

Palpable Findings

Firm but mobile area of increased density approximately 3 cm in diameter in the upper inner quadrant of the right breast.

A well-demarcated lesion could not be identified by palpation.

Sonography

Figure: transverse scan over the mass demonstrating a well-demarcated focal sonographic lesion, 31×14 mm.

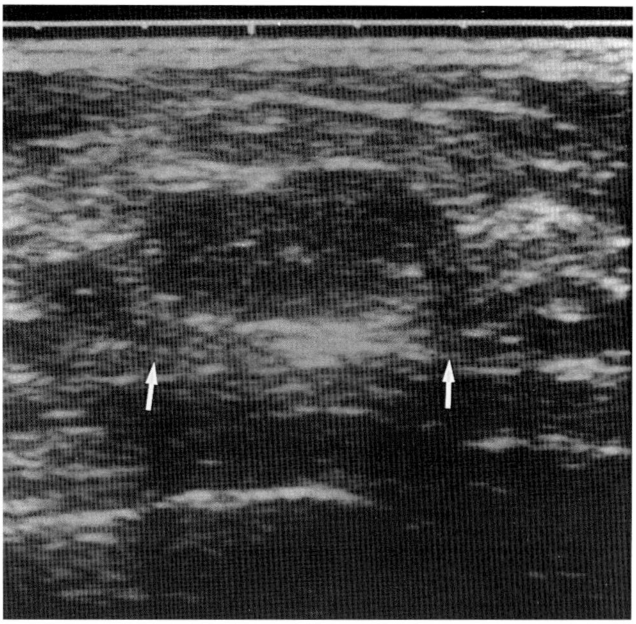

Interpretation

All sonographic criteria suggest a benign tumor. Despite three or four small, bright echoes within the lesion, the internal echo pattern is classified as homogeneous. The lesion is a fibroadenoma by ultrasound.

Histology

Sharply demarcated, 30-mm tumor. Fibroadenoma phylloides. Also fibrocystic mastopathy with intraductal papillomas. No evidence of malignancy or specificity.

Analysis

1. **Margins**	sharp and smooth
2. **Retrotumoral acoustic phenomena**	posterior enhancement and faint bilateral shadowing *(arrows)*
3. **Internal echo pattern**	homogeneous
4. **Echogenicity**	fat-equivalent
5. **Compression effect** on **shape**	no deformation
6. **Compression effect** on **internal echoes**	no change

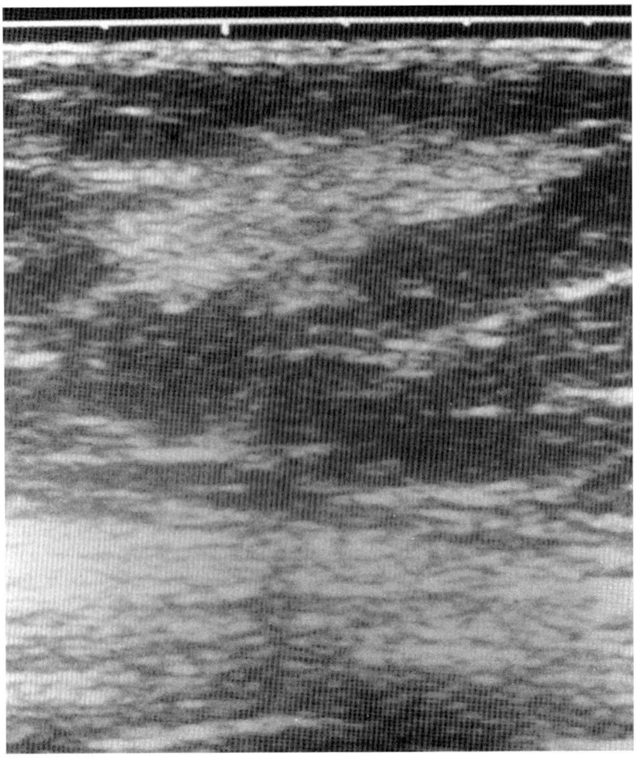

History

The 33-year-old woman was evaluated for right breast pain radiating to the arm.

Palpable Findings

Approximately plum-sized, firm, relatively mobile, knobby mass with ill-defined borders in the upper outer quadrant of the right breast. Marked bilateral macromastia.

Sonography

Figure: sagittal scan over the palpable mass showing a hyperechoic area, approximately 48×23 mm, within the fatty breast. A focal sonographic lesion in the true sense is not present.

Analysis

The analytic criteria cannot be applied.

Interpretation

The fact that a focal sonographic lesion cannot be demonstrated for the impressive palpable mass implies a benign disorder by ultrasound. The most likely sonographic correlate is a circumscribed area of glandular tissue within the fatty breast.

X-ray Mammography

Extensive fatty involution. The palpable mass correlates with a circumscribed density in the upper outer quadrant of the right breast, which may represent residual breast parenchyma.

Histology

Dense parenchyma with no focal abnormalities. Histology reveals diffuse hyperplasia of the mammary lobules, which are bordered by thin strands of fibrous connective tissue. No evidence of malignancy.

Radiographically Dense Breasts

Radiographically dense breasts, which are very difficult or impossible to evaluate by X-ray mammography, usually present optimum conditions for ultrasound examination because of their favorable acoustic properties. This particularly applies to women with significant fibrocystic disease. Sonography can frequently exclude a circumscribed focal lesion in clinically nodular areas and radiodense breasts (Guyer and Dewburry 1985).

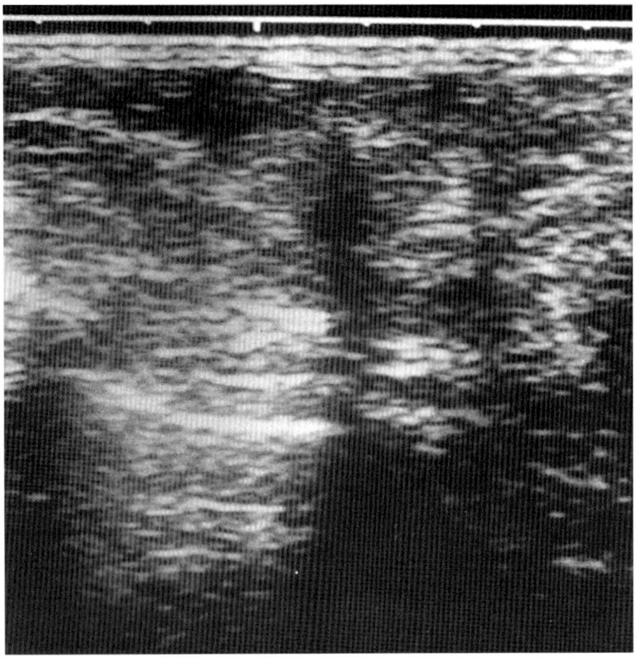
a

History

The 43-year-old woman, who had a known several-year history of fibrocystic disease, was found to have a new lump in the upper quadrant of her right breast. The referring specialist offered a presumptive *sonographic* diagnosis of breast carcinoma.

Palpable Findings

Bilateral fibrocystic mastopathy with coarsely nodular breasts. An approximately 1 cm, demarcated mass was also found in the right breast.

Sonography

Figure **a**: sagittal scan over the palpable right breast mass.

Readability: good.

Focal lesion, 12×10 mm, with posterior shadowing.

Analysis

1. Margins	indistinct, jagged
2. Retrotumoral acoustic phenomena	moderate posterior shadowing
3. Internal echo pattern	few echoes, non-homogeneous
4. Echogenicity	almost anechoic
5. Compression effect on **shape**	no deformation
6. Compression effect on **internal echoes**	no change

Interpretation

All sonographic criteria suggest a malignant process.

X-ray Mammography

Figure **b**: mediolateral projection demonstrating severe dysplasia with disseminated microcalcifications. The palpable mass is not visualized.

Histology

Infiltrating lobular carcinoma with elements of lobular carcinoma in situ (intraoperative size: 15×7 mm).

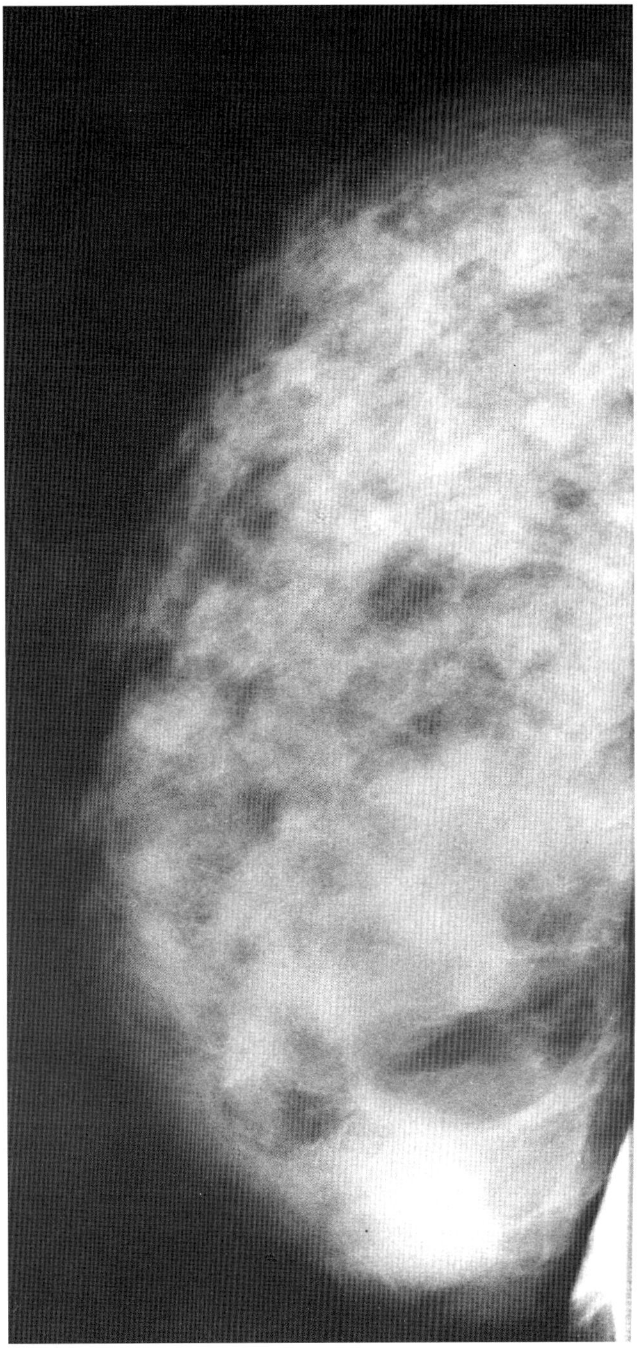

b

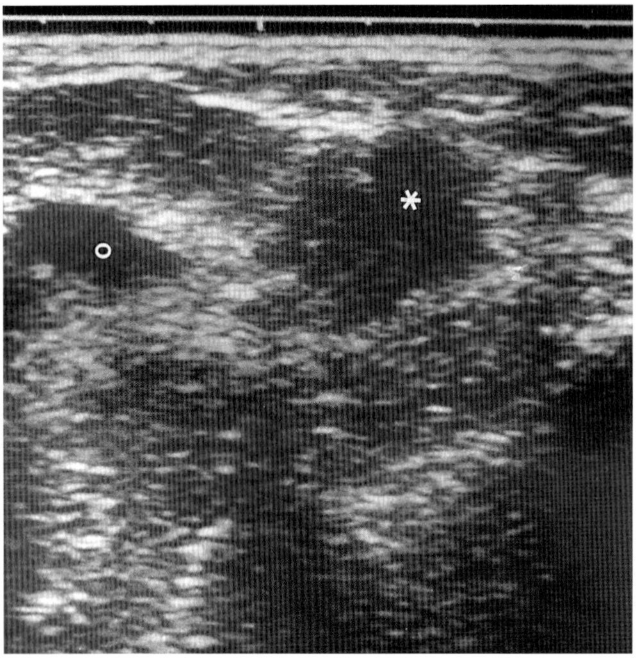

Analysis

	Lesion 1 *
1. **Margins**	indistinct, jagged
2. **Retrotumoral acoustic phenomena**	unchanged echoes
3. **Internal echo pattern**	few echoes, nonhomogeneous
4. **Echogenicity**	almost anechoic
5. **Compression effect** on **shape**	no deformation
6. **Compression effect** on **internal echoes**	no change
	Lesion 2 O
1. **Margins**	sharp, jagged
2. **Retrotumoral acoustic phenomena**	(slight) posterior enhancement
3. **Internal echo pattern**	no echoes
4. **Echogenicity**	anechoic
5. **Compression effect** on **shape**	shape distortion
6. **Compression effect** on **internal echoes**	no change

History

The 47-year-old woman had a known history of cystic breast disease for some years and had undergone repeated cyst aspirations in the past. Mammograms difficult to evaluate.

Palpable Findings

Both breasts nodular. Firm, smooth, relatively fixed mass, 2×3 cm, above the nipple of the right breast at 12 o'clock. A similar mass was palpated in the upper outer quadrant of the left breast.

Sonography

Both breasts harbor multiple cysts ranging from 10 to 30 mm in diameter.
Readability: limited.
Figure: oblique scan over the prominent right breast mass.
Two focal sonographic lesions:
Lesion 1 (*): Suspicious focal lesion, 25×16 mm.
Lesion 2 (O): Indeterminate focal lesion, 18×9 mm, in the immediate vicinity of lesion 1.

Interpretation

Lesion 1: All sonographic criteria suggest a malignant process.
Lesion 2: The sonographic criteria are consistent with a partially deflated cyst.
The contrasting echo characteristics of the two lesions are clearly appreciated in the dynamic examination.

Aspiration Cytology

Cyst aspiration: 1.5 mL of amber-colored fluid. Cytology: Papanicolaou grade I.

Histology

Lesion 1: infiltrating ductal carcinoma with partial tubular differentiation and extensive intraductal carcinoma infiltrates. Histologic size indeterminate, intraoperative size 25×18 mm. Very severe fibrocystic mastopathy with extensive papillomas.

History

The 45-year-old woman with known fibrocystic mastopathy had undergone multiple cyst aspirations in the past and presented now for follow-up examination.

Her mammograms were difficult to interpret.

Palpable Findings

Both breasts coarsely nodular on palpation.

Sonography

Figure: sagittal scan through the lower inner quadrant of the left breast.

Readability: good.

Multiple cystic focal lesions (in both breasts).

Interpretation

All sonographic criteria are highly suggestive of benignancy. The variable degree of acoustic enhancement behind the different cysts is noteworthy.

Aspiration Cytology

Clear, amber-colored fluid. Papanicolaou grades I/II.

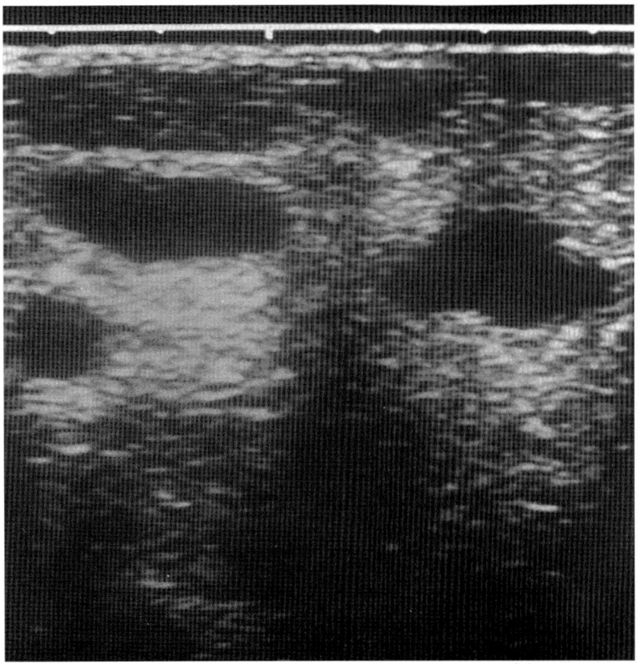

Analysis

1. **Margins**	sharp and smooth
2. **Retrotumoral acoustic phenomena**	posterior enhancement (slight to strong)
3. **Internal echo pattern**	no echoes
4. **Echogenicity**	anechoic
5. **Compression effect** on **shape**	shape distortion
6. **Compression effect** on **internal echoes**	no change

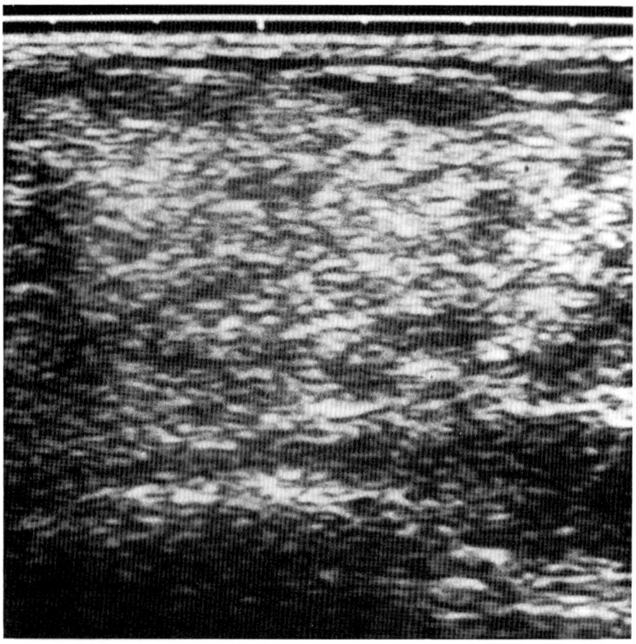
a

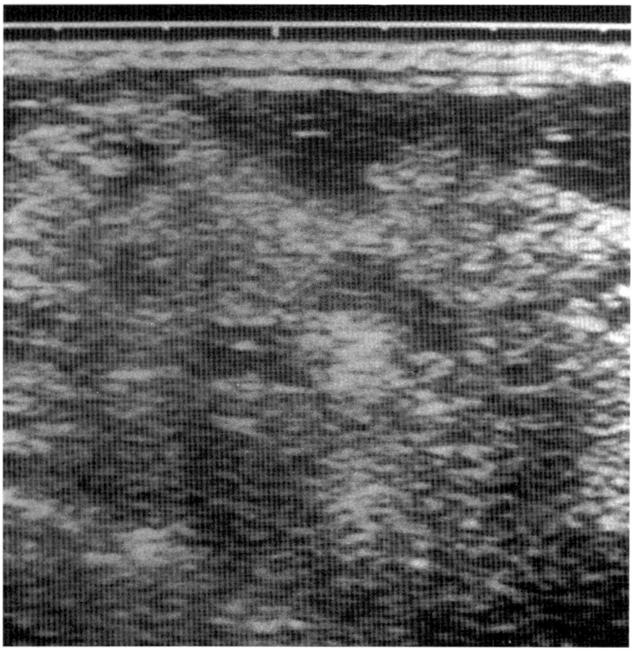
b

History

The 34-year-old woman had complained for years of breast pain, more severe on the right, relating to her menstrual cycle. She recently noticed a lump in her right breast.

Palpable Findings

Both breasts were coarsely nodular. An approximately 2–3 cm, tender mass was found in the right breast at 12 o'clock.

Sonography

Figure **a**: transverse scan over the right breast mass (total gain: 30 dB).

Readability: good.

A focal sonographic lesion is not demonstrated.

Figure **b**: transverse scan over the identical site in the left breast (total gain. 34 dB).

Readability: good.

A focal sonographic lesion is not demonstrated.

There is noc focal lesion, so the analytic criteria cannot be applied.

Interpretation

The sonographic features are consistent with dense fibrocystic disease. The greater radiographic density of the right breast (see X-ray Mammography) is reflected sonographically in the fact that the right breast appears considerably more echogenic at a total gain of 30 dB than does the left breast at a total gain of 34 dB.

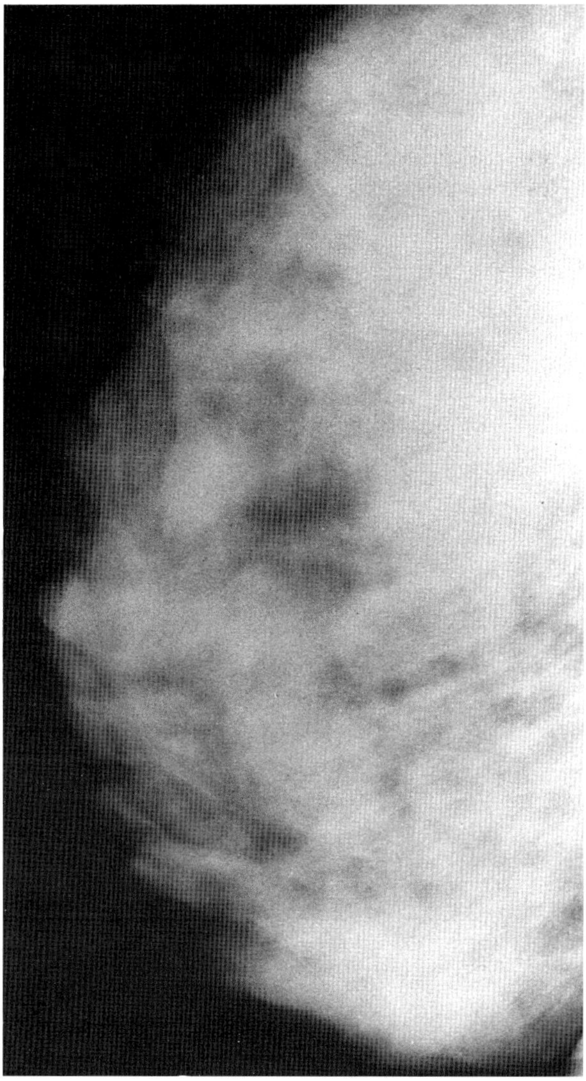

c

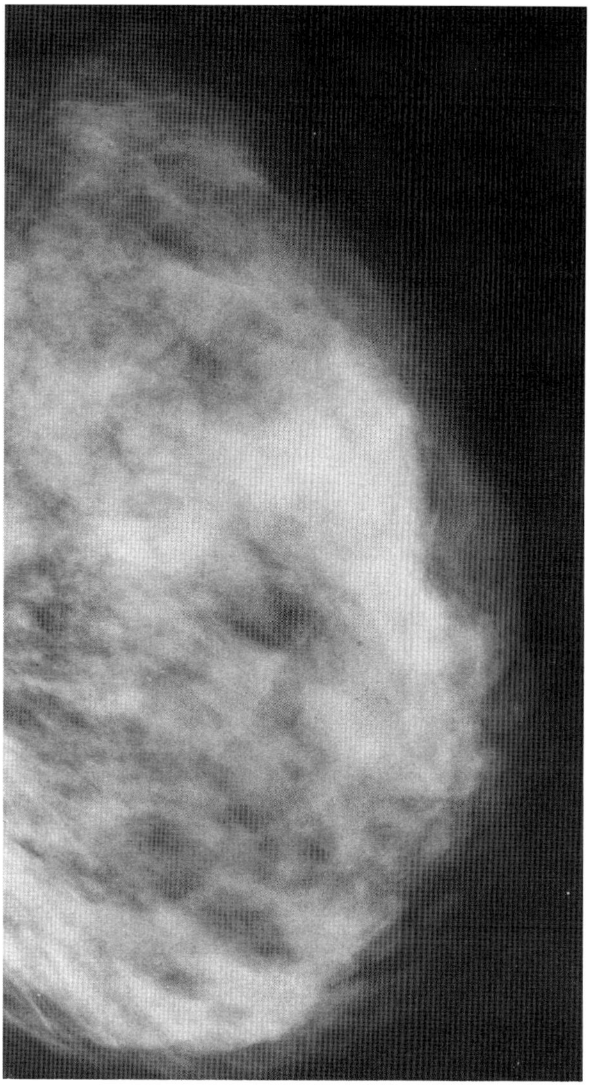

d

X-ray Mammography

Dense fibrocystic mastopathy in both breasts. Interpretation is significantly hampered in the left breast (Fig. **d**) and is not possible in the right breast (Fig. **c**), which shows a particularly marked asymmetric density increase. The palpable right breast mass cannot be characterized as benign or malignant by mammography.

Histology

Excisional biopsy from the right breast encompassed an area of simple fibro(micro)cystic mastopathy.

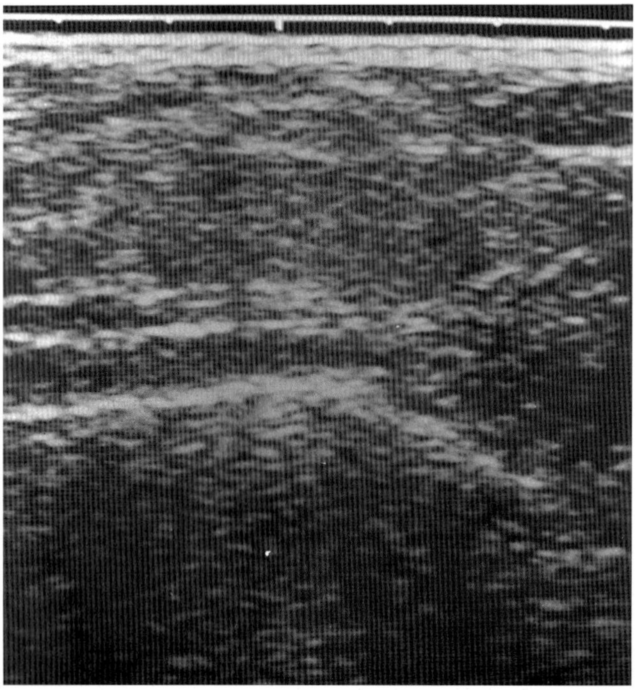

Analysis

1. **Margins**	sharp and smooth
2. **Retrotumoral acoustic phenomena**	unchanged echoes
3. **Internal echo pattern**	homogeneous
4. **Echogenicity**	isoechoic!
5. **Compression effect** on **shape**	shape distortion
6. **Compression effect** on **internal echoes**	become more homogeneous

History

The 34-year-old woman complained of severe premenstrual tension in the breasts and the cyclic appearance of a mass in the left breast.

Palpable Findings

Ill-defined mass in the upper quadrants of the left breast.

Sonography

Figure: transverse scan over the left breast mass.

Readability: good.

Very subtle focal lesion, 33×15 mm.

Interpretation

The sonographic criteria imply a benign disorder. This is a rare instance in which the lesion is *isoechoic* to the breast parenchyma. The compression effects are positive, meaning that the lesion is very likely benign. The sonographic criteria in conjunction with clinical findings support the diagnosis of an isolated area of fibrocystic disease.

X-ray Mammography

Very dense bilateral fibroadenosis with transition to sclerosing adenosis.

Histology

Grade II fibrocystic mastopathy with focal sclerosing adenosis. No evidence of malignancy.

History

The 27-year-old woman with a radiographically dense breast and a family history of breast cancer had multiple excisional biopsies of both breasts, with consistently benign histology (fibrocystic disease, sclerosing adenosis).

Palpable Findings

Both breasts were coarsely nodular with no isolated palpable masses.

Sonography was performed at the patient's request.

Sonography

Figure: survey of the left breast demonstrates a small focal lesion, 8×6 mm, at the areolar border.

Readability: good.

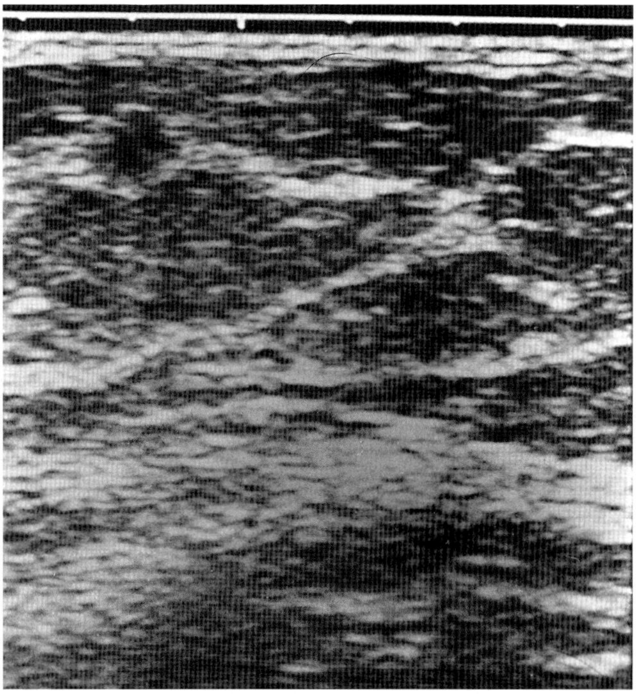

Interpretation

Criteria 1, 3 and 4 imply a malignant lesion, while criteria 2 and 5 suggest benignancy. Indeed, a confident benign/malignant differentiation cannot be made by sonographic analysis. The overall impression of the case does not preclude a cyst. Fine-needle aspiration is indicated in such cases. Aspiration in this case yielded a trace amount of milky fluid, whereupon the lesion was no longer demonstrable by ultrasound. Air insufflation was unnecessary. In cases where aspiration is unsuccessful due to the small size of the lesion, a histologic workup is indicated.

Aspiration Cytology

Papanicolaou grades I/II.

Analysis

1. Margins	indistinct, jagged
2. Retrotumoral acoustic phenomena	faint posterior enhancement
3. Internal echo pattern	few echoes, nonhomogeneous
4. Echogenicity	almost anechoic
5. Compression effect on **shape**	shape distortion
6. Compression effect on **internal echoes**	no change

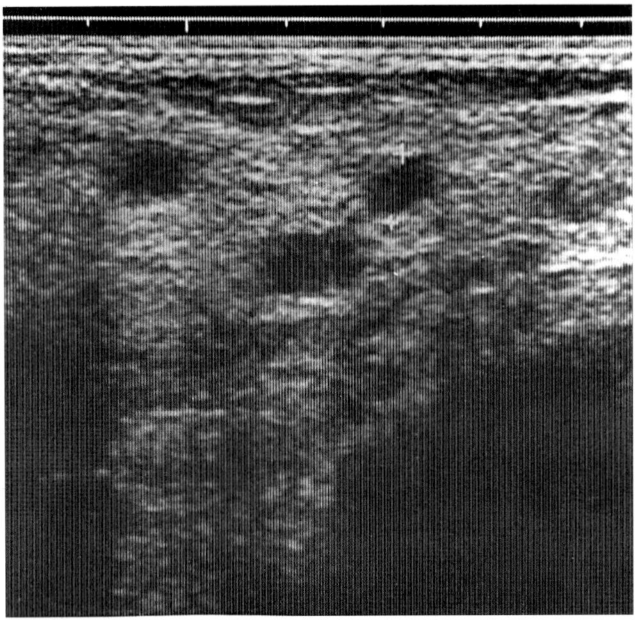

Analysis
(all three lesions)

1. **Margins**	indistinct but smooth
2. **Retrotumoral acoustic phenomena**	slight posterior enhancement
3. **Internal echo pattern**	few echoes, nonhomogeneous
4. **Echogenicity**	almost anechoic
5. **Compression effect** on **shape**	shape distortion
6. **Compression effect** on **internal echoes**	no change

History

The 42-year-old woman with known fibrocystic mastopathy had undergone multiple trials of medical treatment and cyst aspirations. She presented now for follow-up while on low-dosage antiestrogen therapy. Her breasts became softer with the treatment, and her symptoms became regressive.

Palpable Findings

Nodular breasts with no isolated palpable mass.

Sonography

Figure: transverse scan through the upper outer quadrant of the right breast. Multiple small, hypoechoic focal lesions were found in both breasts.

Readability: good.

Three focal sonographic lesions.

Interpretation

The sonographic criteria are inconsistent. It is important to know that the nonhomogeneous echo pattern in this case results mainly from peripheral internal echoes, which may disappear during compression. These focal lesions represent partially deflated cysts with low wall tension. The cysts are known to undergo volume changes during different phases of the menstrual cycle, although their regression may signify positive response to therapy.

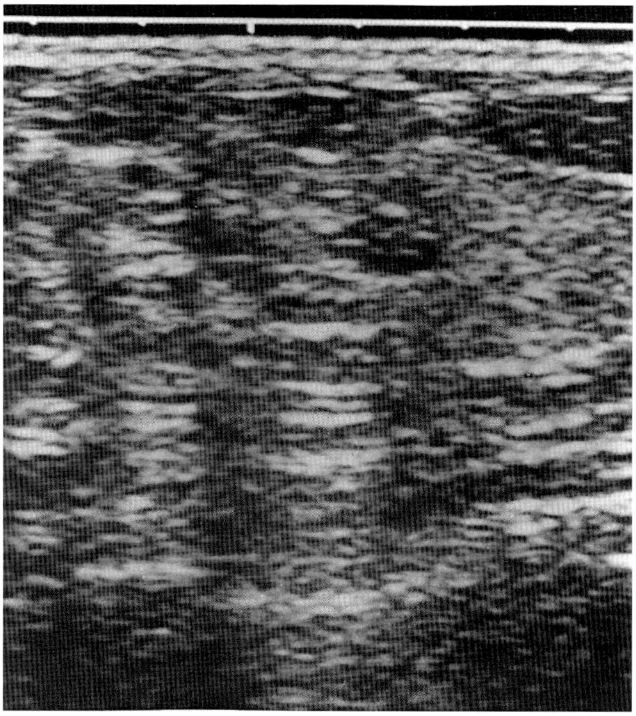

History

The 37-year-old woman had a history of premenstrual tension in both breasts with enlargement. She had no family history of breast cancer.

Palpable Findings

Nodularity in both breasts, most pronounced in the upper outer quadrants.

Sonography

Figure: sagittal scan over the upper outer quadrant showing dense breast parenchyma at the right side of the image whose structure becomes increasingly disordered toward the left. A focal abnormality is not seen.

Analysis

The absence of a focal lesion precludes application of the analytic criteria.

Interpretation

Typical sonographic presentation of a fibrocystic process. At the patient's request, a drill biopsy was performed to determine the degree of proliferation.

Histology

Fibrocystic mastopathy with intraductal papillomas and microcalcifications.

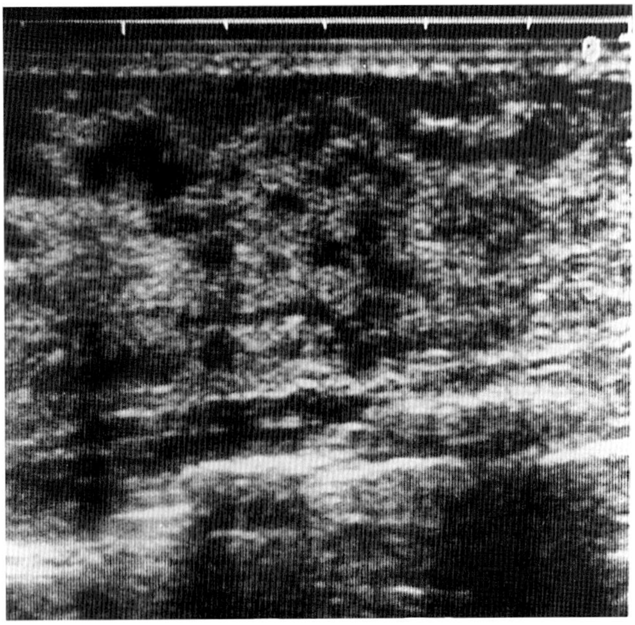

History

The 29-year-old woman had a long history of radiographically dense breasts, had been virtually asymptomatic while using oral contraceptives. The patient requested a breast ultrasound examination.

Palpable Findings

Dense, firm breasts with no discrete palpable masses.

Sonography

Figure: sagittal scan through the upper outer quadrant of the right breast.

Typical appearance of microcystic to small-cystic breast disease.

No focal sonographic lesions, so the analytic criteria cannot be applied.

Interpretation

Multiple small to very small cystic structures are observed within a dense breast. Cysts requiring aspiration were not found. No further diagnostic measures are indicated.

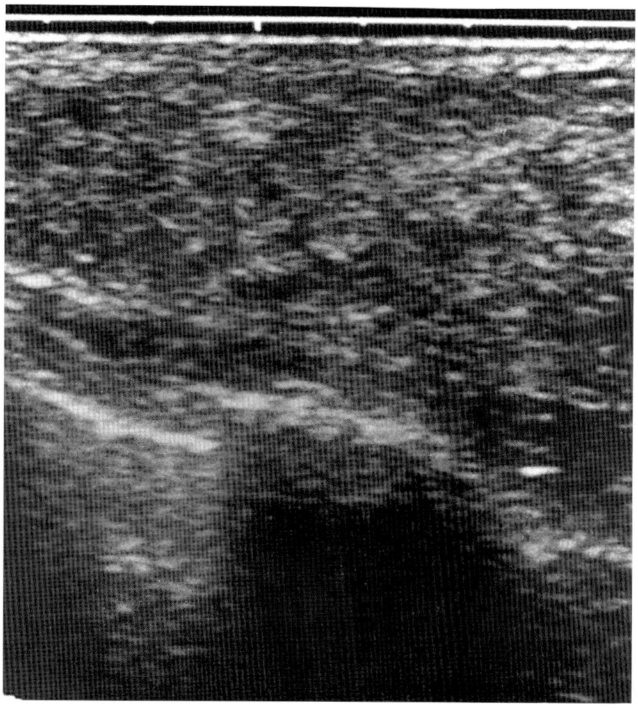

History

The 38-year-old woman had felt a small lump in her right breast 2 weeks before.

Palpable Findings

Firm, mobile mass, 5×5 mm, in the upper outer quadrant of the right breast at the areolar border.

Sonography

Figure: sagittal scan over the palpable mass showing a dense breast with no subcutaneous or retromammary fat.

Readability: good.

There is no focal sonographic lesion, so the analytic criteria cannot be applied.

Interpretation

Sonographic findings indicate dense fibrocystic disease with no focal abnormalities.

The palpable mass was excised.

Histology

Fibrocystic mastopathy with microcalcifications. No evidence of malignancy or specifity.

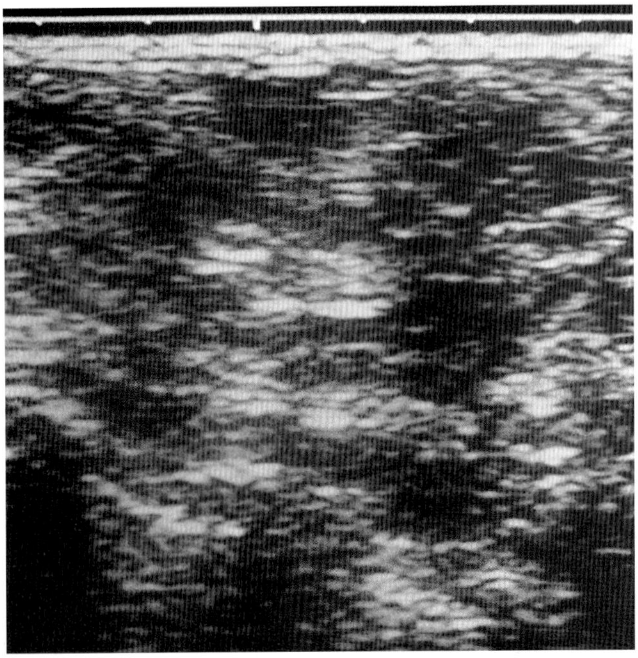

a

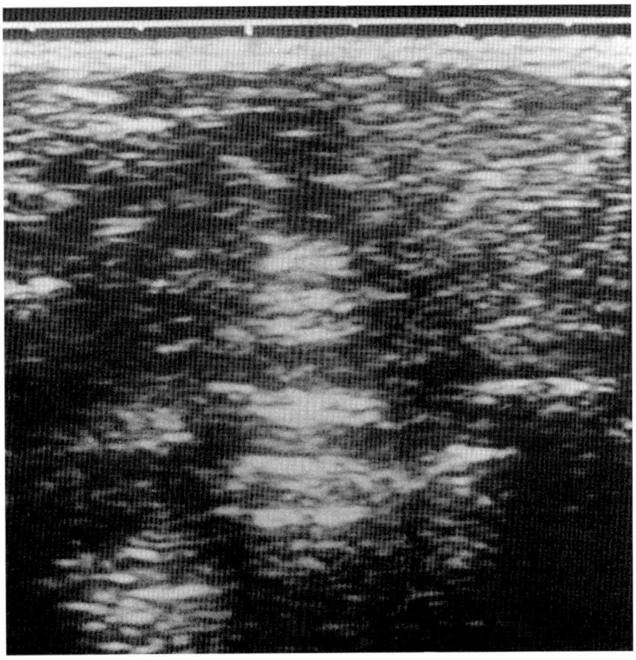

b

History

The 38-year-old woman presented in the second half of her menstrual cycle with pain, more pronounced in the right breast.

Palpable Findings

Increased density in the upper outer quadrant of the right breast.

Sonography

Figure **a**: sagittal scan over the dense area.

Figure **b**: transverse scan over the dense area.

Readability: limited.

A focal sonographic lesion is not demonstrated, so the analytic criteria cannot be applied.

Interpretation

The sonographic picture is completely disordered, with no evidence of a normal glandular architecture. The breast contains adjacent hypoechoic and hyperechoic areas, some with posterior shadowing.

This type of pattern is actually seen only in breasts with severe fibrocystic disease.

Histology

Fibrocystic mastopathy with apocrine metaplasia and intraductal microcalcifications. No evidence of malignancy or specificity.

Mammographically Indeterminate Lesions

Carcinomas are not detected by X-ray mammography in approximately 13% of cases (Dodd 1977). Through the adjunctive use of ultrasound imaging, mammographically indeterminate lesions can be correctly categorized preoperatively as benign or malignant in approximately 70% of cases (Leucht et al. 1985). This can can sometimes result in a modification of the therapeutic approach.

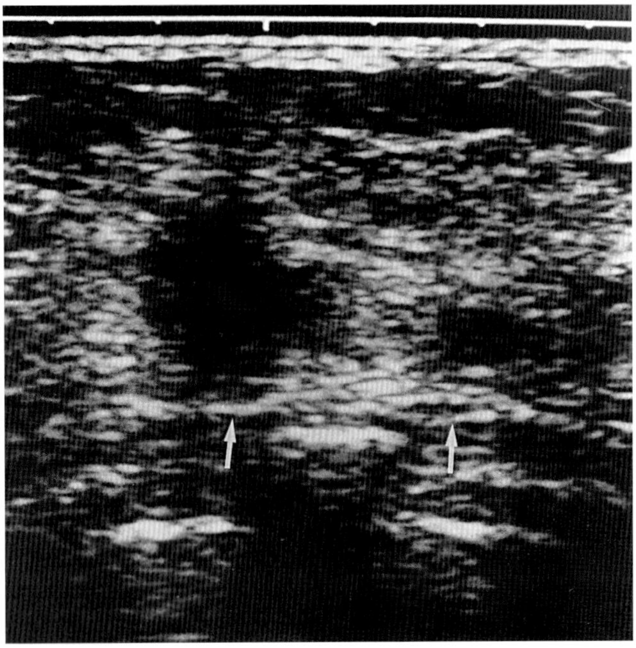

Analysis

1. Margins	indistinct, jagged
2. Retrotumoral acoustic phenomena	unchanged echoes
3. Internal echo pattern	few echoes, non-homogeneous
4. Echogenicity	almost anechoic
5. Compression effect on **shape**	no deformation
6. Compression effect on **internal echoes**	no change

History

The 48-year-old woman had undergone breast-conserving surgery elsewhere 14 days before for a carcinoma of the right breast. Later she felt a lump (lymphoma) in the left axilla.

Palpable Findings

General density of the left breast, especially in the upper outer quadrant.

A discrete breast mass was not identified. Suspicious lymph node in the left axilla.

Sonography

Figure: sagittal scan through the upper outer quadrant of the left breast.

Readability: good.

Focal lesion, 15×12 mm, near the chest wall. Intact pectoral fascia *(arrows)*.

Interpretation

The sonographic criteria are suggestive of a malignant tumor. In this case, a palpable lymph node was the indication for breast ultrasound. The tumor itself was extremely difficult to palpate, even at operation.

X-ray Mammography

Mammography in this patient was unrewarding.

Histology

Partly solid, partly tubular infiltrating ductal carcinoma (approximately 10 mm in diameter). The pectoral fascia is free of tumor infiltration.

History

The 47-year-old woman with a family history of breast cancer noticed enlargement of her right breast 2 months ago. She had undergone bilateral reduction mammoplasty 25 years before.

Palpable Findings

Area, approximately 8×8 cm, with multiple isolated, suspicious nodules in the right breast.

Sonography

Figure **a**: sagittal scan over two palpable masses (*).

Figure **b**: sagittal scan over al larger mass (*) located farther medially.

Readibility: good.

All three of the focal sonographic lesions have a similar appearance and are jointly analyzed.

Interpretation

All the lesions have the same sonographic features. Except for an absence of retrotumoral acoustic effect, the analytic criteria are diagnostic of carcinoma, which here is multifocal or multicentric.

X-ray Mammography

No focal abnormalities other than a density increase in the right breast.

Histology

Multifocal infiltrating ductal carcinoma, with a total extent 60 mm and pronounced intraductal spread.

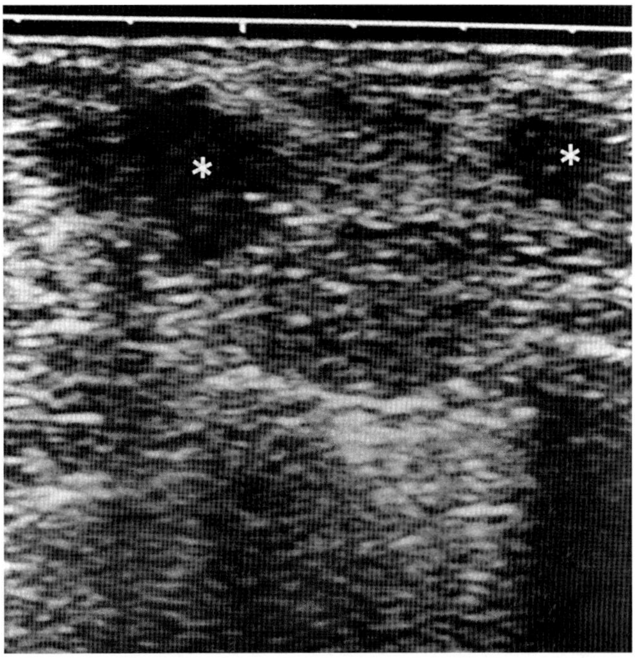

a

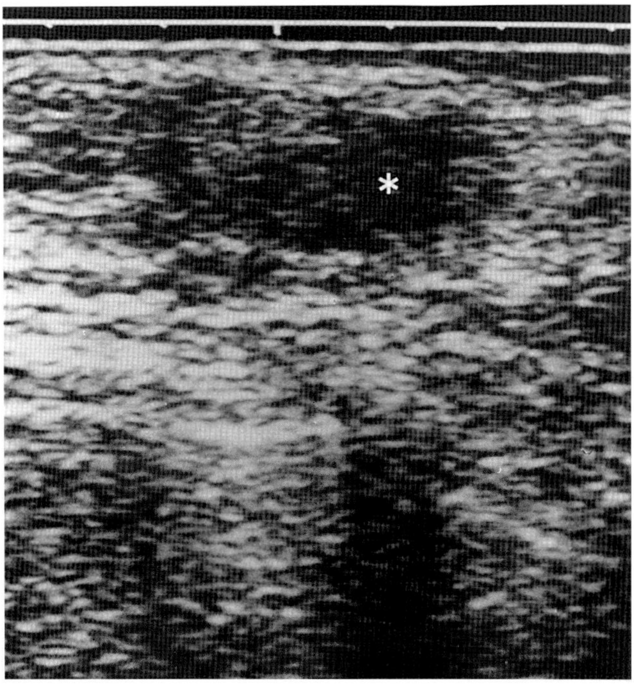

b

Analysis

1. **Margins**	indistinct, jagged
2. **Retrotumoral acoustic phenomena**	unchanged echoes
3. **Internal echo pattern**	few echoes, non-homogeneous
4. **Echogenicity**	almost anechoic
5. **Compression effect** on **shape**	no deformation
6. **Compression effect** on **internal echoes**	no change

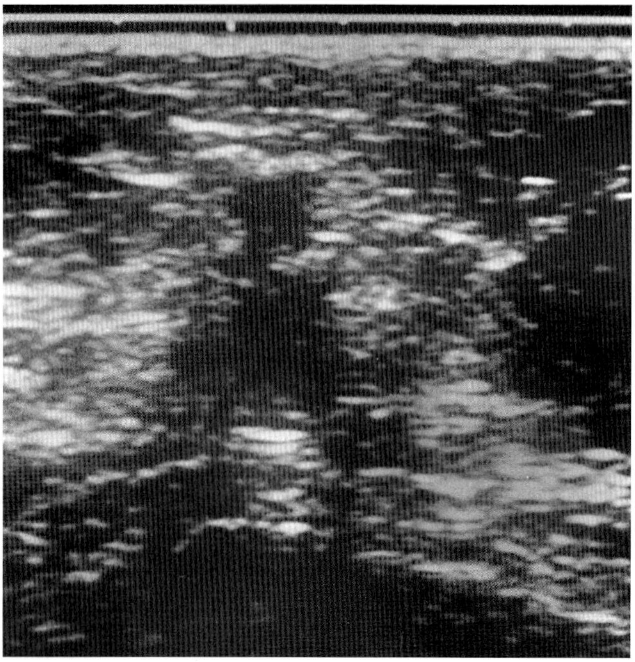

a

Analysis

1. Margins	indistinct, jagged
2. Retrotumoral acoustic phenomena	unchanged echoes
3. Internal echo pattern	few echoes, nonhomogeneous
4. Echogenicity	almost anechoic
5. Compression effect on **shape**	no deformation
6. Compression effect on **internal echoes**	no change

History

The 53-year-old woman had felt a lump in her right breast 2 months before. Prior to that, she had sustained impact trauma to the same breast.

Palpable Findings

Relatively fixed, firm, approximately 3 cm mass near the nipple in the upper outer quadrant of the right breast.

Sonography

Figure **a**: transverse scan over the palpable mass.

Readability: good.

Focal lesion, 16×21 mm.

Interpretation

All sonographic criteria suggest a malignant process.

X-ray Mammography

Figure **b**: mediolateral projection demonstrating a cordlike density in the upper quadrants. No circumscribed abnormality. Same feature is seen in the craniocaudal projection.

Histology

Poorly differentiated infiltrating ductal carcinoma (intraoperative size: 23×20 mm).

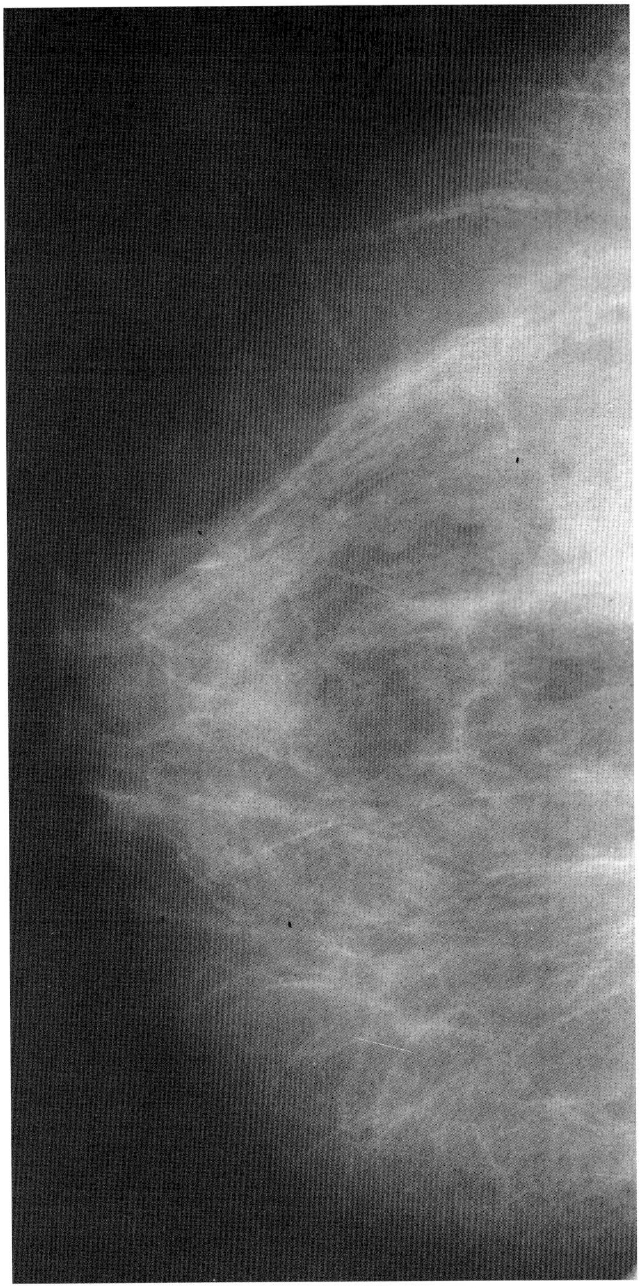

b

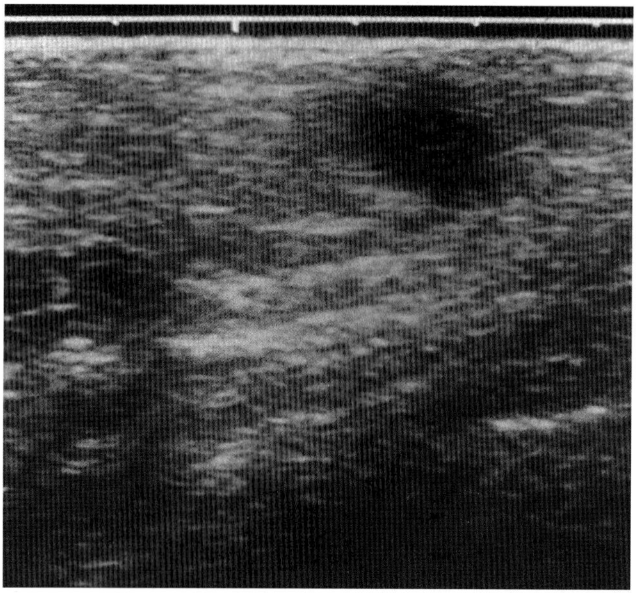

a

Analysis

1. Margins	indistinct, jagged
2. Retrotumoral acoustic phenomena	unchanged echoes
3. Internal echo pattern	few echoes, nonhomogeneous
4. Echogenicity	almost anechoic
5. Compression effect on **shape**	no deformation
6. Compression effect on **internal echoes**	no change

History

The 29-year-old woman felt a lump lateral to the nipple of her left breast. She had a family history of breast cancer.

Palpable Findings

Firm, approximately 1.5 cm subcutaneous mass in the left breast at 3 o'clock.

Sonography

Figure **a**: sagittal scan over the palpable mass (7.5 MHz).

Readability: good.

Suspicious focal lesion located just beneath the skin in mastopathy-altered glandular parenchyma (17×11 mm).

Interpretation

The sonographic criteria suggest a malignant process.

The almost anechoic lesion contrasts markedly with its very dense mastopathic environment.

X-ray Mammography

Figure **c**: craniocaudal projection showing a dense dysplastic breast with no discernible focal abnormality. Same on mediolateral view.

Histology

Poorly differentiated infiltrating ductal carcinoma (diameter approximately 20 mm) with lymphatic invasion.

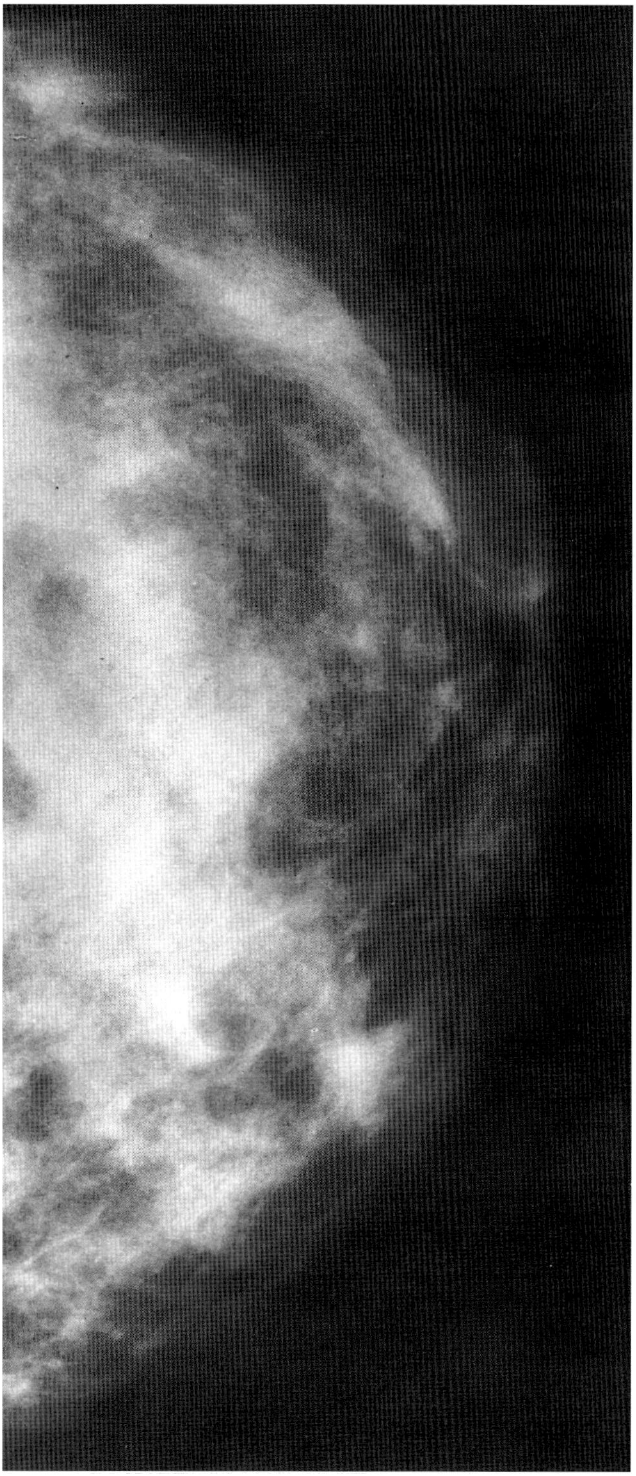

b

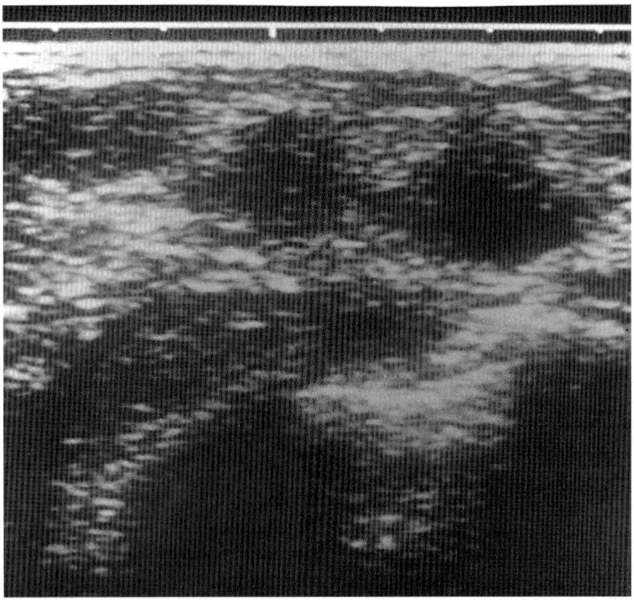
a

Analysis

1. **Margins**	indistinct, jagged
2. **Retrotumoral acoustic phenomena**	unchanged echoes
3. **Internal echo pattern**	few echoes, nonhomogeneous
4. **Echogenicity**	almost anechoic
5. **Compression effect** on **shape**	no deformation
6. **Compression effect** on **internal echoes**	no change

History

This woman, 33 years of age, had a 1-week history of increasing pain in the left breast.

Palpable Findings

Firm, knobby, 3-cm mass in the upper outer quadrant of the left breast. Lateral to it, a suspicious, approximately chestnut-sized lymph node.

Sonography

Figure **a**: sagittal scan over the palpable mass.

Readability: good.

Two suspicious, apparently contiguous focal lesions.

Sonographic size: 37×23 mm.

Interpretation

All sonographic criteria are consistent with multicentric breast carcinoma.

X-ray Mammography

The craniocaudal (Fig. **b**) and mediolateral projections (Fig. **c**) show no features typical of carcinoma.

Histology

Predominantly solid, partly tubular infiltrating duct carcinoma with invasion of small lymph spaces. Histologic tumor size: maximum diameter 50 mm.

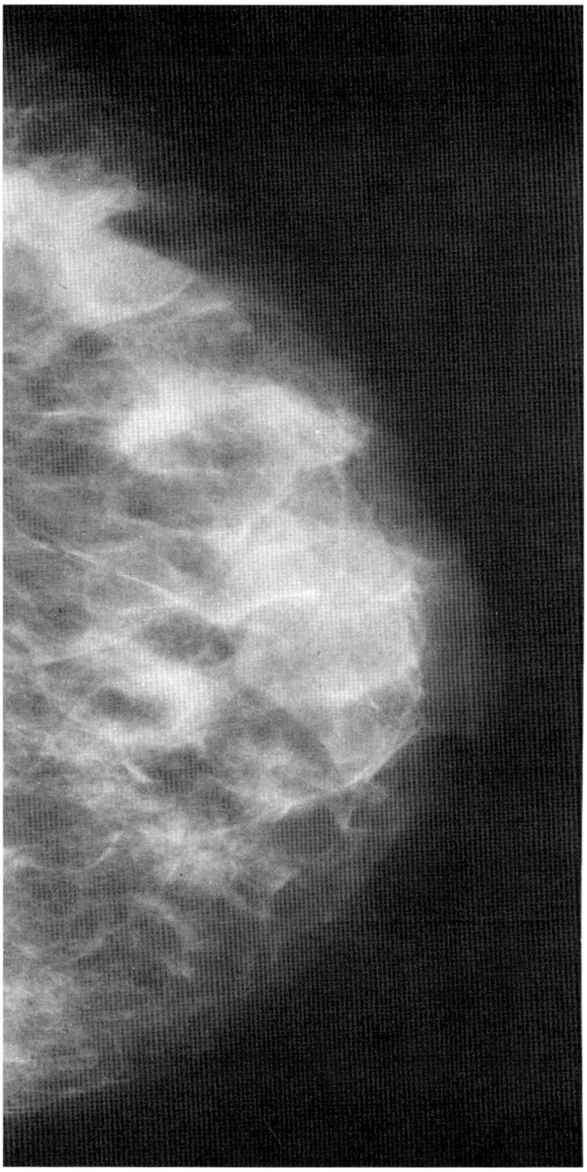

b

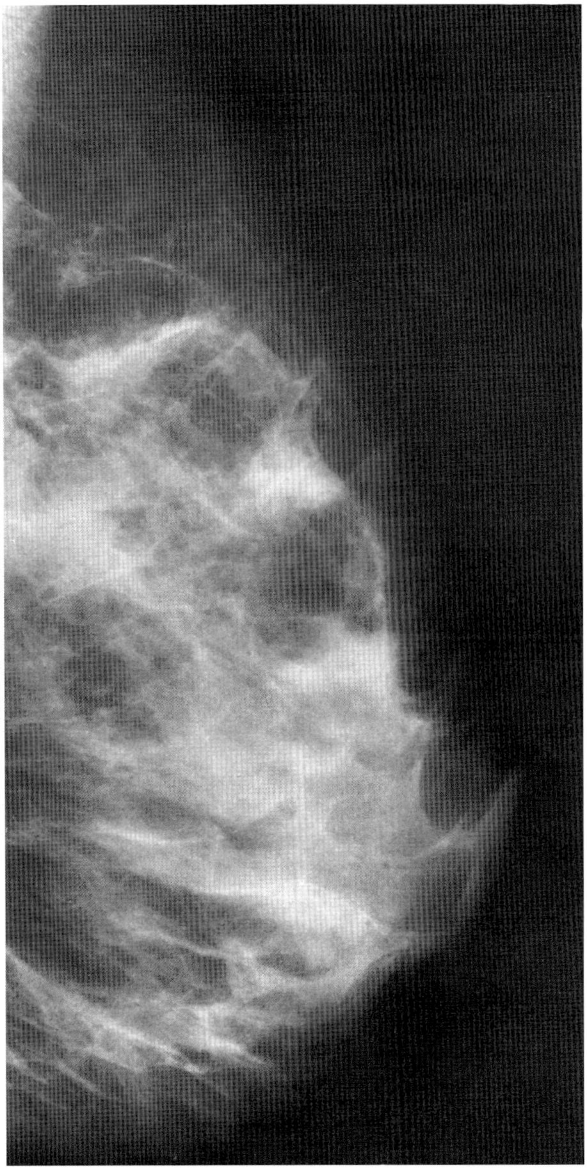

c

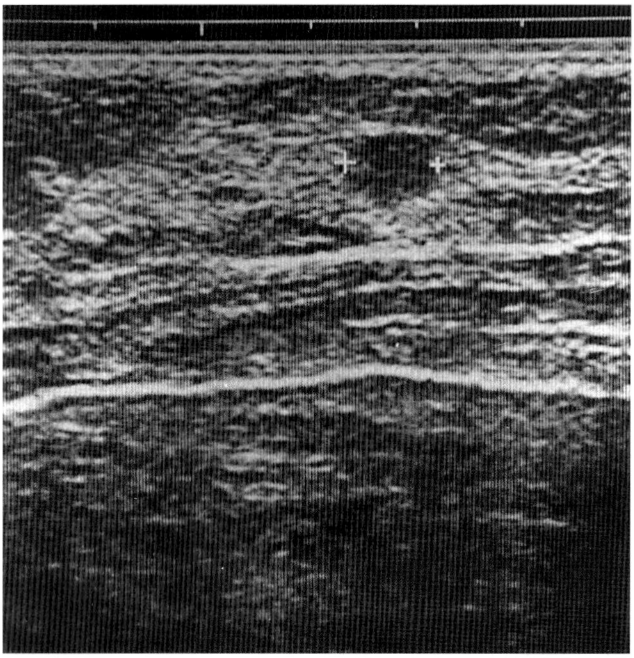

a

Analysis

1. Margins	indistinct, jagged
2. Retrotumoral acoustic phenomena	unchanged echoes
3. Internal echo pattern	homogeneous
4. Echogenicity	almost anechoic
5. Compression effect on **shape**	no deformation
6. Compression effect on **internal echoes**	no change

Note: The internal echo pattern of a very small lesion is often difficult to evaluate.

History

This woman, 43 years of age, had a left breast mass noted by her gynecologist. She had a family history of breast cancer.

Palpable Findings

Mobile, smoothly marginated, 2 cm mass above the left nipple, a nonsuspicious nodule.

Sonography

Figure **a**: transverse scan over the palpable mass.

Readability: good.

Focal sonographic lesion, 9×8 mm, at the center of the glandular region.

Interpretation

Except for internal echo pattern, the sonographic criteria are consistent with a malignant tumor.

X-ray Mammography

Figure **b**: craniocaudal projection. Fibro-adenosis. No focal abnormality.

Histology

Predominantly tubular, 10-mm infiltrating carcinoma with cribriform elements.

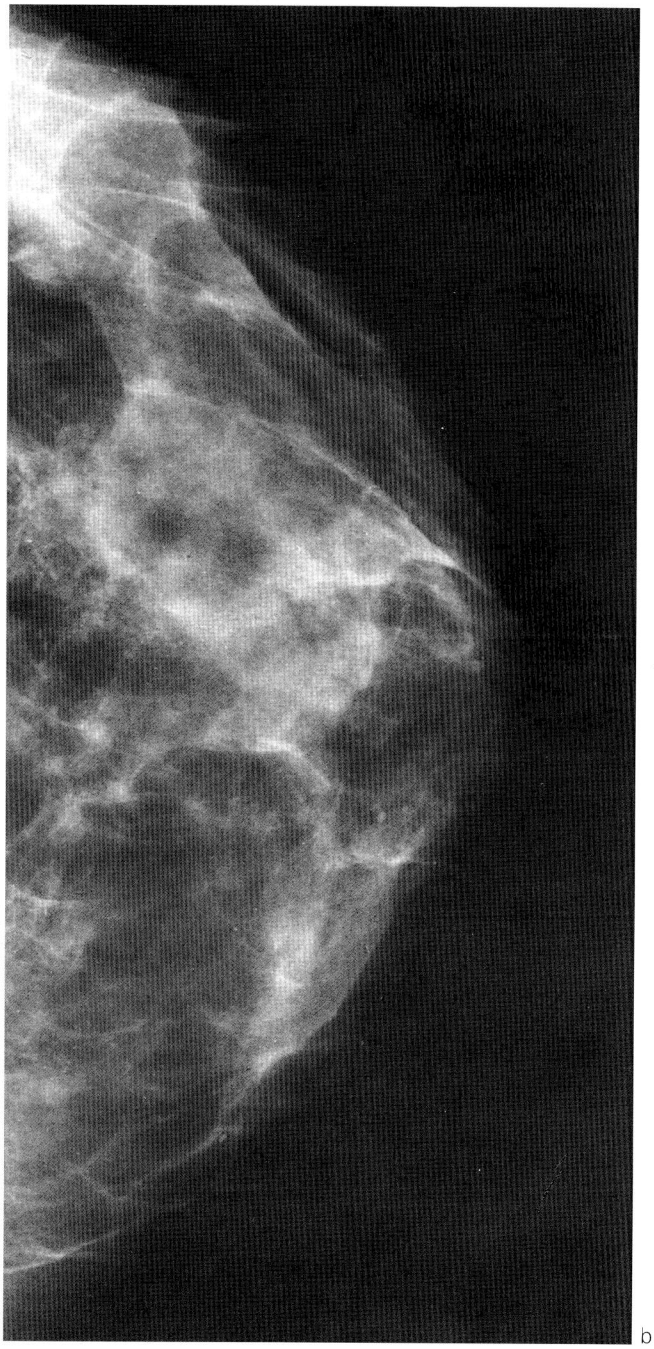

b

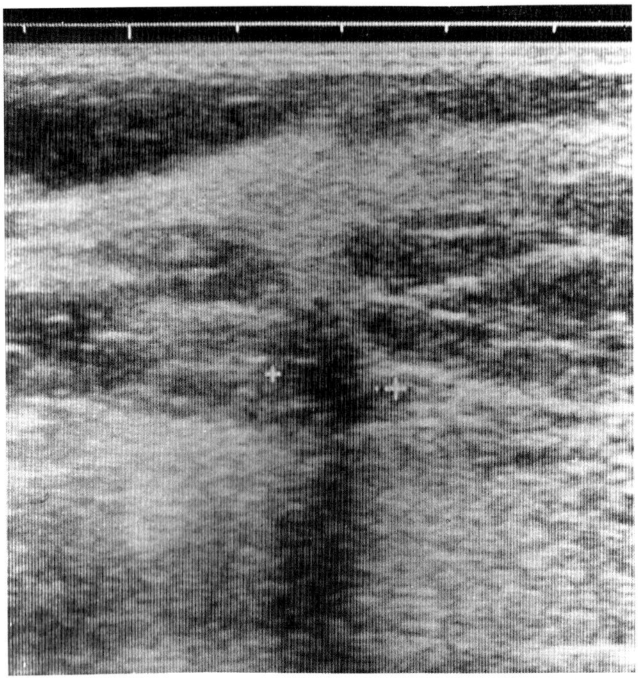

a

Analysis

1. **Margins**	indistinct, jagged
2. **Retrotumoral acoustic phenomena**	moderate posterior shadowing
3. **Internal echo pattern**	few echoes, nonhomogeneous
4. **Echogenicity**	almost anechoic
5. **Compression effect** on **shape**	no deformation
6. **Compression effect** on **internal echoes**	no change

History

The 46-year-old woman presented for her first screening examination.

Palpable Findings

Bilateral macromastia. The large breasts are difficult to evaluate. A palpable mass is not detected.

Sonography

Figure **a**: transverse scan in the upper outer quadrant of the right breast at the edge of the glandular region.

Readability: good.

Focal lesion, 10×14 mm, with posterior shadowing.

Interpretation

All the sonographic criteria suggest a malignant process. Even without a palpable correlate, a conspicuous posterior shadow is seen.

X-ray Mammography

Figure **b** (magnified view): a faintly spiculated density near the chest wall (*) seen at the site of the sonographic lesion in the craniocaudal projection. The benignancy or malignancy of the mass is mammographically indeterminate.

Histology

Scirrhous carcinoma with partial tubular differentiation, 15 mm in diameter.

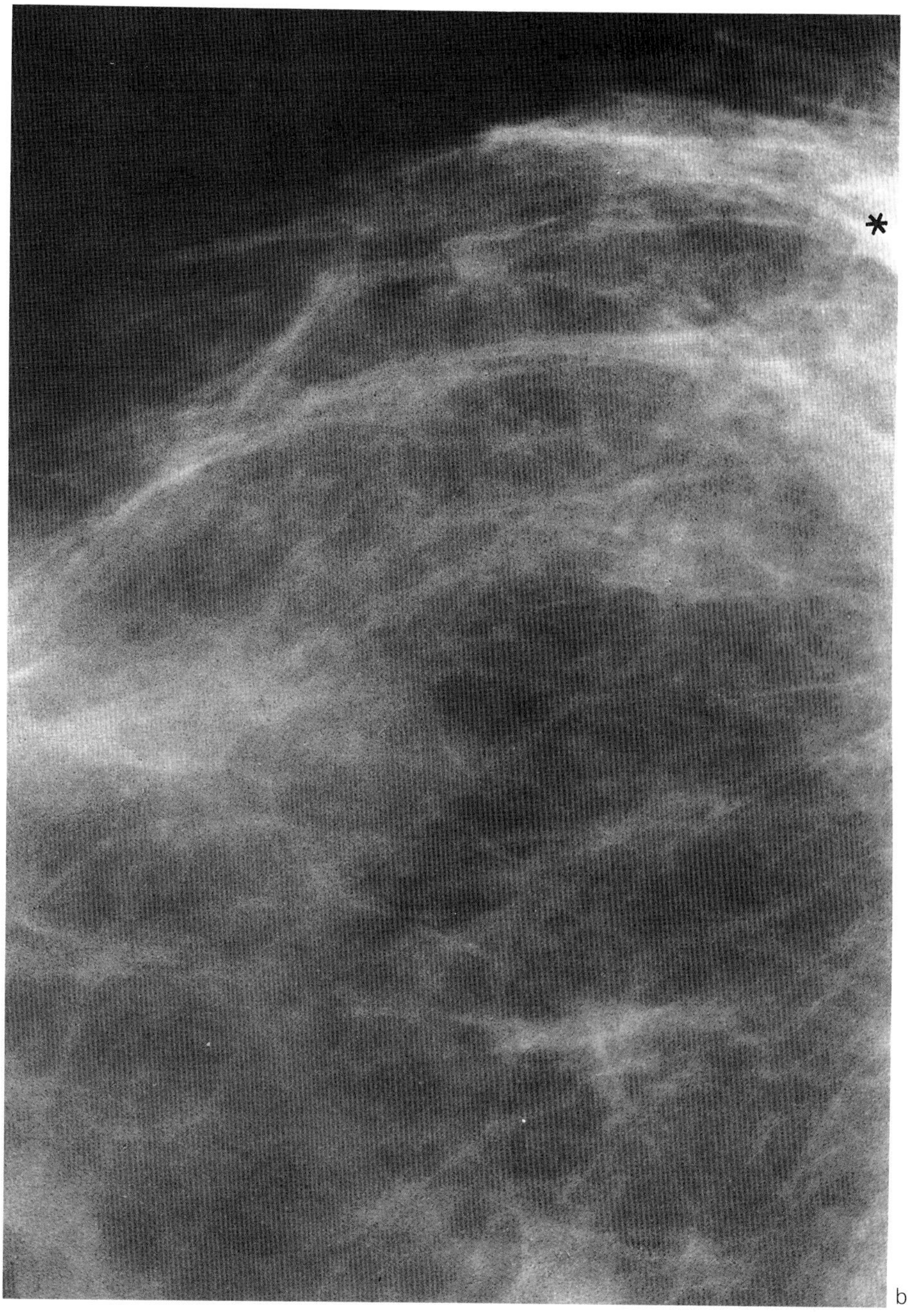
*
b

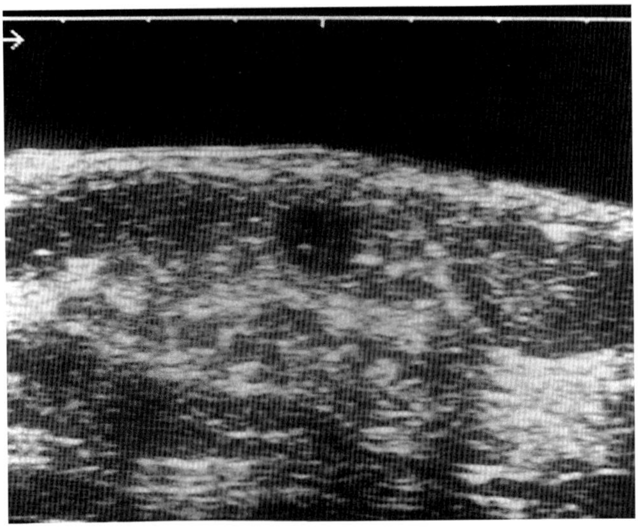

a

Analysis

1. Margins	sharp, jagged
2. Retrotumoral acoustic phenomena	unchanged echoes
3. Internal echo pattern	few echoes, nonhomogeneous
4. Echogenicity	almost anechoic
5. Compression effect on **shape**	no deformation
6. Compression effect on **internal echoes**	no change

History

The 63-year-old woman had noticed a lump in her right breast 3 weeks before.

Palpable Findings

Firm mass, 3×2 cm, in the upper inner quadrant of the right breast.

Sonography

(with standoff)

Figure **a**: sagittal scan over the palpable mass (7.5 MHz).

Readability: good.

Focal sonographic lesion, 8×9 mm.

Interpretation

Only criteria 3 and 4 are suggestive of malignancy. Criteria 2, 5 and 6 are indifferent, although the margins have a benign appearance. A benign/malignant differentiation cannot be made in this case by ultrasound.

X-ray Mammography

Figure **b**: craniocaudal projection showing clustered periareolar microcalcifications with no focal abnormality in a dysplastic breast. Same on mediolateral view.

Mammographic criteria are not sufficient to make a confident benign/malignant differentiation.

Histology

Infiltrating ductal carcinoma with pronounced intraductal tumor spread (pT2).

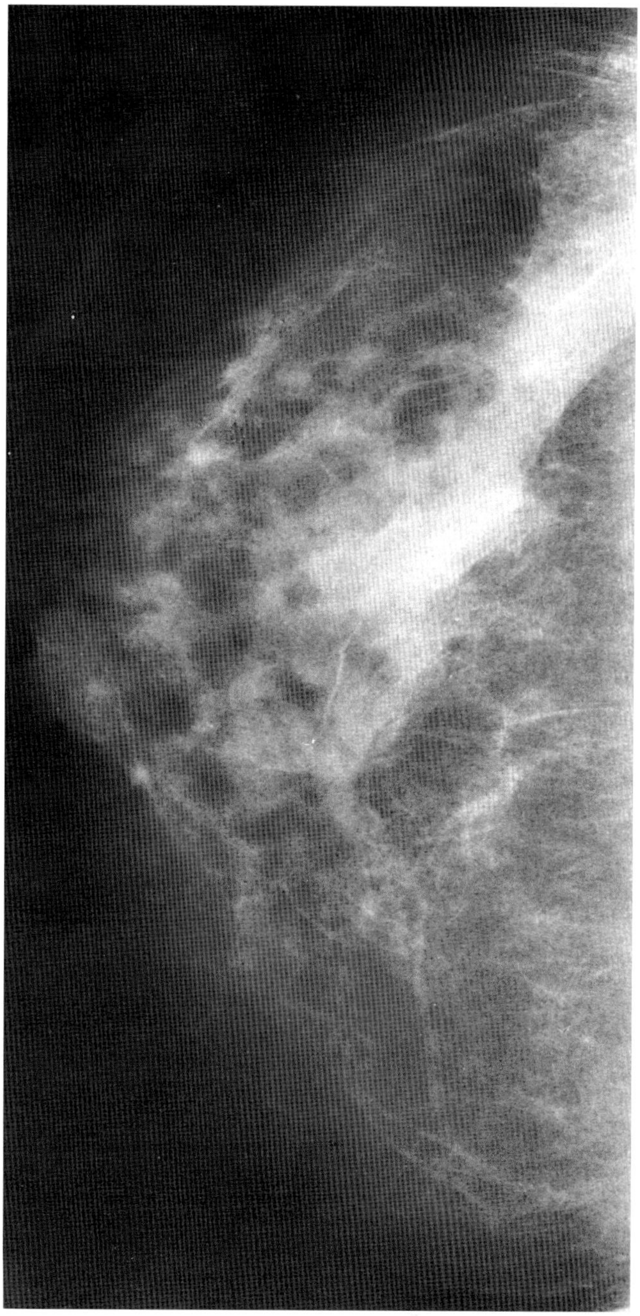

b

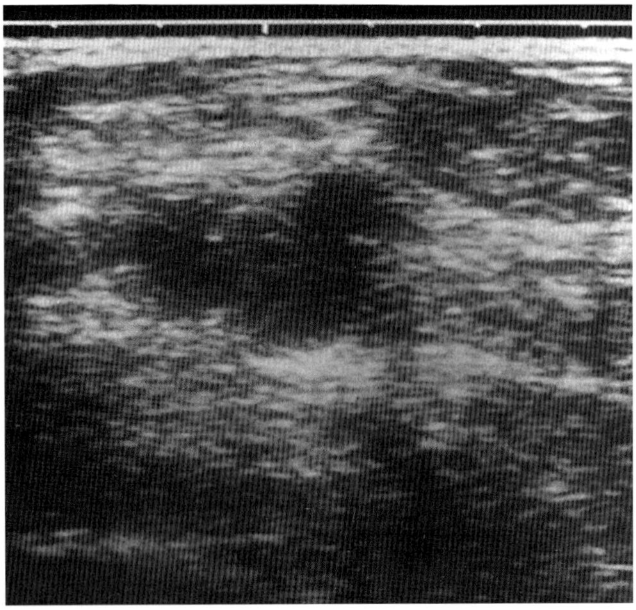

a

Analysis

1. **Margins**	indistinct, jagged
2. **Retrotumoral acoustic phenomena**	unchanged echoes
3. **Internal echo pattern**	few echoes, nonhomogeneous
4. **Echogenicity**	almost anechoic
5. **Compression effect** on **shape**	no deformation
6. **Compression effect** on **internal echoes**	no change

History

The 77-year-old woman had noticed a lump in her left breast 4 weeks ago.

Palpable Findings

Firm, mobile mass, 4×3 cm, with irregular boundaries in the left breast at 3 o'clock.

Sonography

Figure **a**: transverse scan over the palpable mass.

Readability: good.

Lobulated focal lesion, 28×14 mm.

Interpretation

All sonographic criteria suggest a malignant tumor.

X-ray Mammography

Figure **b**: craniocaudal and mediolateral projections showing an asymmetric density increase near the chest wall with no circumscribed focal lesion. Also, two calcified foci of fat necrosis.

Histology

Poorly differentiated, 26-mm infiltrating ductal carcinoma.

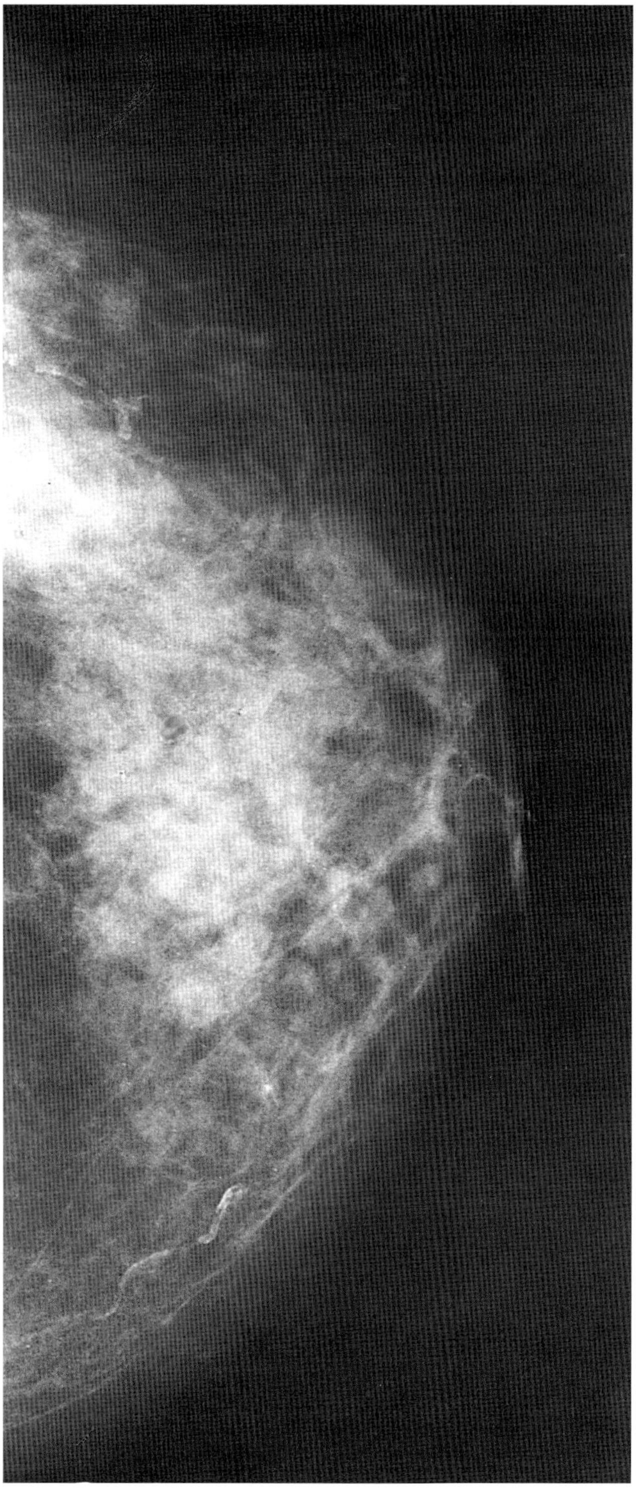

b

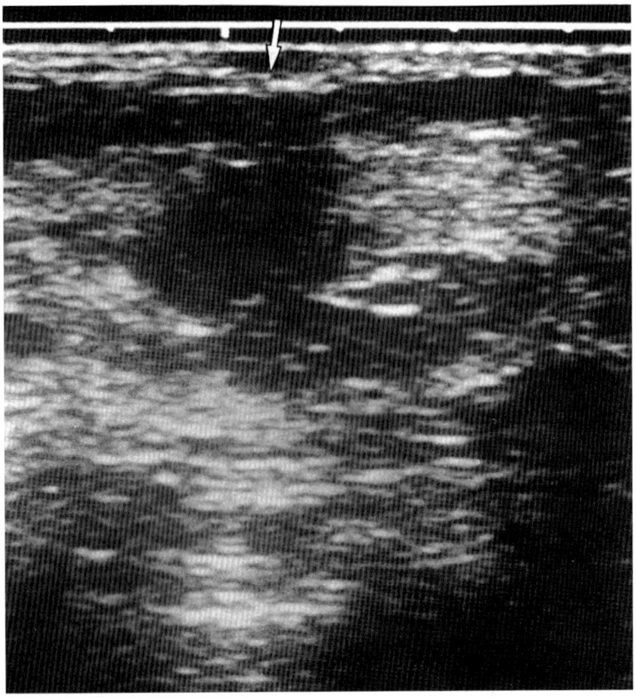
a

Analysis

1. Margins	indistinct, jagged
2. Retrotumoral acoustic phenomena	unchanged echoes
3. Internal echo pattern	few echoes, nonhomogeneous
4. Echogenicity	almost anechoic
5. Compression effect on **shape**	no deformation
6. Compression effect on **internal echoes**	no change

History

The 34-year-old woman had undergone right mastectomy (T2 N1 M0) with right breast reconstruction and y symmetrizing left reduction mammoplasty 1 year before. During subsequent follow-up, a thickened area was discovered at the left areolar border.

Palpable Findings

Clinically indeterminate, firm, relatively fixed thickened a area at the left areolar border.

Sonography

Figure **a**: sagittal scan over the thickened area, which crosses the periareolar scar at right angles *(arrow)*.

Readability: good.

Focal sonographic lesion, 22×18 mm, located beneath the scar.

Interpretation

All sonographic criteria suggest a malignant process. It is noteworthy that this lesion lies directly beneath the periareolar cutaneous scar, which appears sonographically as a hypoechoic discontinuity in the skin.

X-ray Mammography

Both the mediolateral (Fig. **b**) and craniocaudal projections (Fig. **c**) show an edematous fibrocystic breast with no suspicious focal abnormality.

Aspiration Cytology

Papanicolaou grade V (specimen taken under sonographic vision).

Histology

Partly solid, partly scirrhous breast carcinoma with tubular components.

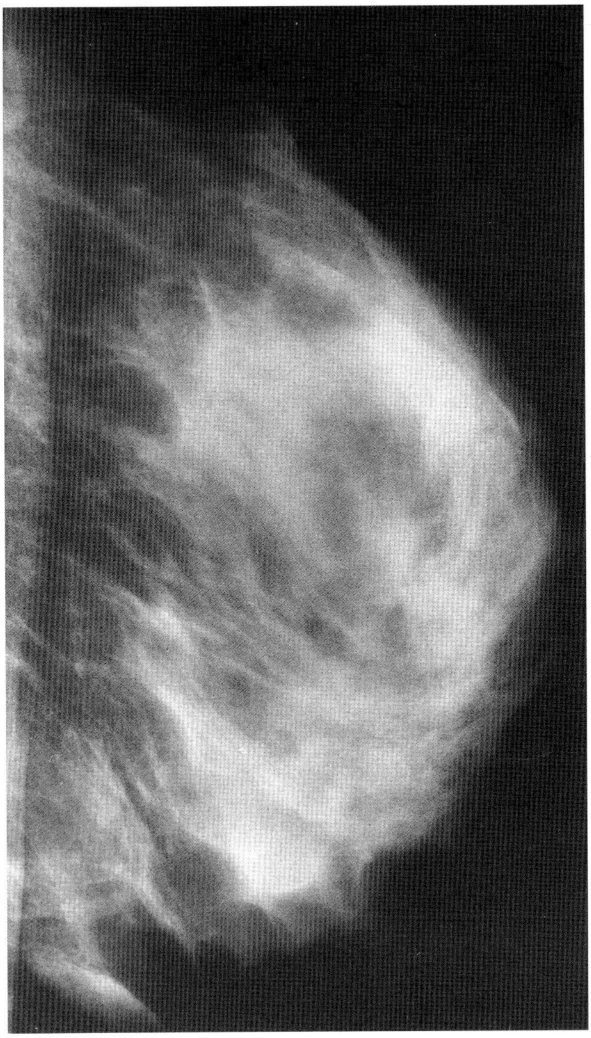

b

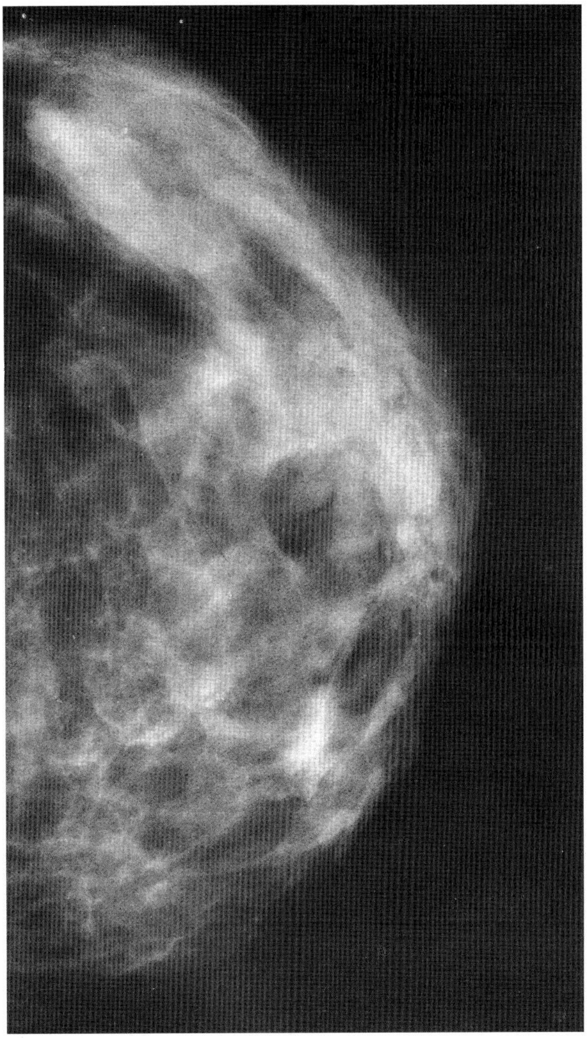

c

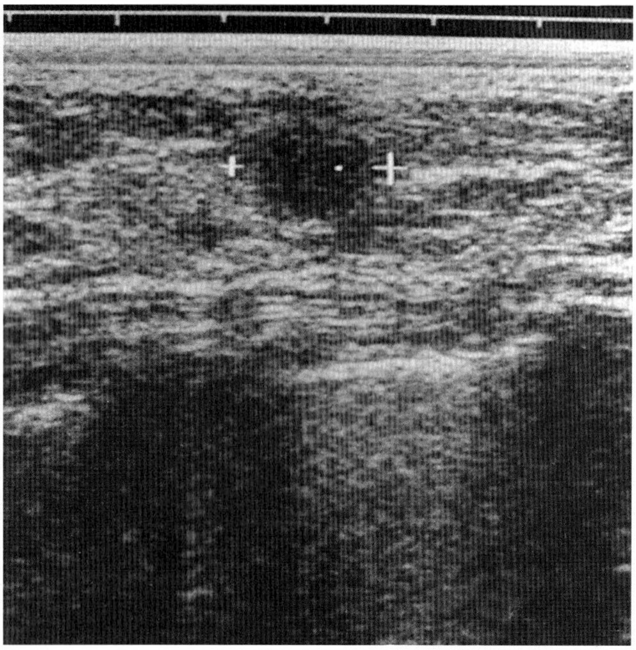

a

Analysis

1. Margins	indistinct, jagged
2. Retrotumoral acoustic phenomena	unchanged echoes
3. Internal echo pattern	nonhomogeneous
4. Echogenicity	almost anechoic
5. Compression effect on **shape**	no deformation
6. Compression effect on **internal echoes**	no change

History

The 38-year-old woman had felt a lump in her right breast 4–6 weeks before.

Palpable Findings

Firm, freely mobile mass about the size of the distal phalanx of the small finger, located directly at the nipple margin between the upper and lower inner quadrants of the right breast.

Sonography

Figure **a**: sagittal scan over the mass.

Readability: good.

Focal sonography lesion, 14×12 mm.

Interpretation

The sonographic criteria are suggestive of malignancy.

X-ray Mammography

Figure **b**: craniocaudal view showing a faint retroareolar density not visible in the mediolateral projection (Fig. **c**). Otherwise the mammograms are normal.

Histology

Predominantly tubular infiltrating ductal carcinoma. Size: 15 mm.

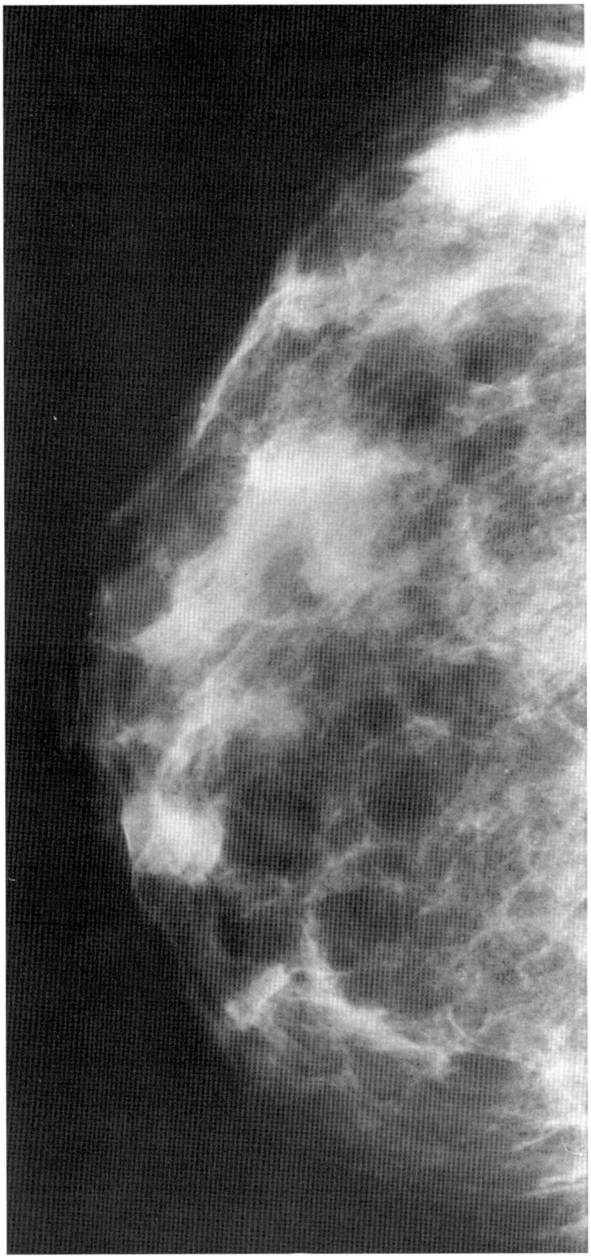
b

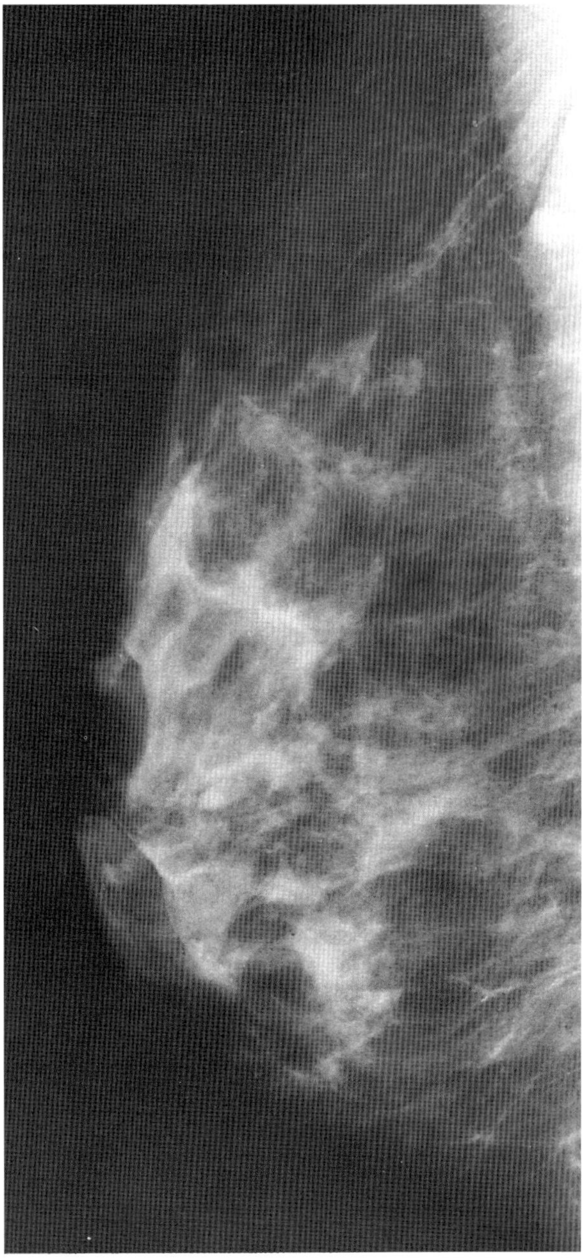
c

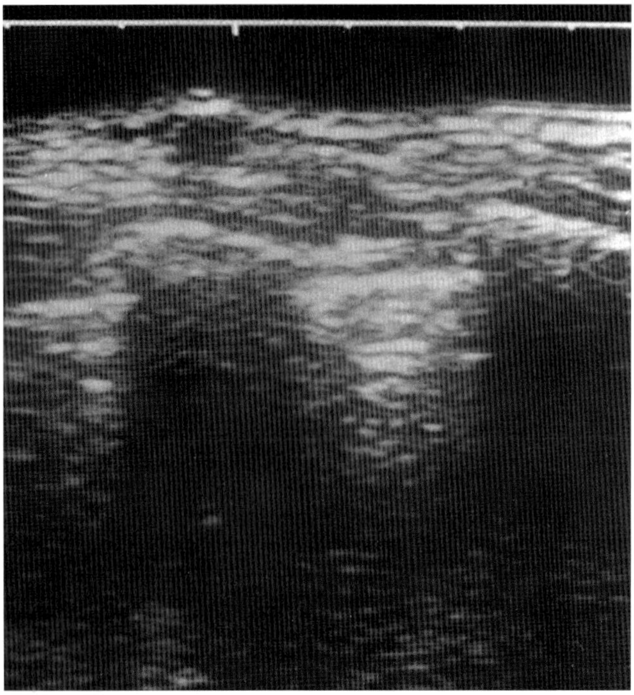
a

Analysis

1. **Margins**	indistinct but smooth
2. **Retrotumoral acoustic phenomena**	unchanged echoes
3. **Internal echo pattern**	homogeneous
4. **Echogenicity**	almost anechoic
5. **Compression effect** on **shape**	no deformation
6. **Compression effect** on **internal echoes**	no change

History

The 52-year-old woman had a lentil-sized nodule in the axillary tail of the right breast noted on routine examination.

Palpable Findings

See above.

Sonography

(with water path)

Figure **a**: sagittal scan over the palpable mass.

Readability: good.

Focal sonographic lesion, 5×4 mm, just below the skin.

Interpretation

Although most of the sonographic criteria suggest a benign lesion, the abrupt structural discontinuity is suspicious for an invasive process. A confident benign/malignant differentiation cannot be made by ultrasound. Biopsy is definitely indicated.

X-ray Mammography

Figure **b** (magnified view): mediolateral view of the right breast demonstrating microcystic mastopathy with scattered microcalcifications. At the edge of the glandular region is a smoothly marginated round lesion, approximately 8 mm in diameter, with a central microcalcification not typical of carcinoma.

The round lesion does not appear on the mediolateral projection. Benignancy or malignancy is indeterminable by mammography.

Histology

Small infiltrating lobular carcinoma 4 mm in diameter. Fibrocystic mastopathy: Prechtel stage II with focal sclerosing adenosis.

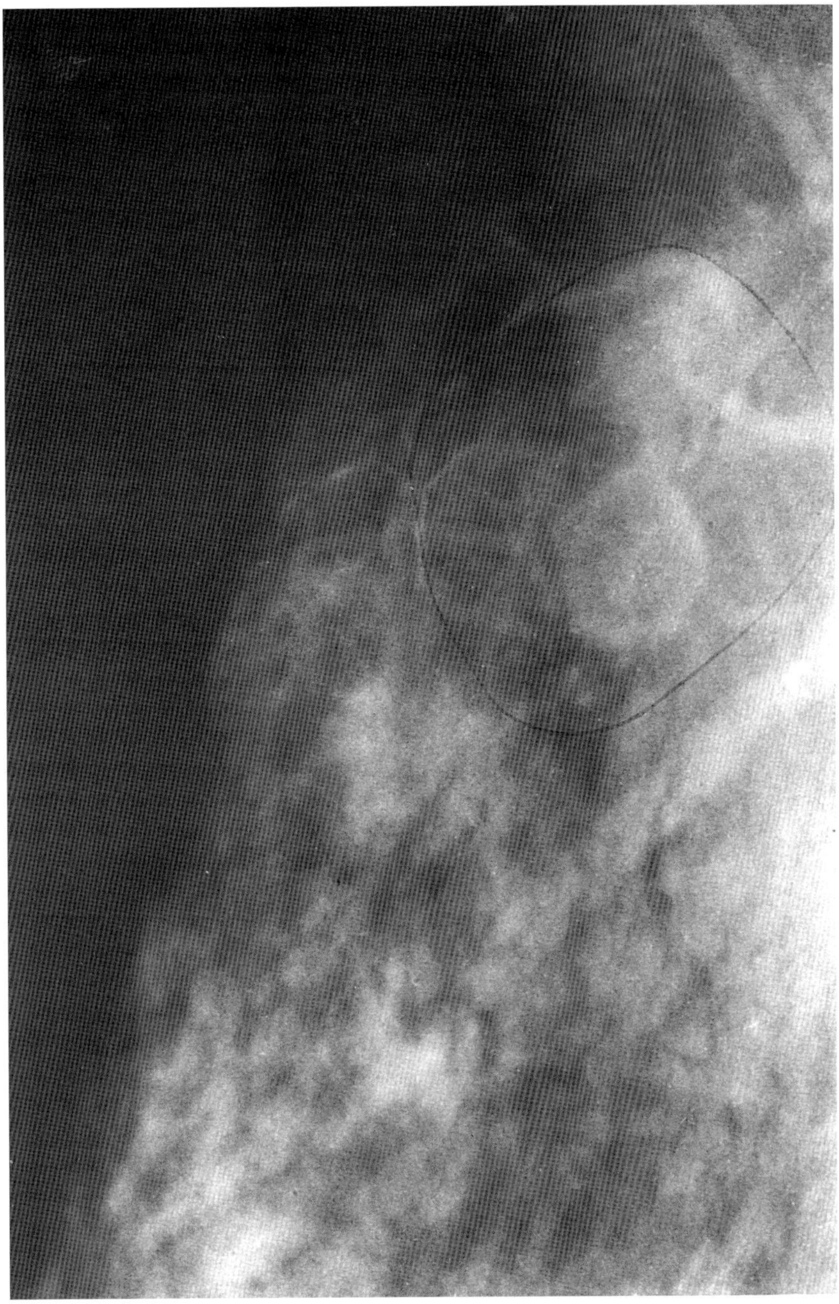

b

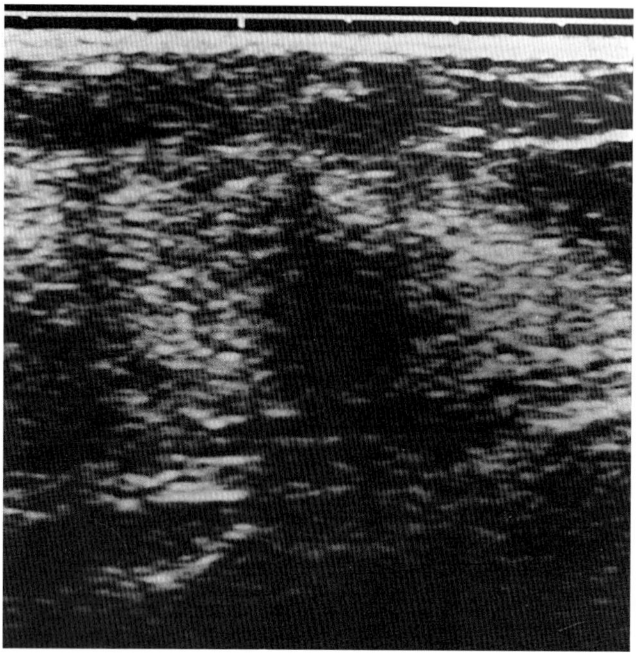

a

History

The 60-year-old woman who had had ovarian carcinoma 3 years before was noted at follow-up to have a poorly demarcated but relatively firm mass with subtle skin changes in the dense, coarsely nodular left breast.

Sonography

Figure **a**: transverse scan over the mass.

Readability: good.

Focal sonographic lesion, 20×20 mm.

Interpretation

The sonographic criteria strongly suggest a malignant process.

Analysis

1. **Margins**	indistinct, jagged
2. **Retrotumoral acoustic phenomena**	cannot be assessed
3. **Internal echo pattern**	few echoes, nonhomogeneous
4. **Echogenicity**	almost anechoic
5. **Compression effect** on **shape**	no deformation
6. **Compression effect** on **internal echoes**	no change

X-ray Mammography

Figure **b**: craniocaudal projection showing a faintly spiculated area of fibrosis with scattered microcalcifications and marked proliferation.

Histology

Infiltrating lobular carcinoma with predominantly scirrhous differentiation pattern, 20 mm in diameter.

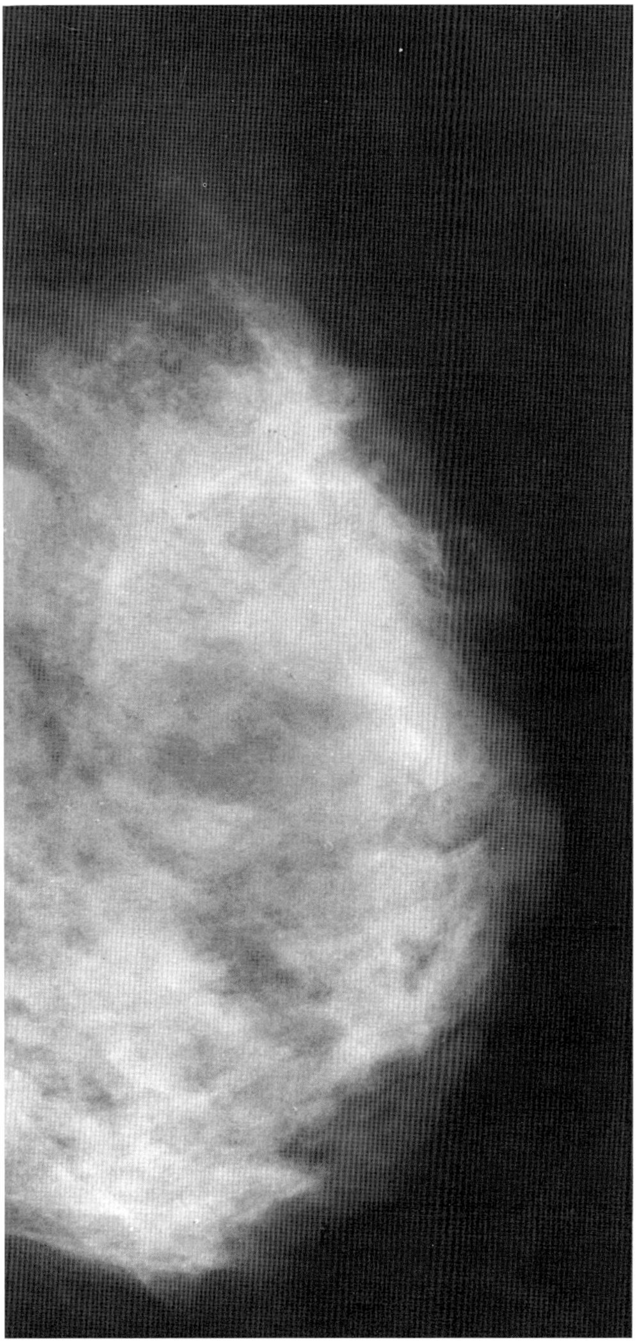

b

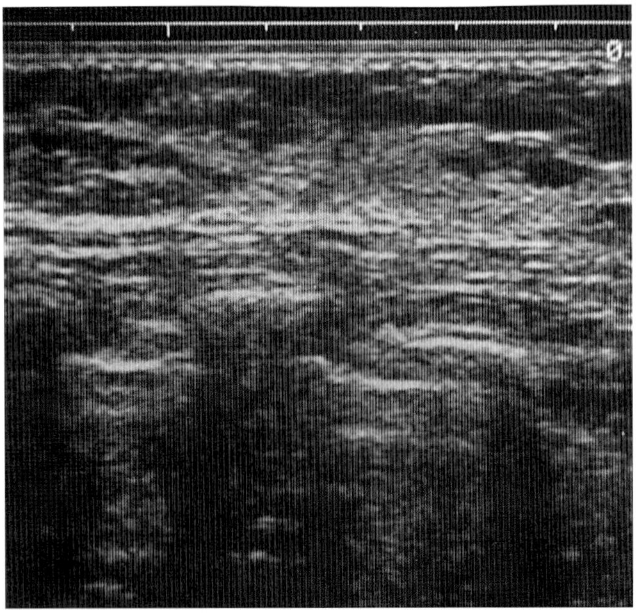

a

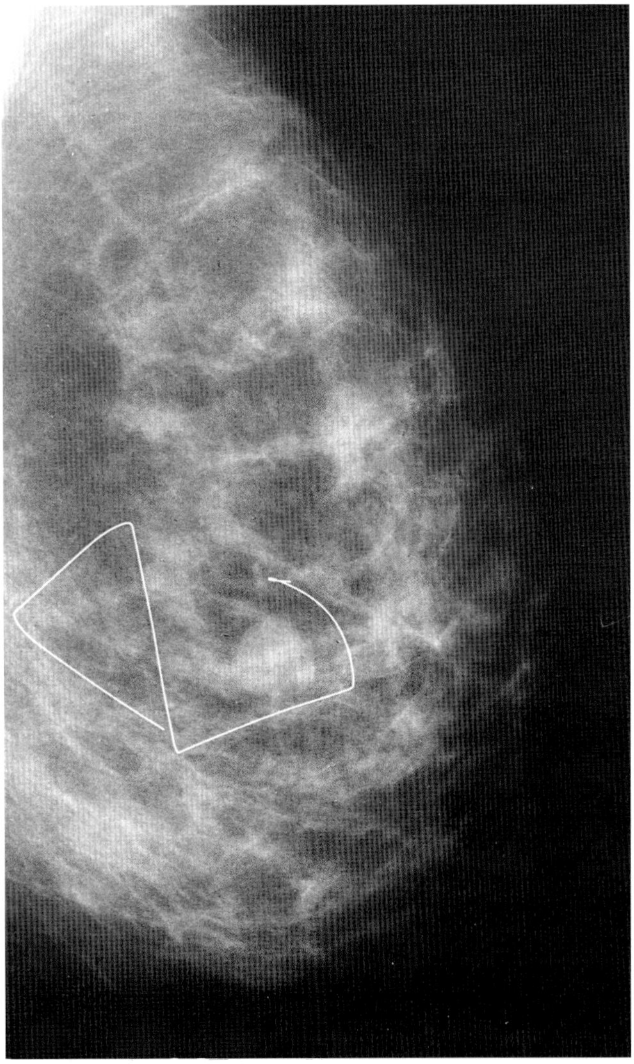

b

History

The 34-year-old woman had complained of tenderness in the upper outer quadrant of the left breast for 1 year. Premenstrual syndrome.

Palpable Findings

Palpable density at 3 o'clock in the left breast. All lymphatic drainage areas appeared free of disease.

Sonography

Figure **a**: sagittal scan of the left breast in the area of the palpable density and roentgen correlate.

Readability: good.

Normal mammary tissue with no evidence of a focal sonographic abnormality.

Analysis

Not possible without a focal lesion.

Interpretation

Sonographic diagnosis: no evidence of disease.

X-ray Mammography

Figure **b**: mediolateral projection showing a circumscribed, round to oval, 12-mm lesion of low radiopacity. Localization wire in situ. Same on craniocaudal view.

Mammographic diagnosis: inconclusive.

Histology

Simple fibrocystic mastopathy with intraductal papillomas. No evidence of malignancy or specificity.

History

The 45-year-old woman had her first screening mammograms; the craniocaudal film showed a smoothly marginated round lesion in the right breast. She was referred for differential diagnostic evaluation (cystic or solid lesion?).

Palpable Findings

No palpable masses in either breast.

Sonography

Figure: sagittal scan demonstrating a focal lesion, 15×10 mm, laterally at 9 o'clock in the right breast.

Interpretation

The focal lesion displays all the criteria of a benign cystic mass.

Aspiration Cytology

Aspiration yielded 1.5 mL of a clear, amber-colored fluid. Papanicolaou grades I/II.

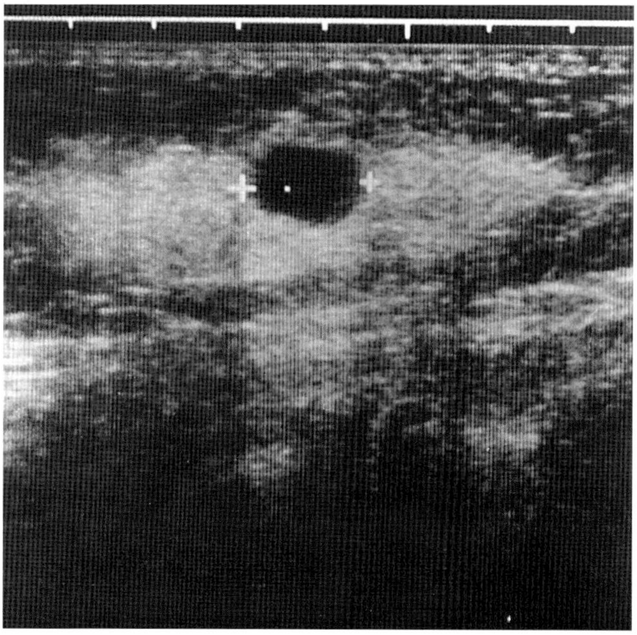

Analysis

1. **Margins**	sharp and smooth
2. **Retrotumoral acoustic phenomena**	posterior enhancement, bilateral shadowing phenomena
3. **Internal echo pattern**	no echoes
4. **Echogenicity**	anechoic
5. **Compression effect** on **shape**	shape distortion
6. **Compression effect** on **internal echoes**	no change

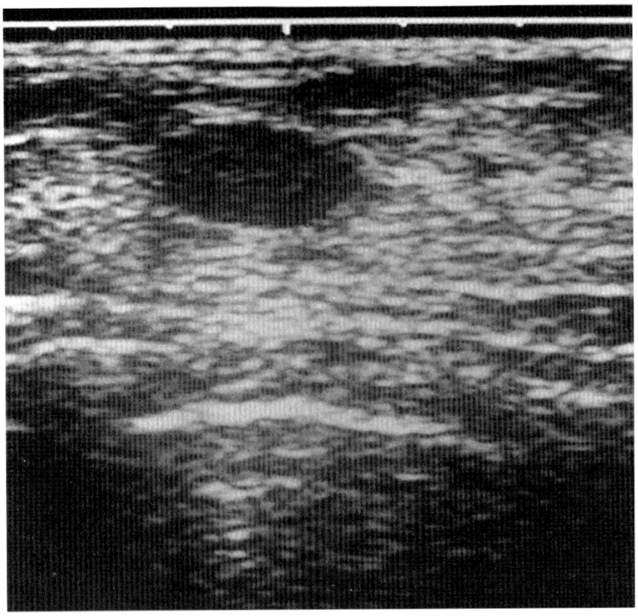

Analysis

1. **Margins**	sharp and smooth
2. **Retrotumoral acoustic phenomena**	unchanged echoes
3. **Internal echo pattern**	homogeneous
4. **Echogenicity**	fat-equivalent
5. **Compression effect** on **shape**	no deformation
6. **Compression effect** on **internal echoes**	no change

History

During a screening mammography, the 41-year-old woman was noted to have a round lesion in her right breast.

Palpable Findings

A definite palpable correlate to the radiographic lesion could not be found.

Sonography

Figure: transverse scan through the upper inner quadrant of the right breast.

Readability: good.

Conspicuous focal lesion, 16×9 mm.

Interpretation

The sonographic criteria give the overall impression of a fibroadenoma.

X-ray Mammography

Smoothly marginated round lesion.

Histology

Pericanalicular fibroadenoma.

History

The 43-year-old woman had undergone bilateral subcutaneous mastectomy with subpectoral augmentation 3 years earlier for ductal carcinoma in situ. The left prosthesis was removed 1 year ago. Follow-up mammography demonstrated a stellate density 4 cm deep to the nipple of the left breast, raising the suspicion of an infiltrating carcinoma.

Palpable Findings

No palpable mass.

Sonography

Figure **a**: sagittal scan in the nipple area (* = areola).

Readability: good.
The subareolar region is plainly demonstrated.
There is no focal sonographic lesion, only a sharply marginated, rectangular hyperechoic area within the pectoral muscle *(arrows)*.

Interpretation

No focal sonographic lesion. The hyperechoic area can be interpreted as a scar. Ultrasound alone does not provide an indication for surgical excision.

X-ray Mammography

Figure **b**: craniocaudal and mediolateral projections showing an asymmetric density increase near the chest wall with no circumscribed focal lesion. Also, two calcified foci of fat necrosis.

Histology

Poorly differentiated, 26-mm infiltrating ductal carcinoma.

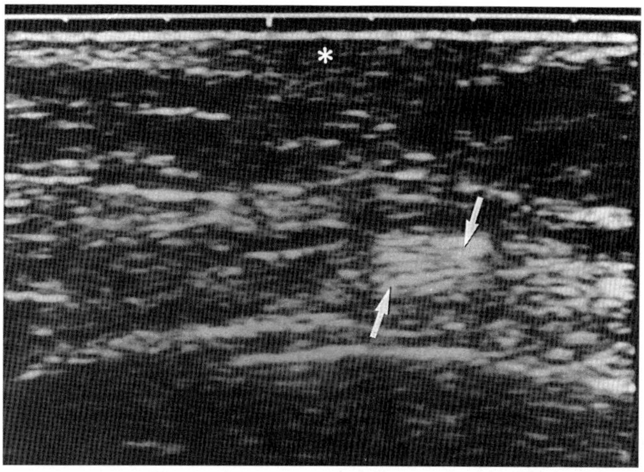

a

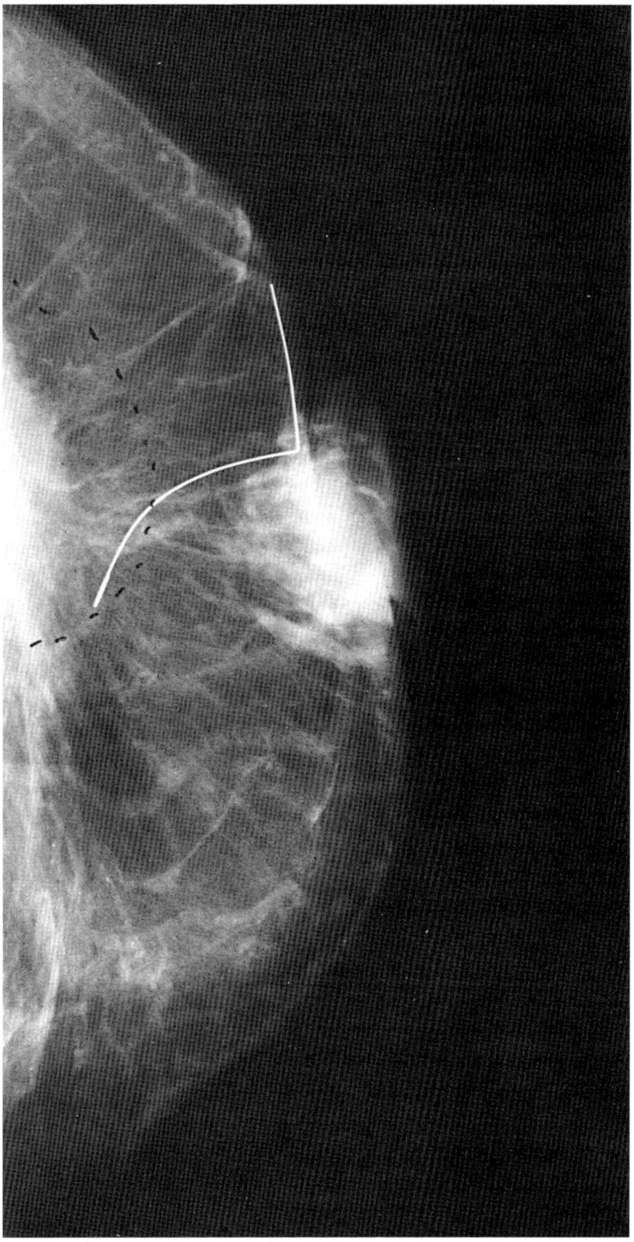
b

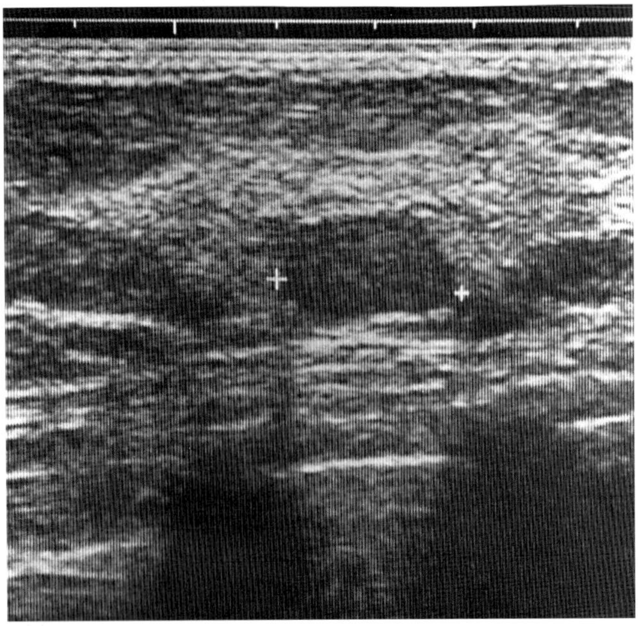

Analysis

1. Margins	sharp and smooth
2. Retrotumoral acoustic phenomena	slight posterior enhancement, bilateral shadowing phenomena
3. Internal echo pattern	homogeneous
4. Echogenicity	fat-equivalent
5. Compression effect on **shape**	no deformation
6. Compression effect on **internal echoes**	no change

History

During a screening mammography, the 42-year-old woman was noted to have a smooth-margined round lesion in the upper outer quadrant of her left breast. Breast ultrasound was performed for cystic/solid differentiation.

Palpable Findings

No palpable masses were found in either breast.

Sonography

Figure: sagittal scan through the upper outer quadrant.

A conspicuous focal lesion, 18×10 mm, is seen at the posterior border of the glandular region.

Interpretation

The sonographic criteria are benign, and the sonographic features are those of a fibroadenoma. The "fat-equivalent" areas that flank the focal lesion are retromammary fat.

Histology

Pericanalicular fibroadenoma, 20 mm in diameter.

History

The 35-year-old woman had noted a lump in her left breast 3 weeks before.

Palpable Findings

Firm mass, approximately 1×1 cm, within the (soft) glandular region in the lower inner quadrant of the left breast.

Sonography

Figure **a**: sagittal scan over the mass.

Readability: good.

A focal lesion is not defined. The overall impression corresponds most closely to fibrocystic mastopathy.

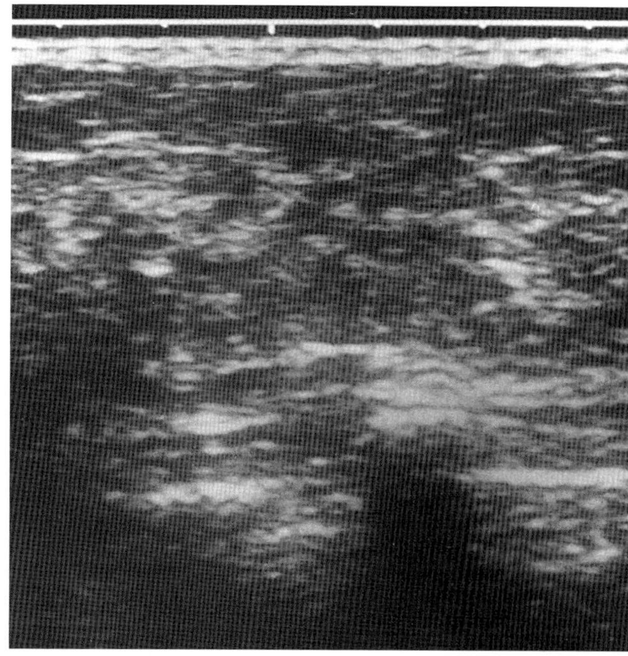

a

Analysis

Not possible without a focal lesion.

Interpretation

The palpable mass is not visualized.

X-ray Mammography

(magnified view of the lower quadrants)

Figure **b**: mediolateral projection showing a suspicious stellate density inferiorly, corresponding to the palpable mass. Same on the craniocaudal view. This lesion is mammographically indeterminate but is somewhat suspicious for malignancy.

Histology

Chronic granulating, nonspecific mastitis.

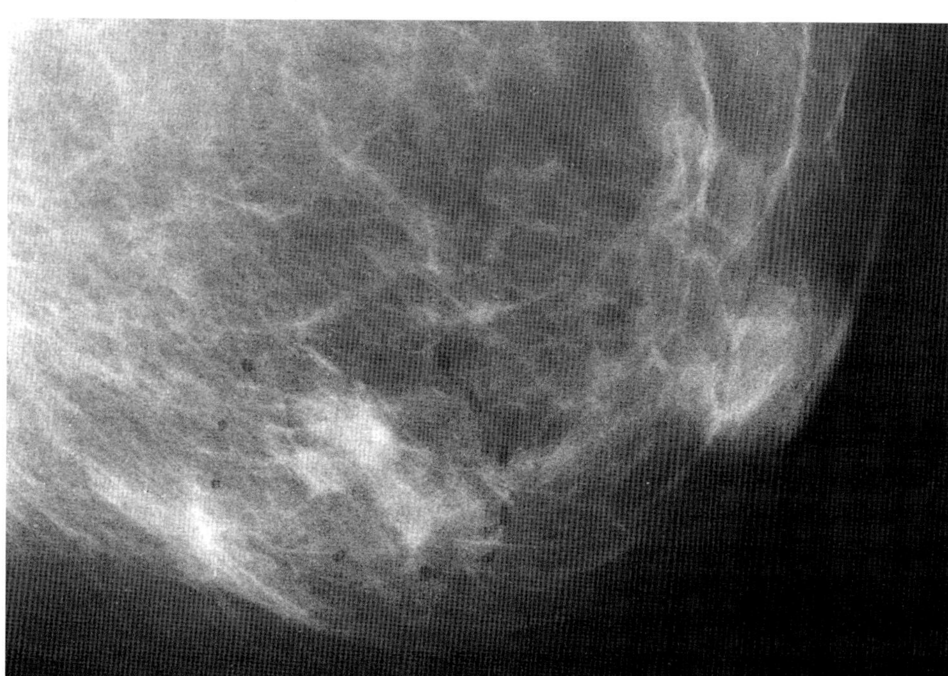

b

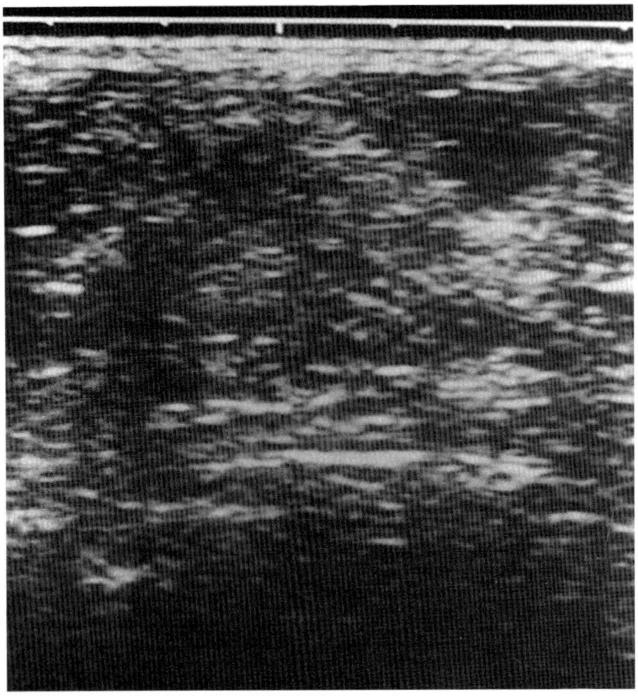

a

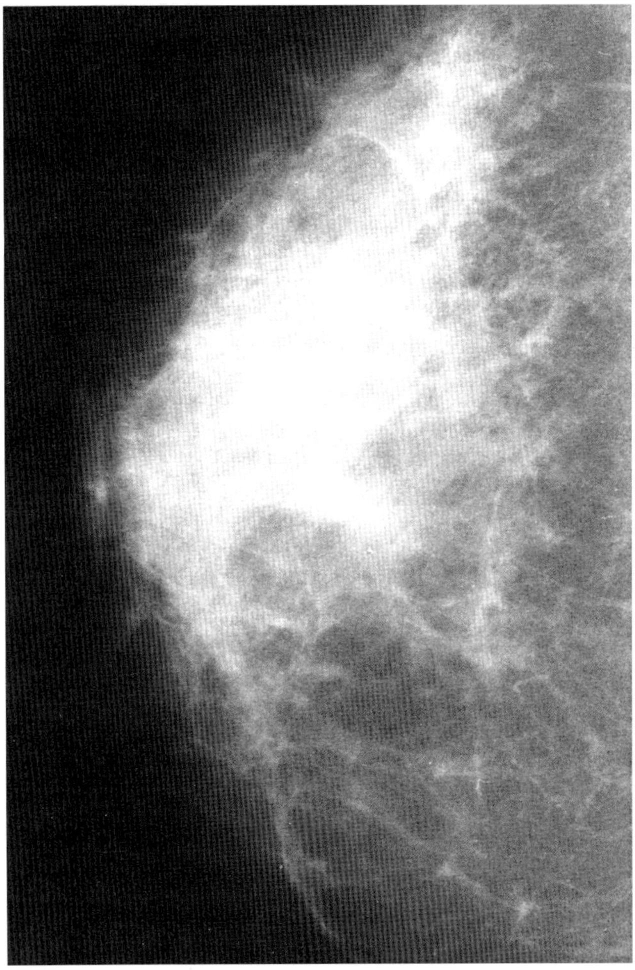

b

History

The 44-year-old woman had noticed retraction of her right nipple 10 days before, followed 2 days later by heat and tenderness. She had had puerperal mastitis 10 years earlier.

Palpable Findings

Knobby, chestnut-sized, suspicious mass in the lower outer quadrant of the right breast, accompanied by yellowish discharge from a milk duct.

Sonography

Figure **a**: transverse scan over the palpable mass.

Readability: limited.

A circumscribed focal lesion is not defined. The glandular structure appears disordered, with alternating hyperechoic and hypoechoic zones.

Analysis

Without a focal lesion, the criteria cannot be applied.

Interpretation

The absence of a focal sonographic lesion combined with extreme structural irregularity over a palpable mass should direct suspicion toward an inflammatory process (without abscessation).

X-ray Mammography

Figure **b**: craniocaudal projection of the right breast showing a cloudy density with nipple retraction. Same on the mediolateral view.

A confident assessment of benignancy or malignancy cannot be made on the basis of roentgen findings.

Histology

Pronounced duct ectasia, retained secretions with chronic, nonspecific periductal granulomatous inflammation. No evidence of malignancy or specificity.

Pregnancy and Lactation

It is wise to avoid the use of X-rays during pregnancy, so ultrasound is the modality of choice when breast imaging is required. The lactation period, which offers the same favorable physical acoustic conditions as pregnancy, is considered another important area of application for breast ultrasound.

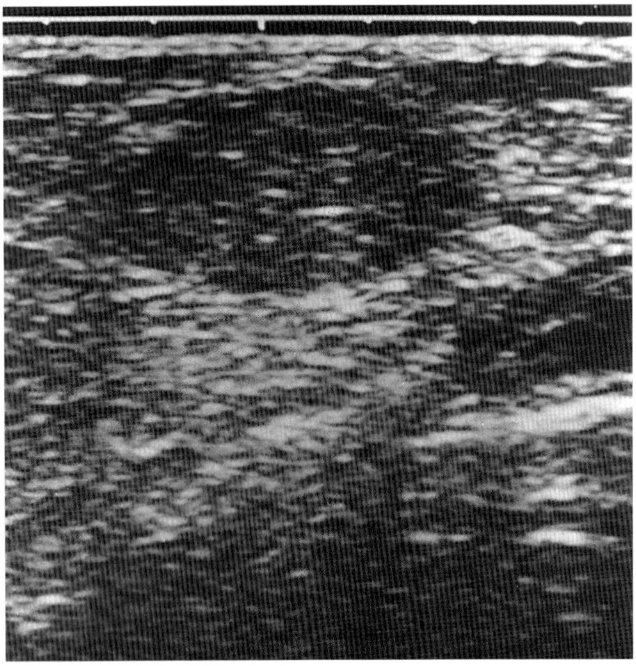

a

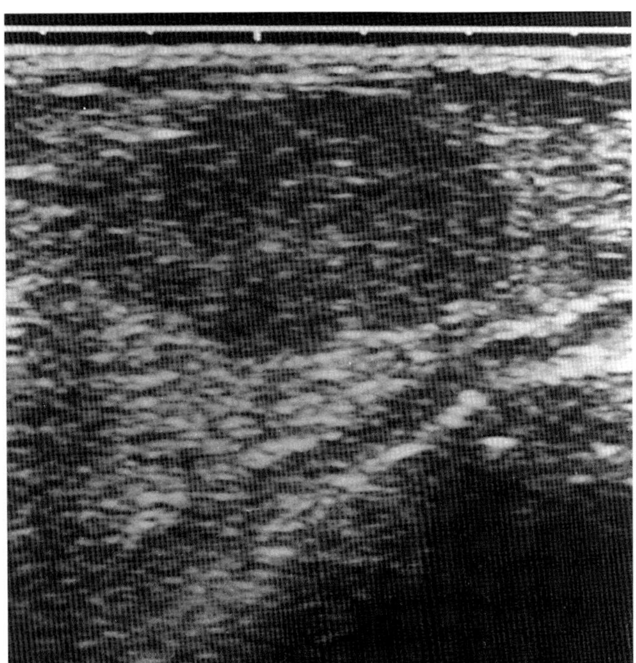

b

History

The 29-year-old woman noticed a firm lump in her left breast during the 27th week of pregnancy.

Palpable Findings

Approximately walnut-sized, smooth-bordered, mobile mass in the lower inner quadrant of the left breast. At follow-up 3 weeks later, the mass appeared clinically to have enlarged.

Sonography

Figure **a**: transverse scan over the palpable mass.

Readability: good.

Focal lesion, 39×17 mm.

Figure **b**: same view as in Figure **a**, 3 weeks later. Sonogram confirms enlargement of the mass to 42×22 mm.

Interpretation

All sonographic criteria are consistent with a benign tumor (e.g., fibroadenoma).

X-ray mammography was withheld due to pregnancy.

The mass was excised in the 32nd week of pregnancy.

Histology

Sharply marginated tumor with a very firm consistency and lobular architecture. Histology established tubular adenoma (adenoma purum) with no evidence of malignancy or specificity.

Note: A subtle, scalloped intratumoral structure is visible on image **b**.

Analysis

1. **Margins**	sharp and smooth
2. **Retrotumoral acoustic phenomena**	posterior enhancement
3. **Internal echo pattern**	homogeneous
4. **Echogenicity**	hypoechoic
5. **Compression effect** on **shape**	no deformation
6. **Compression effect** on **internal echoes**	no change

History

The 23-year-old woman noticed a bloody discharge from her left breast in the 30th week of pregnancy.

Palpable Findings

No palpable masses were found in either breast. Compression of the left nipple elicited a watery discharge.

Sonography

Figure **a**: sagittal scan over the left areolar region.

Readability: good.

Dilated milk ducts *(arrows)* cut longitudinally by the scan.

Figure **b**: sagittal scan over the left nipple.

Readability: good.

Nipple shadow. On the left side of the image is an oblique section of a dilated milk duct with an intraductal process *(arrow)*. The glandular region shows pregnancy-specific alterations.

Analysis

An analysis of diagnostic criteria is not significant in this case.

Interpretation

Although sonography is not the method of choice for evaluating a breast with nipple discharge, it is sometimes possible to demonstrate papillomas in dilated glandular ducts. In this case, galactography was withheld due to pregnancy. Although smear cytology was negative, further diagnostic procedures should be initiated at least in the postpartum period.

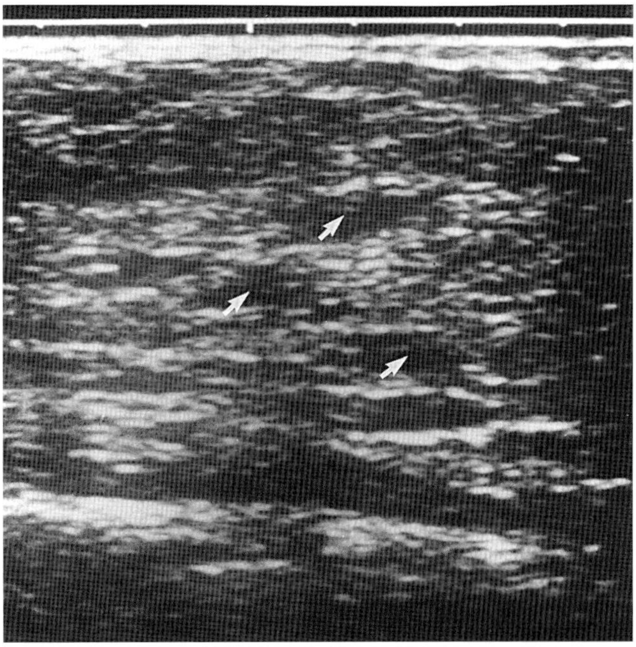

a

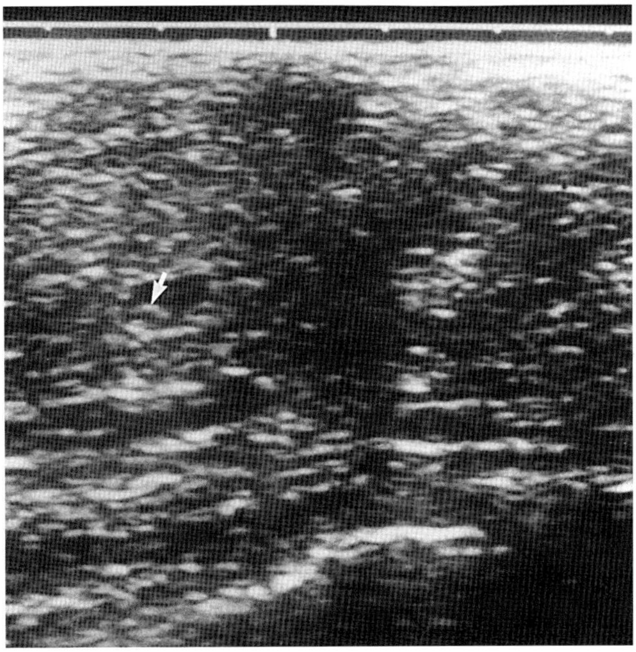

b

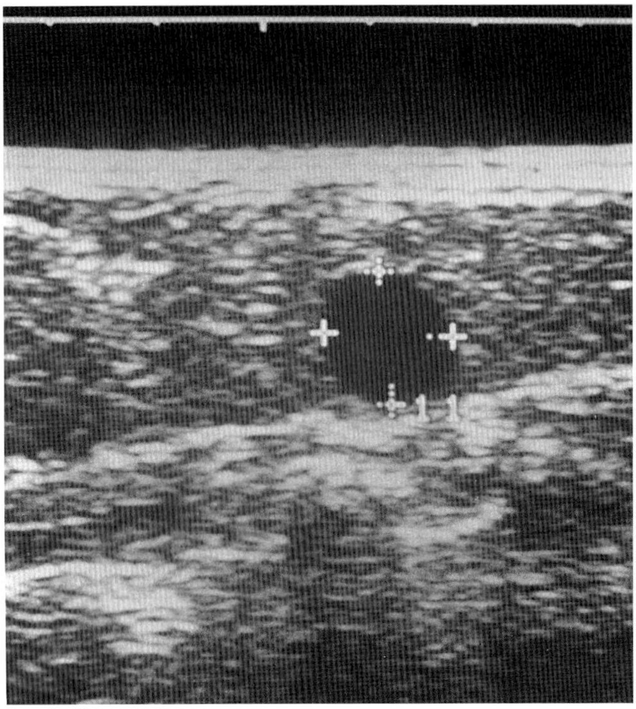

Analysis

1. Margins	sharp and smooth
2. Retrotumoral acoustic phenomena	unchanged echoes
3. Internal echo pattern	no echoes
4. Echogenicity	anechoic
5. Compression effect on **shape**	shape distortion
6. Compression effect on **internal echoes**	no change

History

The 33-year-old woman, who gave birth 4 months ago and is still nursing, noticed a painful mass in her left breast.

Palpable Findings

After nursing, a mass about the size of the distal phalanx of a finger was palpated in the lower outer quadrant of the left breast.

Sonography

with water path)

Figure: sagittal scan over the palpable mass.

Readability: good.

A focal sonographic lesion is noted in the homogeneous-appearing lactating breast.

Interpretation

The sonographic criteria indicate a benign cystic lesion.

Aspiration Cytology

Aspiration yielded 3 mL of a clear, slightly greenish fluid. Papanicolaou grades I/II.

History

The 30-year-old woman noticed a lump in the upper inner quadrant of her left breast in the 34th week of pregnancy.

Palpable Findings

Poorly circumscribed mass about as large as the ball of the thumb in the upper inner quadrant of the left breast.

Sonography

Figure **a**: sagittal scan over the mass in the upper inner quadrant.

Readability: good.

Multiple cystic masses.

Figure **b**: sagittal scan in the lower inner quadrant of the left breast.

Readability: good.

Generally loose but homogeneous structure of the glandular region. No focal sonographic lesion.

Analysis

An analysis of diagnostic criteria is not significant in this case.

Interpretation

The parenchymal pattern in Figure **b** is typical of a lactating breast. The cystic masses in Figure **a** represent congested milk ducts.

Aspiration Cytology

(from a cystic mass)

Milky fluid; Papanicolaou grade I.

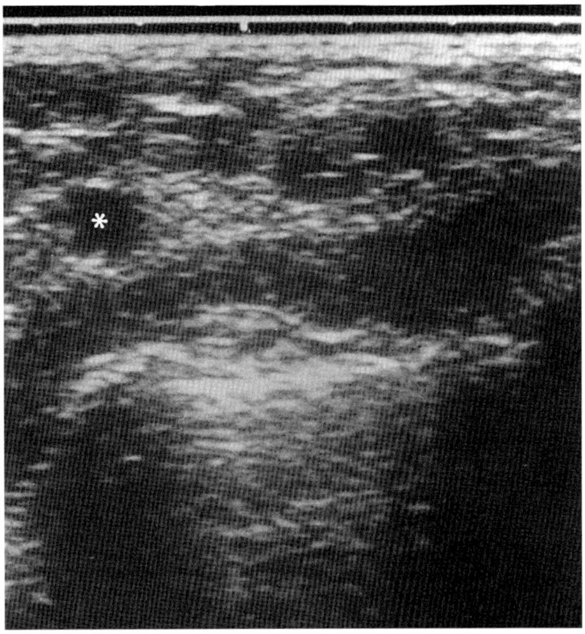

a

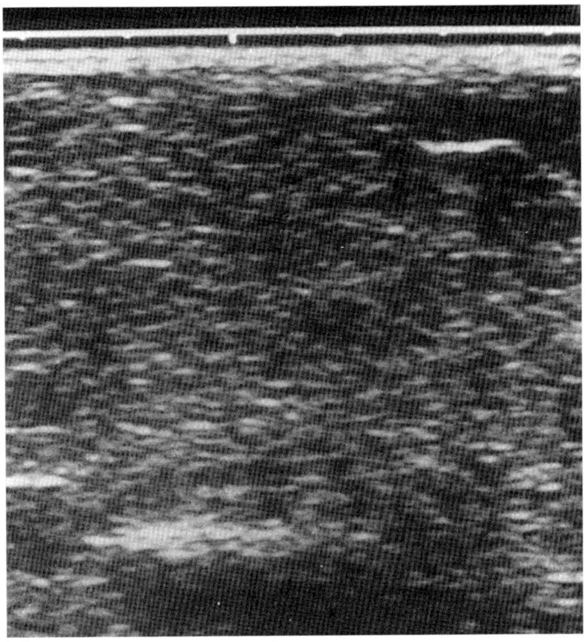
b

Oncologic Follow-Up

In the follow-up care of breast cancer patients, ultrasound is useful for evaluating the chest wall and the partially resected breast.

Chest-Wall Evaluation after Mastectomy

Sonography is currently the only acceptable paraclinical method for evaluation of the chest wall. In these cases, approximately 80% of palpable masses can be correctly identified as benign or malignant by ultrasound, as opposed to only 36% by palpation (Rabe et al. 1987). Even when clinical findings are unequivocal, ultrasound is extremely useful for ascertaining the extent of disease (infiltration depth) and its relationship to neighboring structures (vessels, bone, pleura).

History

The 63-year-old woman had undergone left mastectomy 14 years before for infiltrating ductal carcinoma (T1 N2 M0) and right mastectomy 2 years before for a similar cancer (T1 N2 M0) with postoperative irradiation. Now she was evaluated for a possible chest-wall recurrence on the right side.

Palpable Findings

A firm, fixed, approximately bean-sized mass was palpable in the intercostal space above the mastectomy scar.

Sonography

Figure: sagittal scan over the palpable mass.

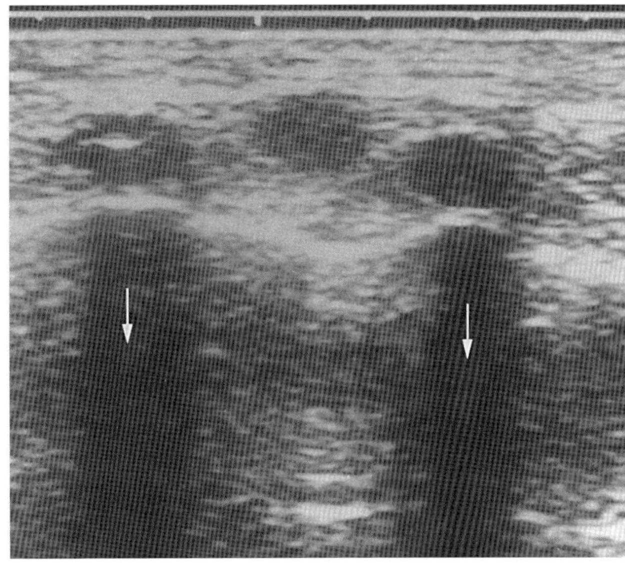

The scan shows a conspicuous focal lesion between two ribs (*arrows* indicate rib shadows) within the intercostal muscle.

Analysis

Not possible due to poor image quality (excessive gain).

Interpretation

Intercostal chest-wall recurrence.

Histology

Metastasis from a poorly differentiated, solid carcinoma.

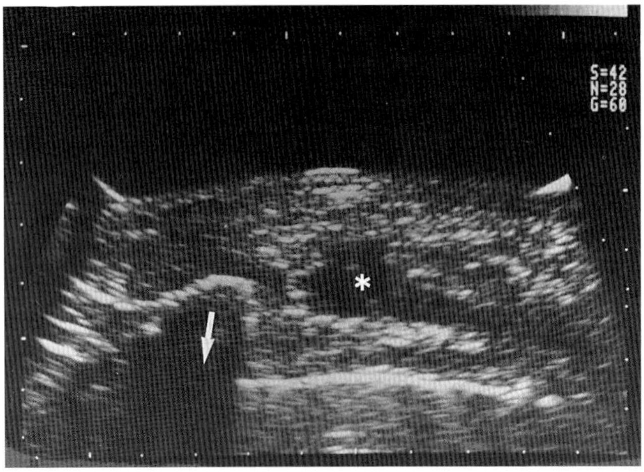

Analysis

1. **Margins**	indistinct, jagged
2. **Retrotumoral acoustic phenomena**	unchanged echoes
3. **Internal echo pattern**	few echoes, nonhomogeneous
4. **Echogenicity**	almost anechoic
5. **Compression effect** on **shape**	no deformation
6. **Compression effect** on **internal echoes**	no change

History

The 63-year-old woman had undergone right mastectomy 14 years before (T2 N0 M0) and had subsequently developed a skin recurrence of small-cell carcinoma in the area of the mastectomy scar, treated by radiation. At follow-up, an indurated area was again noted over the chest wall.

Palpable Findings

Fixed, hazelnut-sized mass in close proximity to a rib was found in the region of the right anterior axillary line at the edge of the former irradiation field.

Sonography

(with standoff)

Figure: sagittal scan over the palpable mass.

A focal sonographic focal (*), 17×12 mm, is seen above a rib, which casts an acoustic shadow *(arrow)*.

Interpretation

Analysis of the sonographic criteria suggests another recurrence. The lesion is in very close proximity to a rib. Neither the intercostal muscle nor pleura are involved by tumor.

Histology

Recurrence of infiltrating lobular carcinoma.

History

The 40-year-old woman had undergone right mastectomy for infiltrating ductal carcinoma (T2 N1 M0) 3 years before. During a subsequent follow-up examination, three small nodules were discovered on the chest wall.

Palpable Findings

Three firm, fixed, pea-sized nodules on the right chest wall above the mastectomy scar.

Sonography

(with water path)

Figure **a**: transverse scan over two of the palpable nodules demonstrating two focal sonographic lesions measuring 6×8 mm and 9×6 mm.

Figure **b**: transverse scan over the third nodule demonstrating a focal sonographic lesion, 6×8 mm.

Interpretation

All three lesions meet the sonographic criteria for malignancy.

Histology

Multiple chest-wall recurrences of infiltrating ductal carcinoma.

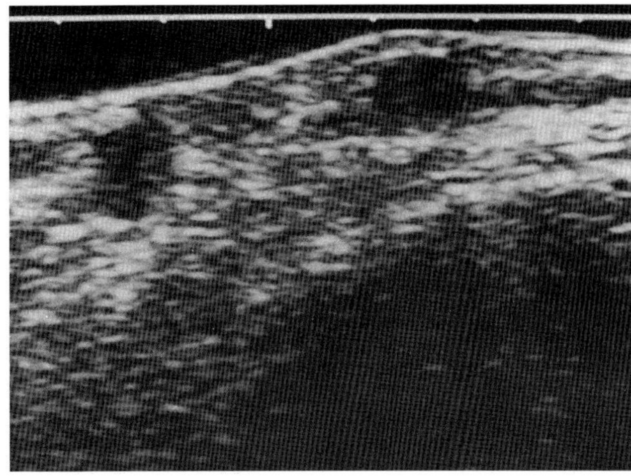

a

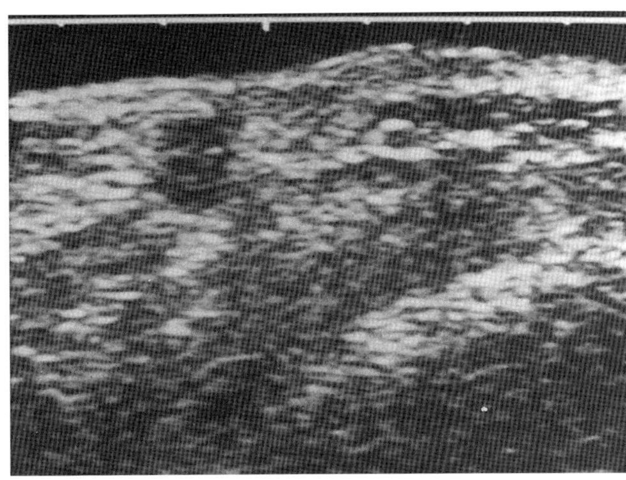

b

Analysis (all 3 lessions)

1. **Margins**	indistinct, jagged
2. **Retrotumoral acoustic phenomena**	unchanged echoes
3. **Internal echo pattern**	few echoes, nonhomogeneous
4. **Echogenicity**	almost anechoic
5. **Compression effect** on **shape**	no deformation
6. **Compression effect** on **internal echoes**	no change

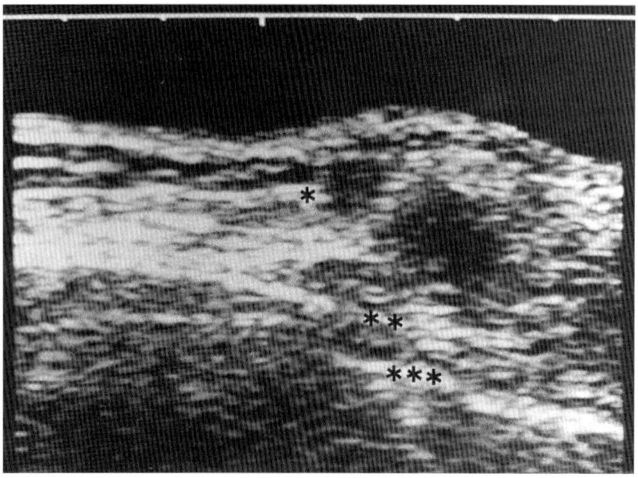

Analysis

1. Margins	indistinct, jagged
2. Retrotumoral acoustic phenomena	unchanged echoes
3. Internal echo pattern	few echoes, non-homogeneous
4. Echogenicity	almost anechoic
5. Compression effect on **shape**	no deformation
6. Compression effect on **internal echoes**	no change

History

The 50-year-old woman had undergone right mastectomy for breast carcinoma (T2 N1 M0) 3 years before. A chest-wall mass was noted on subsequent follow-up.

Palpable Findings

Firm, fixed, hazelnut-sized mass above the mastectomy scar.

Sonography

(with water path)

Figure: transverse scan over the palpable mass demonstrating two focal lesions that appear to be interconnected.

Skin protrusion above the lesions is visible owing to the elastic compliance of the water bag.

Interpretation

All sonographic criteria are suggestive of a recurrence. There is also evidence of pectoralis infiltration at this site (* = anterior pectoral fascia, ** = posterior pectoral fascia, *** = pleura).

Histology

Recurrence of infiltrating lobular carcinoma with fanlike infiltration of a portion of the pectoral muscle.

History

The 51-year-old woman had undergone right mastectomy for infiltrating ductal carcinoma (T1 N0 M0) 3 years before.

Palpable Findings

A clinically indeterminate, rather benign-appearing mass was noted beneath the mastectomy scar during a follow-up examination.

Sonography

Figure: sagittal scan over the suspicious area.

Focal lesion, 8×8 mm, suspicious for malignancy.

Interpretation

The sonographic criteria are suggestive of a recurrence. The lesion is located in the intercostal space but does not involve the pleura (* = ribs).

Histology

Undifferentiated carcinoma with partial necrotic degeneration.

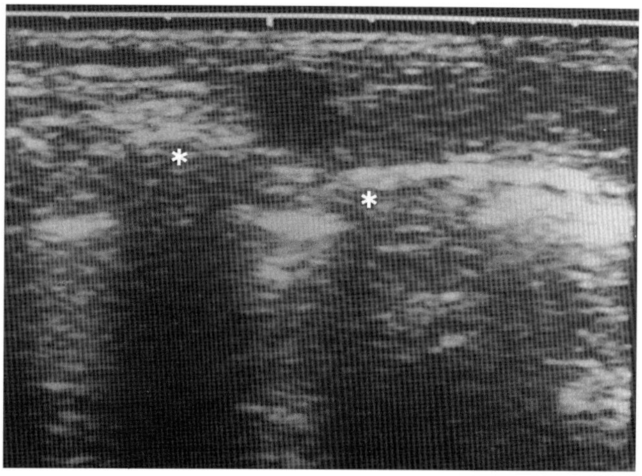

Analysis

1. **Margins**	indistinct, jagged
2. **Retrotumoral acoustic phenomena**	unchanged echoes
3. **Internal echo pattern**	few echoes, nonhomogeneous
4. **Echogenicity**	almost anechoic
5. **Compression effect** on **shape**	no deformation
6. **Compression effect** on **internal echoes**	no change

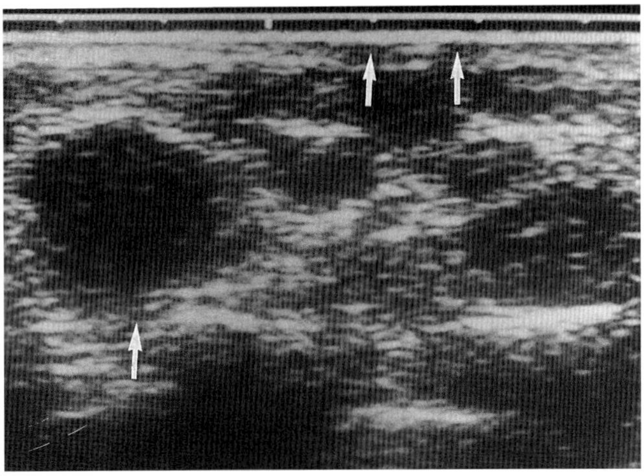

Analysis

1. Margins	indistinct, jagged
2. Retrotumoral acoustic phenomena	unchanged echoes
3. Internal echo pattern	few echoes, nonhomogeneous
4. Echogenicity	almost anechoic
5. Compression effect on **shape**	no deformation
6. Compression effect on **internal echoes**	no change

History

The 60-year-old woman had undergone right mastectomy 10 years before. Primary tumor stage unknown. She now presented with clinical suspicion of an extensive chest-wall recurrence.

Palpable Findings

Approximately palm-sized area with multiple firm, fixed nodules on the right chest wall.

Sonography

Figure: transverse scan over the palpable mass showing multiple adjacent focal abnormalities.

Interpretation

The focal sonographic lesions exhibit malignant features. The large lesion on the left side of the image is infiltrating the pleura *(arrow)*. On the right, two nodular tumor extensions are invading the skin *(arrows)*.

Computed tomography showed nodular extensions of recurrent tumor penetrating the costal muscles and invading the pleura.

Aspiration Cytology

Invasive carcinoma.

Note: The presence or absence of pleural infiltration by recurrent tumor is an important consideration in treatment planning. In the present case, primary surgical resection was not an appropriate option due to pleural infiltration; treatment began with radiation to the chest wall.

History

The 60-year-old woman had undergone left mastectomy for adenocarcinoma (T2 N0 M0) and postoperative irradiation 3 years before. An indeterminate mass was noted above the mastectomy scar during a follow-up examination.

Sonography

Figure: sagittal scan over the palpable mass demonstrating a subcutaneous focal lesion invading the pectoral muscle.

Interpretation

Except for criterion 4, all the sonographic criteria suggest a malignant process.

Histology

Fat-tissue metastasis from a solid carcinoma.

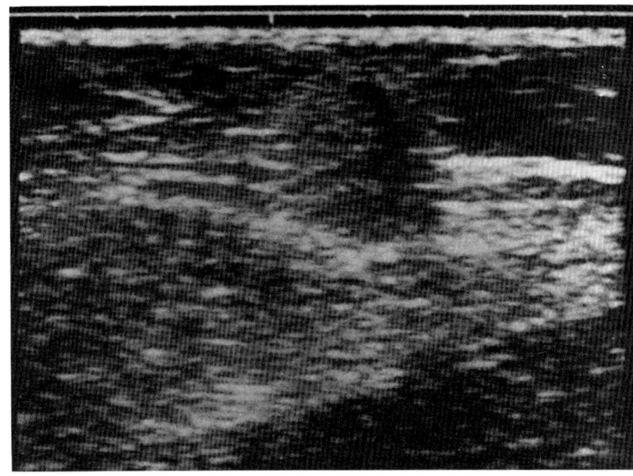

Analysis

1. **Margins**	indistinct, jagged
2. **Retrotumoral acoustic phenomena**	unchanged echoes
3. **Internal echo pattern**	nonhomogeneous
4. **Echogenicity**	fat-equivalent
5. **Compression effect** on **shape**	no deformation
6. **Compression effect** on **internal echoes**	no change

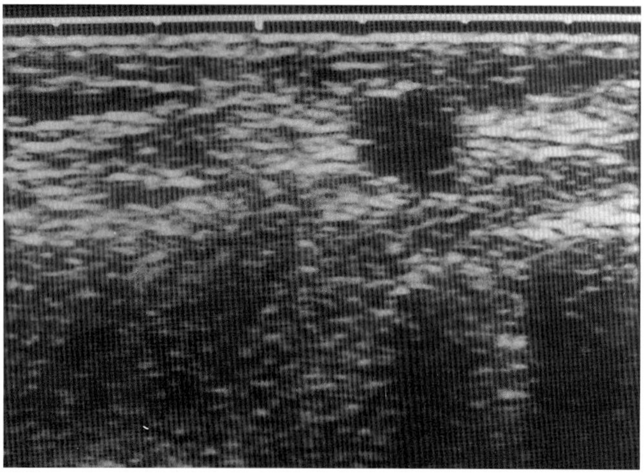

Analysis

1. Margins	sharp, jagged
2. Retrotumoral acoustic phenomena	unchanged echoes
3. Internal echo pattern	few echoes, nonhomogeneous
4. Echogenicity	almost anechoic
5. Compression effect on **shape**	no deformation
6. Compression effect on **internal echoes**	no change

History

The 73-year-old woman had undergone right mastectomy for infiltrating ductal carcinoma (T2 N1 M0) 2 years before. A follow-up examination revealed a firm, fixed nodule on the chest wall.

Sonography

Figure: sagittal scan over the nodule demonstrating a conspicuous focal lesion.

Interpretation

Except for the sharp margins, all sonographic criteria imply a malignant process.

Histology

Soft-tissue metastasis from an undifferentiated infiltrating ductal carcinoma.

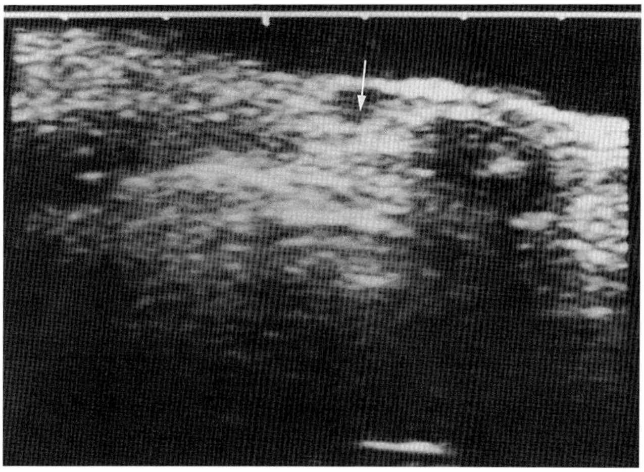

History

The 53-year-old woman had undergone right mastectomy for breast carcinoma (T3 N2 M0) 7 years before. Follow-up prompted referral for a sonographic examination.

Palpable Findings

Unremarkable.

Sonography

(with water path)

Figure: parasternal sagittal scan showing a small hypoechoic focal lesion *(arrow)*, 4×4 mm, above a rib (with shadow).

Analysis

With a very small focal sonographic lesion, the analytic criteria are not reliable.

Interpretation

The small lesion with ill-defined, jagged margins over the rib looked suspicious to the sonographer. Guided by the ultrasound findings, the examiner was able to palpate a small mass directly over the scar.

Histology

Poorly differentiated solid carcinoma.

Note: In this case, the ultrasound examination provided the only evidence for the presence of a recurrence.

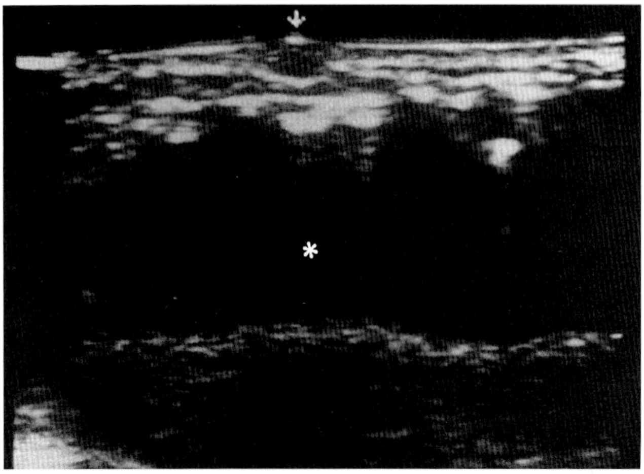

History

The 40-year-old woman had undergone breast-conserving surgery for infiltrating ductal carcinoma (T1 N0 M0) 1 year before. She subsequently developed a multicentric intramammary recurrence, necessitating a left mastectomy with primary subpectoral reconstruction. At follow-up, a pea-sized nodule was noted over the prosthesis.

Sonography

(with water path)

Figure: sagittal scan over the nodule demonstrating an intradermal focal sonographic lesion *(arrow)*, 6×4 mm.

Analysis

With a very small focal lesion, the analytic criteria are difficult or impossible to apply.

Interpretation

The focal lesion over the prosthesis (*) is made conspicuous by its disruption of the skin lines. A confident benign/malignant differentiation cannot be made by ultrasound.

Histology

Metastatic infiltrating ductal carcinoma.

History

The 29-year-old woman had undergone right mastectomy for breast carcinoma (T3 N1 M0) 2 years before with subsequent implantation of a subpectoral prosthesis. At follow-up, a pea-sized nodule was noted above the scar.

Sonography

Figure: transverse scan over the nodule demonstrating a focal lesion *(arrow)*, 5×7 mm, between the skin and the echo-free prosthesis (*).

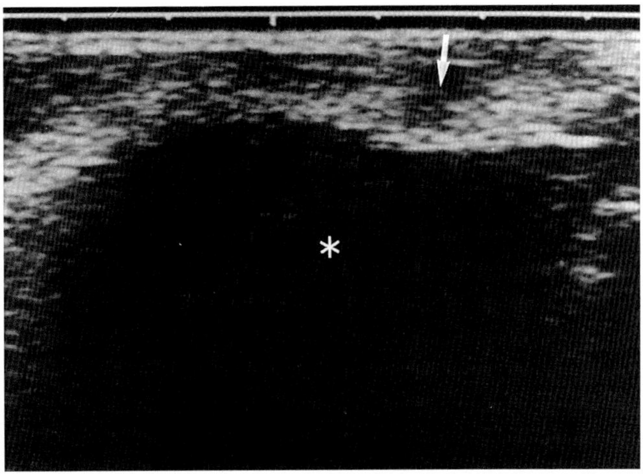

Interpretation

Sonographic criteria 1 and 3 suggest a malignant process. Criteria 5 and 6 are indeterminate due to the underlying prosthesis.

The sonogram also shows a skin discontinuity above the focal lesion. Ultrasound indicates a very high index of suspicion of a recurrence.

Histology

Skin recurrence of a small-cell carcinoma, approximately 5 mm in diameter.

Analysis

1. Margins	indistinct, jagged
2. Retrotumoral acoustic phenomena	unchanged echoes
3. Internal echo pattern	nonhomogeneous
4. Echogenicity	fat-equivalent
5. Compression effect on **shape**	cannot be tested
6. Compression effect on **internal echoes**	cannot be tested

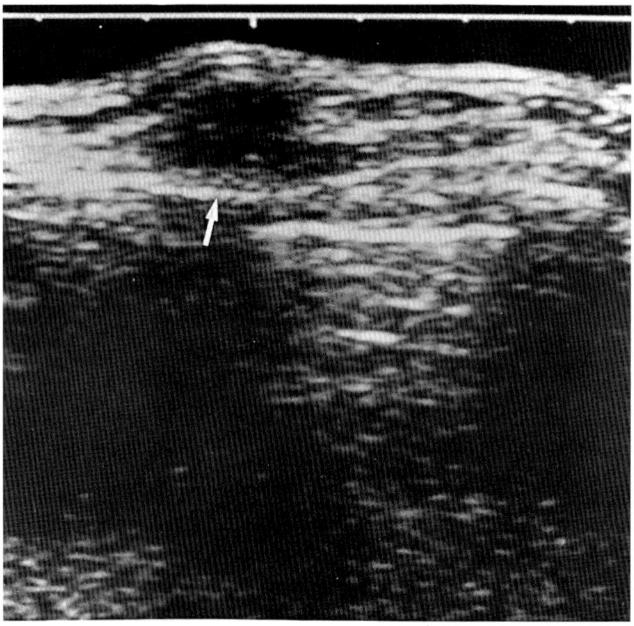

a

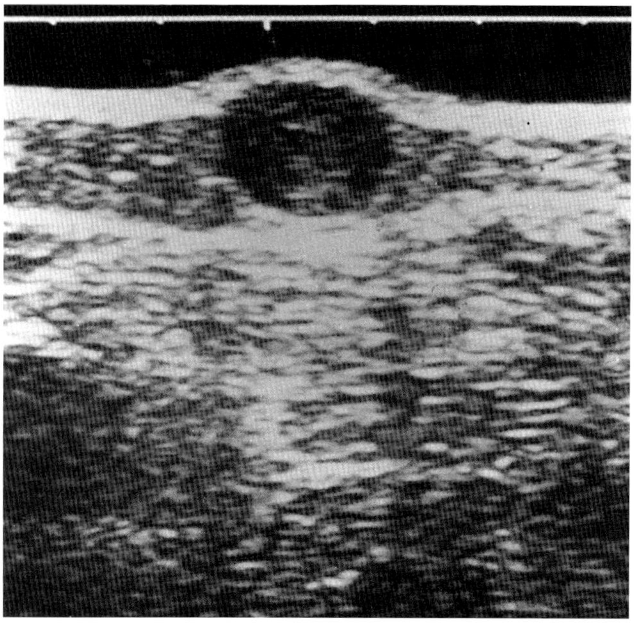

b

History

The 44-year-old woman had undergone left mastectomy 5 years before.

Palpable Findings

Mobile, smooth-bordered mass the size of the distal phalanx of the thumb located, below the mastectomy scar on the midclavicular line. Also a smooth-bordered, cherry sized paravertebral mass at the L5 level resembling the palpable mass on the chest wall.

Sonography

(with water path)

Figure **a**: sagittal scan over the palpable mass on the chest wall demonstrating a bulging, hypechoic focal lesion, 20×9 mm.

Figure **b**: sagittal scan over the palpable mass on the back showing a smoothly marginated focal lesion, 16×12 mm.

Analysis

	a	b
1. **Margins**	indistinct, jagged	sharp and smooth
2. **Retrotumoral acoustic phenomena**	unchanged echoes	slight posterior enhancement, bilateral shadowing
3. **Internal echo pattern**	few echoes, nonhomogeneous	nonhomogeneous
4. **Echogenicity**	almost anechoic	fat-equivalent
5. **Compression effect** on **shape**	no deformation	no deformation
6. **Compression effect** on **internal echoes**	no change	no change

Interpretation

Both lesions closely resemble each other clinically, but their sonographic features are quite different. The criteria for lesion 1 strongly suggest a malignant process, whereas the criteria for lesion 2 are obviously benign. With lesion 1, it is noteworthy that the fascia of the pectoralis major muscle is intact *(arrow)* but is in contact with the deep surface of the mass.

Histology

Lesion **a**: chest-wall recurrence of infiltrating lobular carcinoma, 15×20 mm.

Lesion **b**: 20-mm atheroma.

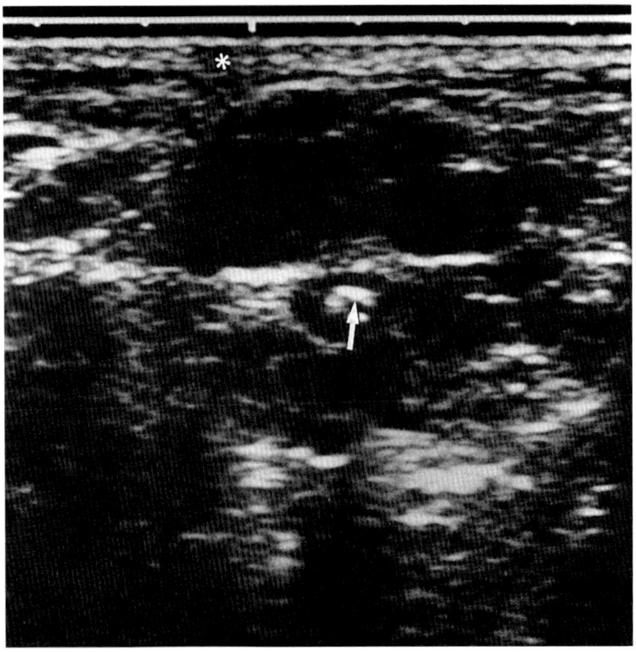

a

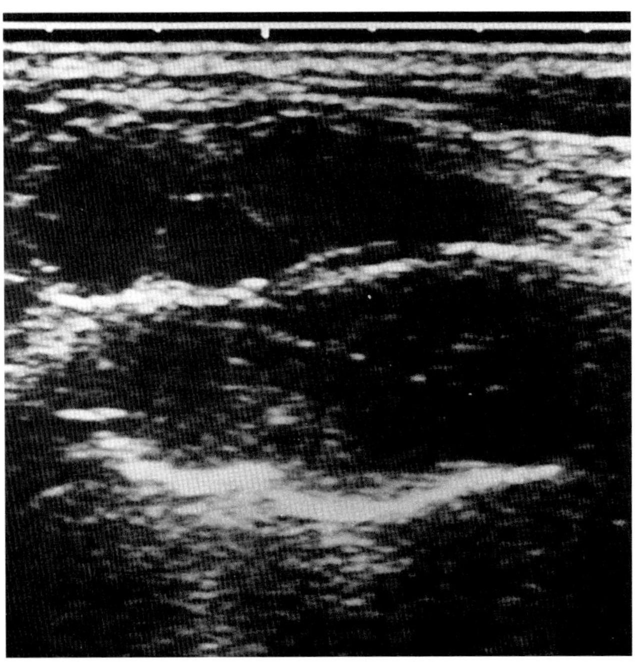

b

History

The 53-year-old woman had undergone right mastectomy with axillary lymphadenectomy 11 months before. For 6 weeks she was aware of a painful mass over the right chest wall.

Palpable Findings

A firm, fixed, disk-shaped subcutaneous mass was palpated above the transverse mastectomy scar in the midline region. The overlying skin was smooth.

Sonography

Figure **a**: sagittal scan over the palpable mass. The small subcutaneous shadow in the left half of the image originates from the mastectomy scar (*). Adjacent to it is a focal lesion, 46×44×36 mm.

Figure **b**: transverse scan over the palpable mass. Intact pectoral muscle is visible on the right side of the image, deep to the subcutaneous fat; to the left of it, the whole field is occupied by a focal sonographic lesion.

Analysis

The usual analytic criteria cannot be applied to this large lesion.

Interpretation

The sagittal scan shows a local recurrence based on the chest wall. At the center is a rib *(arrow)* with portions of the pectoral fascia still partly intact. The crescent-shaped, almost anechoic area below the rib represents ingrowth of the recurrence into the chest cavity.

The transverse scan, which cuts the intercostal space, presents similar findings. The impression is of a recurrent tumor that has invaded the chest cavity without penetrating the pleura.

Histology

Chest-wall recurrence of a poorly differentiated tumor with muscle infiltration. The bone (rib) contains nodular tumor infiltrates spreading from the soft tissue to perichondral areas.

History

This woman, 38 years of age, had a difficult prior history (breast-conserving resection of left breast cancer, local recurrence with secondary mastectomy, extensive local-regional chest-wall recurrence necessitating wide excision and reconstruction by rectus abdominis transfer).

Palpable Findings

Bean-sized mass in the area of the transposed flap, very suspicious for a new recurrence.

Sonography

Figure **a**: sagittal scan over the palpable mass. Readability: limited to unreadable.

The palpable mass is not visualized.

Figure **b**: sagittal scan at an identical site in the right breast, for comparison.

Readability: good.

Analysis

Not possible due to absence of a focal lesion.

Interpretation

The palpable mass is not demonstrable by ultrasound, apparently due to a lack of sonographic contrast in the transposed muscle tissue (rectus abdominis). This profoundly limits the ability of ultrasound to evaluate the musculocutaneous flap for recurrent disease.

By comparison, the sonogram of the right breast is far more readable because of the superior contrast.

Histology

Local recurrence of breast carcinoma.

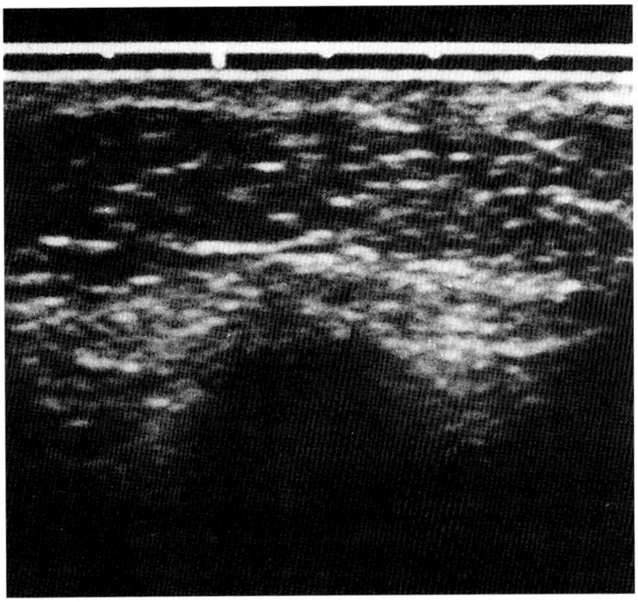

a

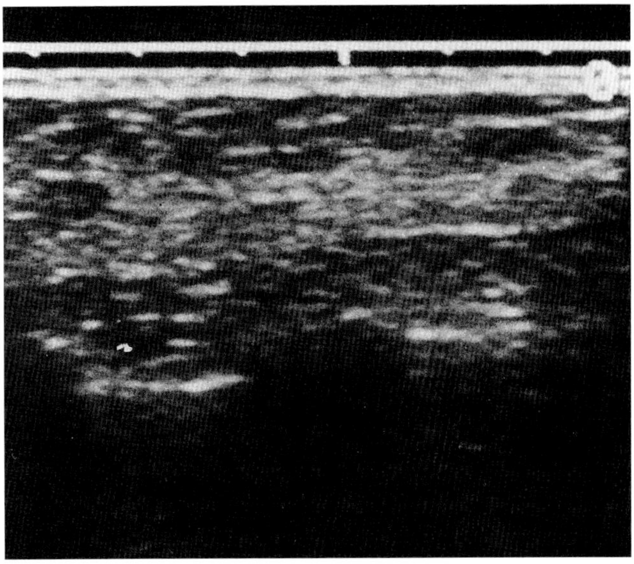

b

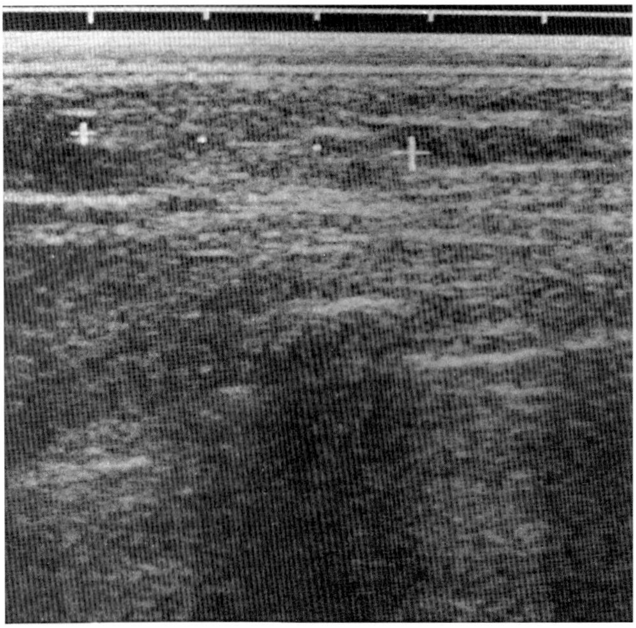

History

The 41-year-old woman had undergone breast-conserving surgery on the right 1 month before. Examination prior to the institution of radiotherapy disclosed an indeterminate palpable mass on the lateral chest wall.

Palpable Findings

Clinically very suspicious mass, 2×3 mm, on the anterior axillary line in the region of the scar.

Sonography

Figure: sagittal scan over the palpable mass.

Readability: good.

Hyperechoic area 28 mm in size; no focal sonographic lesion.

Analysis

Not possible due to the absence of a focal lesion.

Interpretation

The palpable mass is not demonstrated sonographically as a focal lesion; only a hyperechoic area is seen. Such changes are commonly found in association with a freshly operated region.

Histology

Skin-covered tissue specimen showed chronic scarring and inflammation in the subcutaneous tissue with inclusion of suture granulomas. No evidence of malignancy.

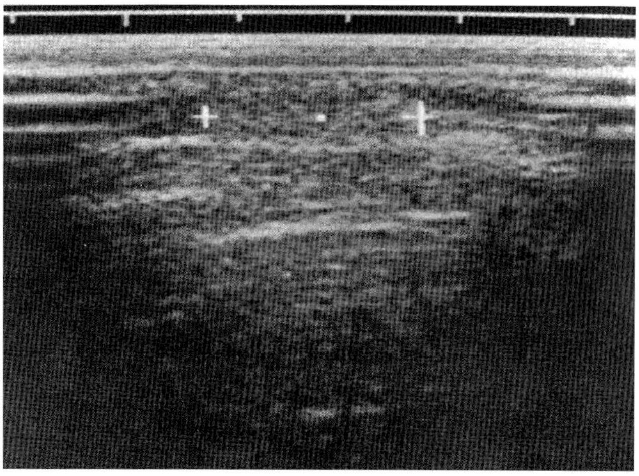

History

The 60-year-old woman had undergone right mastectomy 7 years before and had had excision of a scar recurrence and postoperative radiation 3 years before. Follow-up showed a possible new recurrence in the area of the mastectomy scar.

Palpable Findings

Firm, clinically very suspicious subcutaneous mass, 1×2 cm, in the area of the mastectomy scar.

Sonography

Figure: sagittal scan over the palpable mass showing a hyperechoic area but no focal lesion.

Analysis

Not possible due to the absence of a focal lesion.

Interpretation

Ultrasound demonstrates the palpable mass as an innocent-appearing, hyperechoic area—most likely scar tissue.

Histology

Mildly scarred, hyalinized skin with fibrotic connective tissue, normal-appearing subcutaneous fat, and scattered lymphocytic infiltration. No evidence of malignancy.

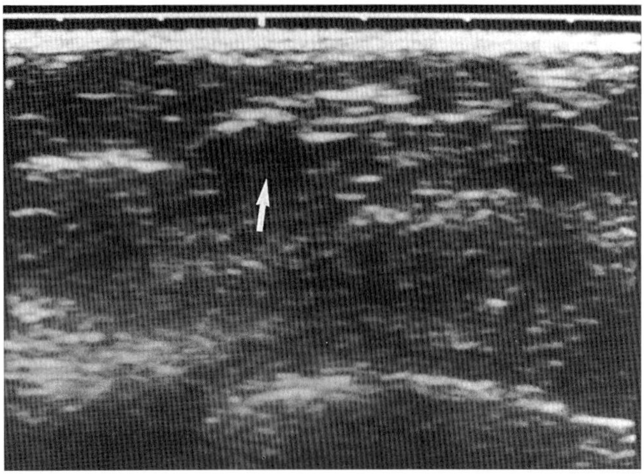

History

The 63-year-old woman had undergone left mastectomy 2 years before for infiltrating lobular breast cancer (T2 N0 M0). At follow-up, a clinically indeterminate mass was noted above the mastectomy scar.

Sonography

Figure: sagittal scan over the questionable mass demonstrating a somewhat hypoechoic area *(arrow)* which, however, cannot be definitely regarded as a focal lesion.

Analysis

After the dynamic examination showed that the mass practically disappeared under digital compression, further analytic evaluation was whithheld.

Interpretation

Lesions that are very radically distorted by compression are usually caused by more or less randomly occurring echo phenomena. Hence the finding was considered to be benign.

Histology

Fatty tissue with mild cicatricial fibrosis. No evidence for recurrence of the original cancer.

Oncologic Follow-Up after Breast-Conserving Surgery

Follow-Up after Breast-Conserving Cancer and Postoperative Radiation

Clinical and mammographic examination are frequently difficult in patients who have had breast-conserving surgery and postoperative radiotherapy. The irradiated breast, which often is radiographically dense for a time due to radiation-induced fibrosis, offers an ideal environment for ultrasonography in the search for recurrent disease (Leucht and Rabe 1988). A knowledge of the acoustic phenomena that may occur in the operated and irradiated breast is essential for the evaluation of this patient group. Besides breasts with identical densities (Fig. 6.**1**, p. 152), scans will frequently show radiation fribrosis in the irradiated breast (Fig. 6.**2**), requiring a reduction in the total gain setting (Fig. 6.**3**). Other common postirradiation changes are skin thickening (Fig. 6.**4**) and icreased density of the subcutaneous fat (Fig. 6.**5**) or breast parenchyma (Fig. 6.**6**). Other sequelae include the destruction of the normal parenchymal architecture (Fig. 6.**7**) or the appearance of hyperechoic striations (Fig. 6.**8**).

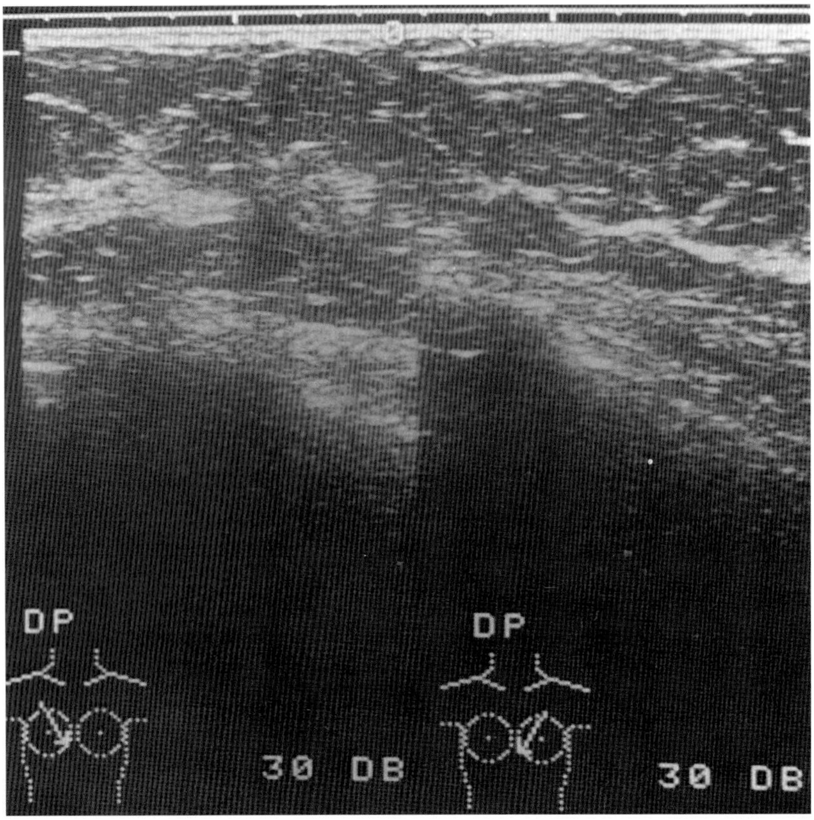

Fig. 6.**1** Woman, 59 years of age, who underwent right quadrantectomy and subsequent irradiation. Scans through the upper inner quadrant show that the irradiated breast has the same sonographic appearance as the untreated left breast. Most notably, the irradiated breast shows no increase in density. X-ray mammography likewise showed no radiation-induced changes

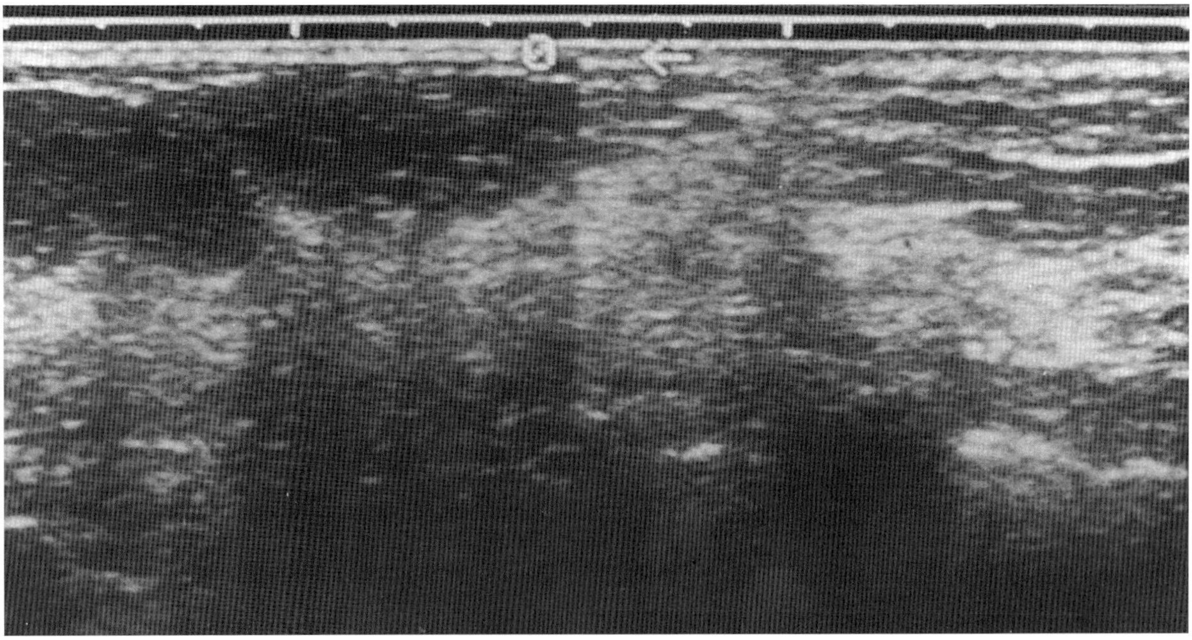

Fig. 6.**2** Woman, 49 years of age, who underwent left segmentectomy and subsequent irradiation. Radiotherapy was terminated 8 months ago

a Sagittal scan over the nonirradiated right breast. Total gain = 32 dB

b Sagittal scan over the irradiated left breast. Total gain = 32 dB a 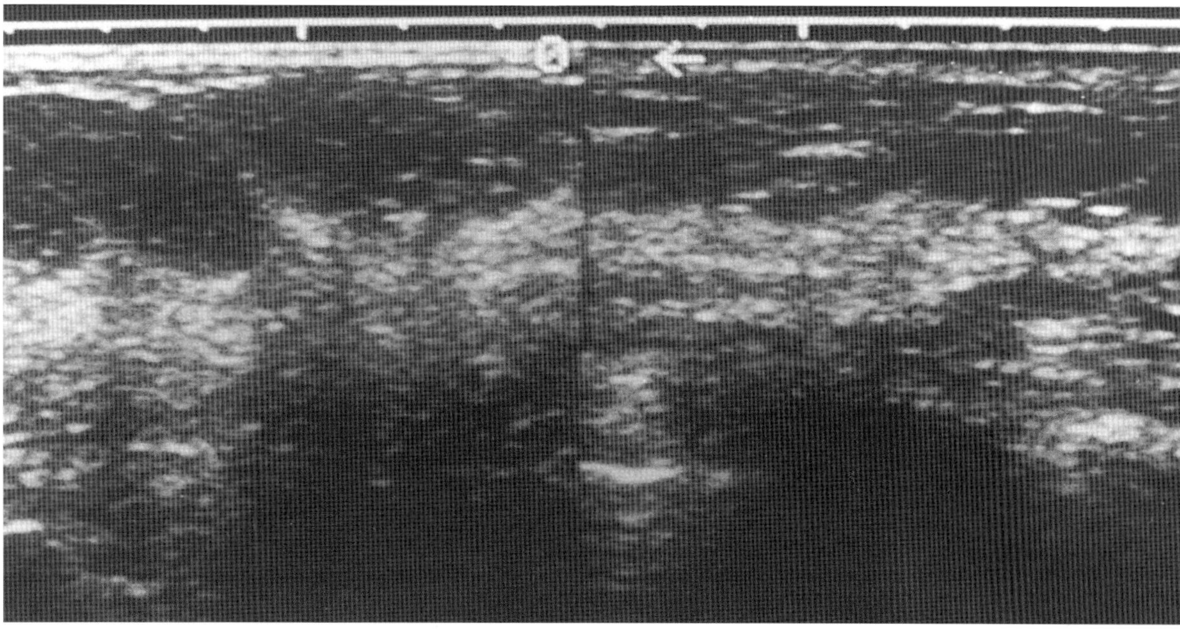 b

Fig. 6.**3** Woman, 49 years of age
a Same image as in Fig. 6.**2a**
b Sagittal scan over the irradiated left side, with total gain reduced by 6 dB

Fig. 6.**4** Woman, 50 years of age, who underwent right quadrantectomy and subsequent irradiation. Radiotherapy was terminated 10 months ago
a Sagittal scan over the irradiated right side. Note that the skin thickness is more than twice that on the nonirradiated side (**b**). There are no other apparent differences between the sides
b Sagittal scan over the nonirradiated left side

a 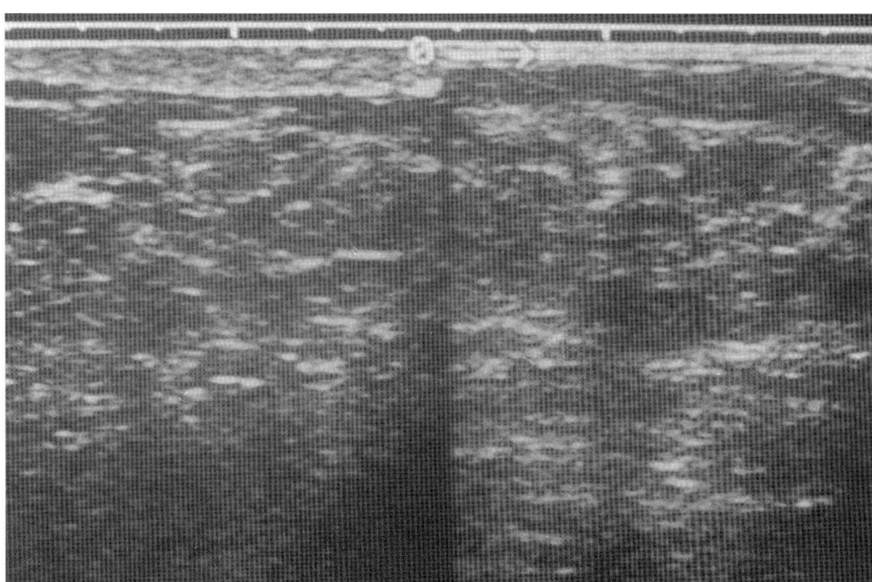 b

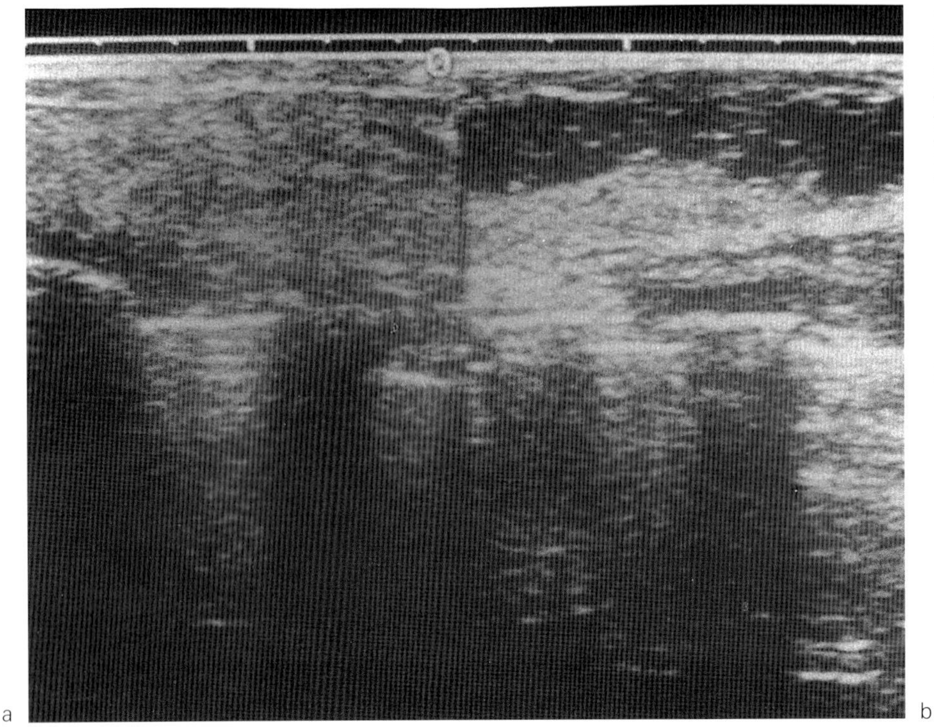

Fig. 6.**5** Woman, 43 years of age, who underwent right quadrantectomy and post-operative radiation. Radiotherapy was terminated 4 1/2 months ago
a Sagittal scan over the irradiated right side. Cutaneous edema. Marked fibrosis of the subcutaneous fat (increased sonodensity) obscures normal contrast between the glandular region and fat
b Sagittal scan over the nonirradiated side shows a normal-appearing tissue composition

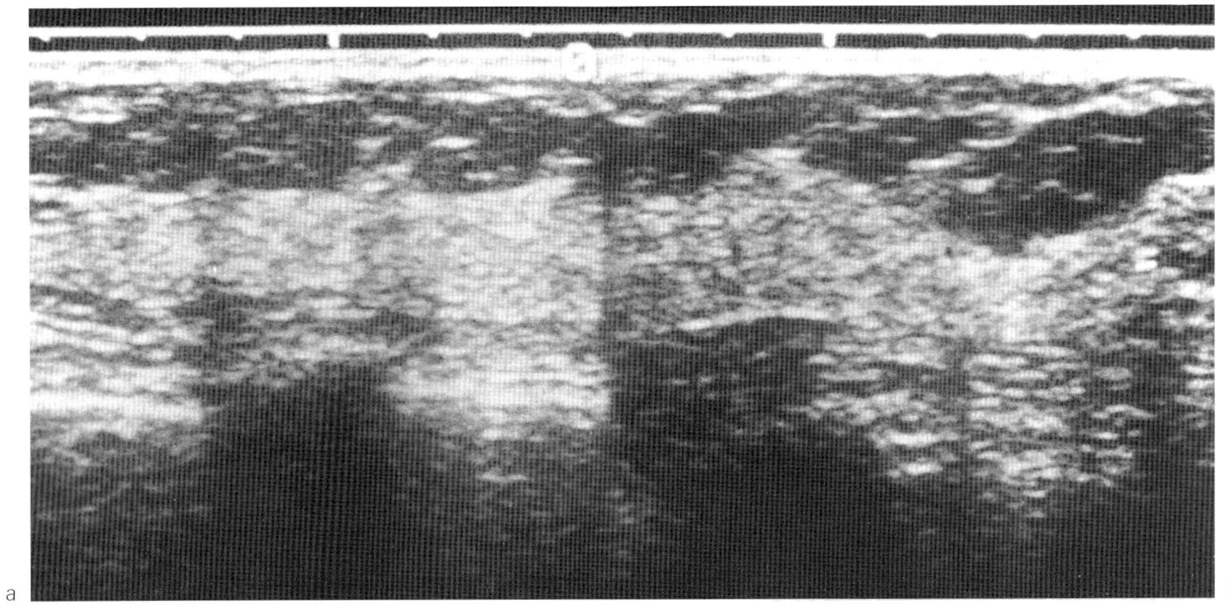

Fig. 6.**6** Woman, 46 years of age, who underwent right quadrantectomy and subsequent irradiation. Radiotherapy was terminated 32 months ago. Total gain on both sides is 28 dB
a Sagittal scan over the irradiated right breast
b Sagittal scan at the identical site on the nonirradiated left breast. Increased sonodensity in the glandular region of the irradiated (right) side, with slight fibrosis of the overlying subcutaneous fat

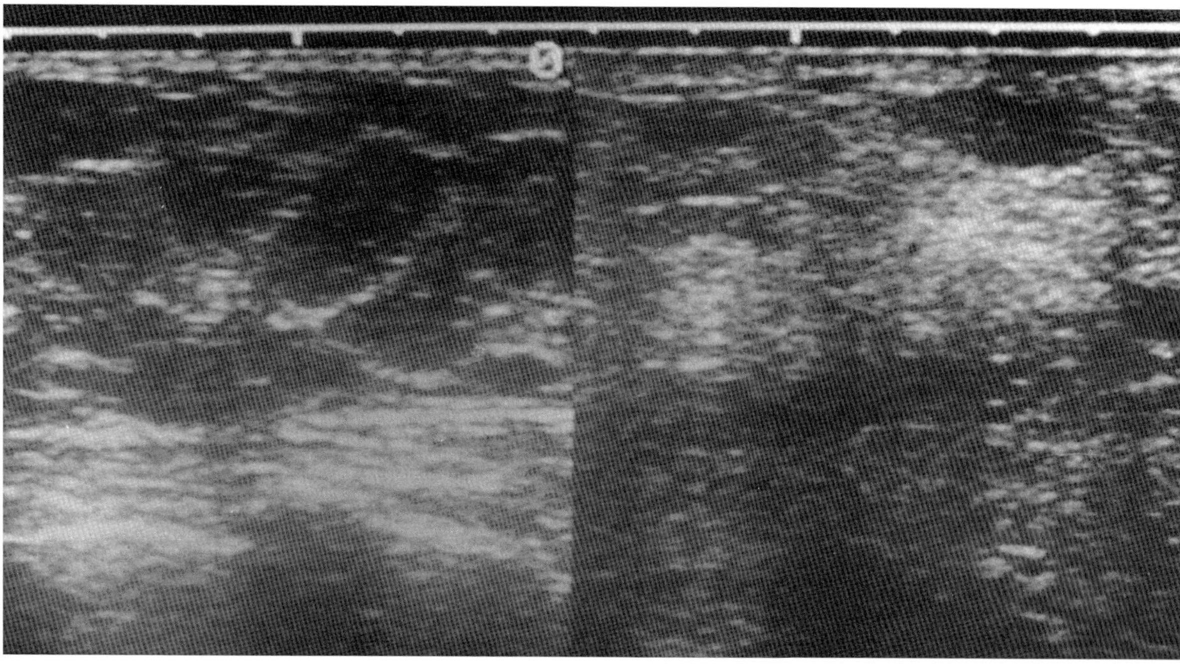

a b

Fig. 6.**7** Woman, 48 years of age, who underwent left quadrantectomy and subsequent irradiation. Radiotherapy was terminated 2 months ago

a Sagittal scan over the nonirradiated right side. Normal-appearing parenchymal pattern

b Sagittal scan at the identical site on the irradiated breast. Mild cutaneous edema. Increased tissue density. Above all, note the destruction of normal parenchymal architecture as seen in the contralateral breast

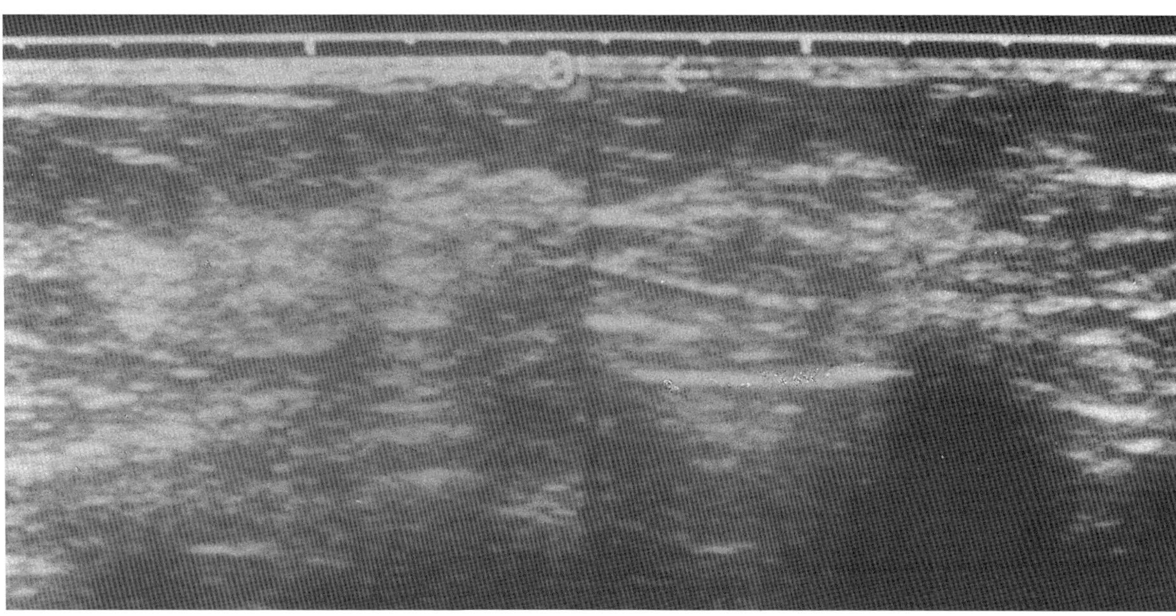

a b

Fig. 6.**8** Woman, 51 years of age, who underwent left quadrantectomy and subsequent irradiation. Radiotherapy was terminated 4 1/2 years ago

a Sagittal scan over the nonirradiated right breast. Normal-appearing parenchymal pattern

b Sagittal scan at the identical site on the left breast, showing conspicuous hyperechoic striations ("striping") in the irradiated breast

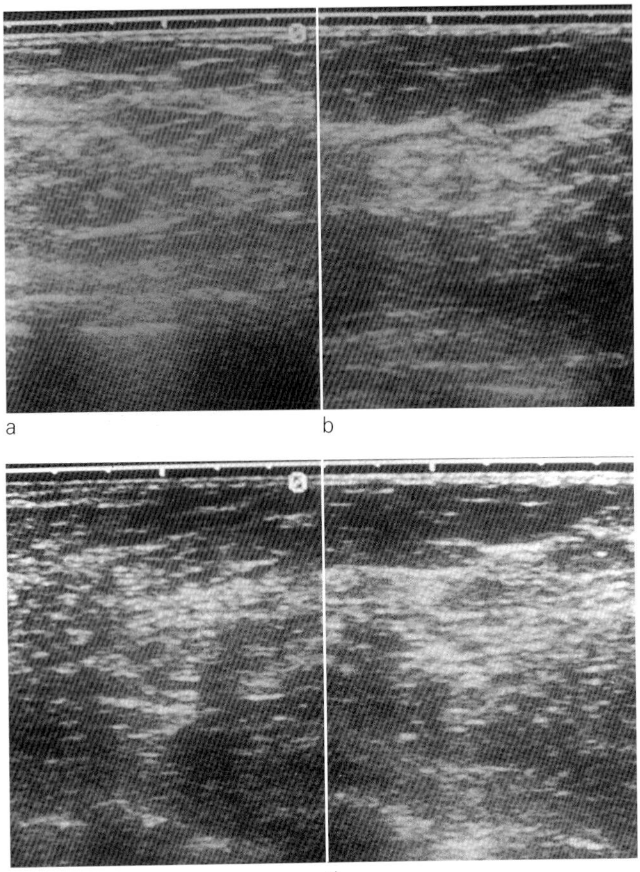

a b c d

History

The 46-year-old woman had undergone breast-conserving surgery on the right with postoperative irradiation terminated 14 months before. At follow-up she was referred for ultrasound of the right breast, made radiographically dense by radiation-induced fibrosis.

Palpable Findings

Slight, generalized induration of the right breast. No palpable masses.

Sonography

Total gain of 34 dB on both sides:

Figure **a**: sagittal scan over the outer quadrants of the right breast.

Figure **b**: sagittal scan over the outer quadrants of the left breast.

Total gain 29 dB on right side, 34 dB on left side:

Figure **c**: sagittal scan over the outer quadrants of the right breast.

Figure **d**: sagittal scan over the outer quadrants of the left breast.

Readability: good.

No detectable focal sonographic lesions.

Interpretation

The scans demonstrate pronounced radiation fibrosis of the right breast. X-ray mammograms of this breast are not readable. Scans taken at a constant gain (34 dB) show significantly higher echogenicity in the irradiated breast than at an identical site in the nonirradiated breast. This increased sonodensity permits a total gain reduction of 5 dB to achieve equal densities on both sides. No evidence of recurrent disease.

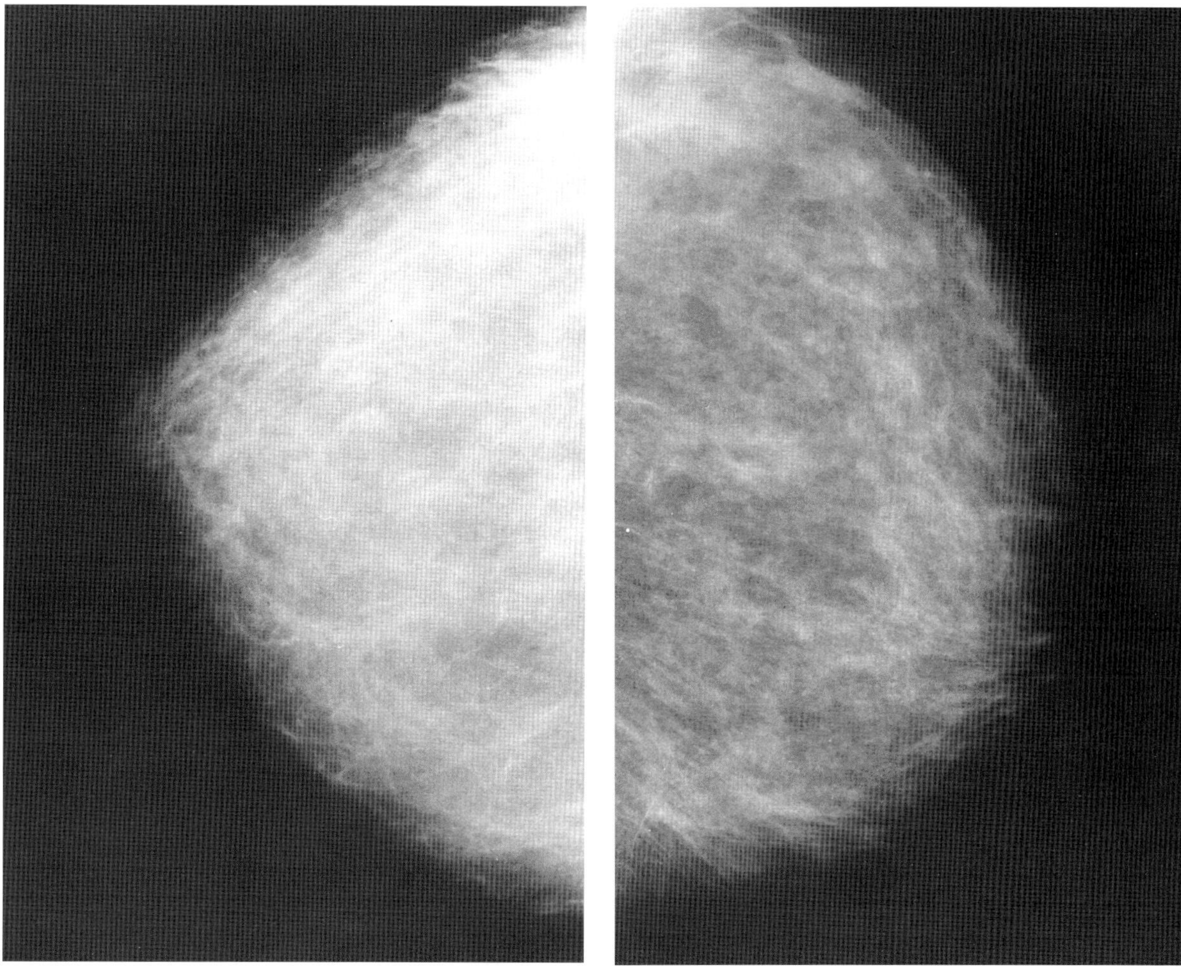

a b

X-ray Mammography

Figure **a**: craniocaudal projection of the irradiated right breast showing marked fibrosis with no focal abnormalities.

Figure **b**: mediolateral projection of the non-irradiated left breast showing a dysplastic breast pattern with no focal abnormalities.

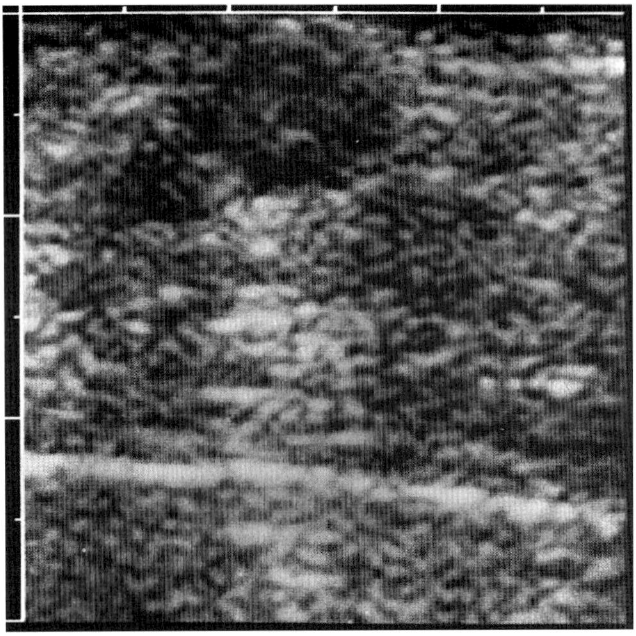

a

Analysis

1. **Margins**	indistinct but smooth
2. **Retrotumoral acoustic phenomena**	slight posterior enhancement
3. **Internal echo pattern**	nonhomogeneous
4. **Echogenicity**	almost anechoic
5. **Compression effect** on **shape**	no deformation
6. **Compression effect** on **internal echoes**	no change

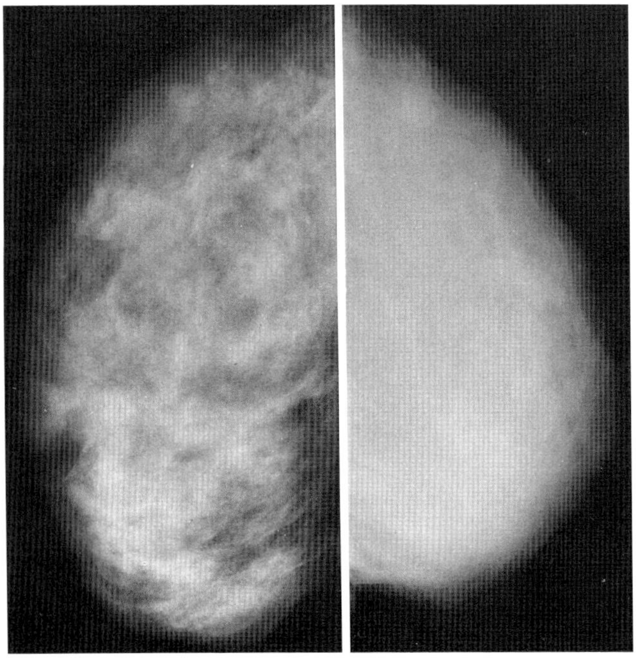

b c

History

The 43-year-old woman had undergone a breast-conserving operation for carcinoma of the left breast. Her radiotherapy had been terminated 5 months before.

Palpable Findings

A firm, fixed, poorly demarcated mass, clinically suspicious for a recurrence, was palpated just beneath the skin in the area of the scar.

Sonography

Figure **a**: sagittal scan over the palpable mass.

Readability: limited.

Focal sonographic lesion, 19×17 mm.

Interpretation

Except for the smooth margins and posterior enhancement, the analytic criteria suggest a recurrence. From a clinical standpoint as well, this is the most likely diagnosis.

X-ray Mammography

Mediolateral projections of the right and left breasts.

Figure **b**: nonirradiated right breast. Pronounced fibrocystic disease.

Readability: limited.

Figure **c**: irradiated left breast. Pronounced radiation response.

Readability: profoundly limited. In the upper part of the breast there is faint evidence of a smooth-margined round lesion, but it does not correspond to the palpable mass demonstrated by ultrasound. This lesion was identified sonographically as a cyst and was aspirated.

Histology

Recurrence of infiltrating ductal carcinoma in the left breast. Diameter: 20 mm.

History

The 40-year-old woman had undergone a breast-conserving operation for breast carcinoma. Radiotherapy had been terminated 3 years ago.

Palpable Findings

During a follow-up examination, an approximately hazelnut-sized, mobile mass was discovered below the nipple in the area of the surgical scar.

Sonography

Figure: oblique scan over the mass.

Readability: good.

Focal sonographic lesion, 11×10 mm.

Interpretation

Although the sonographic criteria are inconsistent, a recurrence of carcinoma must be presumed.

X-ray Mammography

Both projections demonstrate a focal density, 15×20 mm, with microcalcifications. The nature of the lesion is indeterminate.

Histology

Moderately well-differentiated, 15 mm infiltrating duct carcinoma with intraductal extensions.

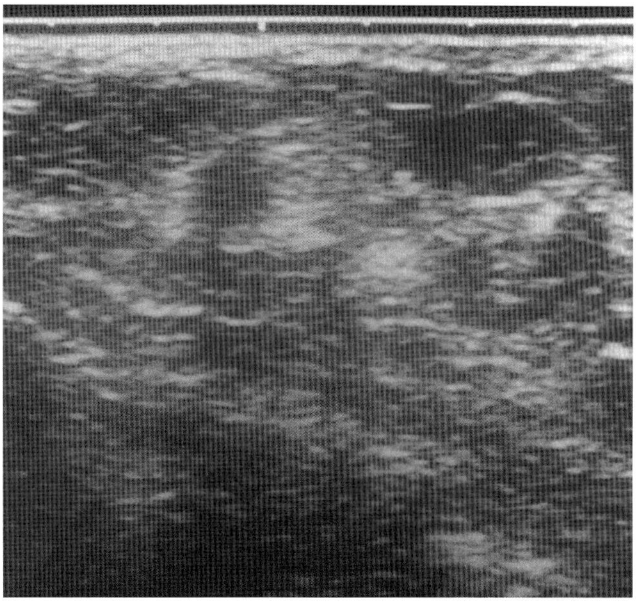

Analysis

1. **Margins**	indistinct, jagged
2. **Retrotumoral acoustic phenomena**	unchanged echoes
3. **Internal echo pattern**	nonhomogeneous
4. **Echogenicity**	fat-equivalent
5. **Compression effect** on **shape**	no deformation
6. **Compression effect** on **internal echoes**	no change

Note: The hyperechoic "halo," occasionally observed, is also seen here.

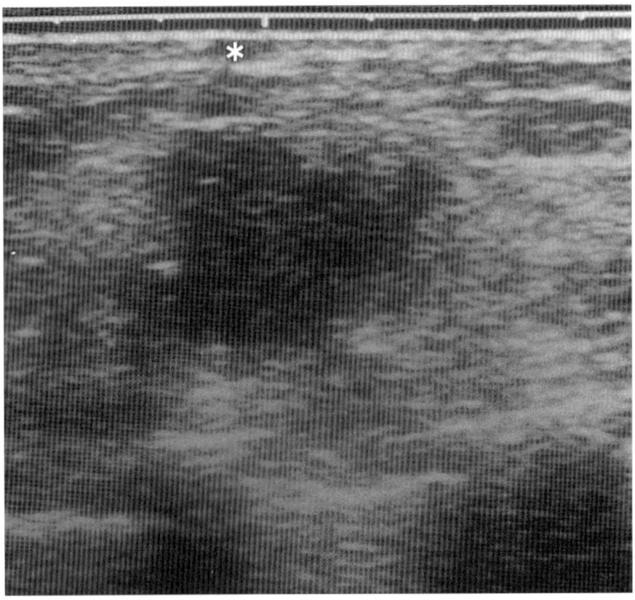

a

Analysis

1. **Margins**	indistinct, jagged
2. **Retrotumoral acoustic phenomena**	unchanged echoes
3. **Internal echo pattern**	few echoes, nonhomogeneous
4. **Echogenicity**	almost anechoic
5. **Compression effect** on **shape**	no deformation
6. **Compression effect** on **internal echoes**	no change

History

The 50-year-old woman had undergone left quadrantectomy with postoperative radiation (T1 N1 M0). Histology identified the tumor as infiltrating duct carcinoma with a predominantly intraductal component. Radiotherapy was concluded 10 months before.

Palpable Findings

During a follow-up examination, a firm, approximately plum-sized mass was noted in the upper outer quadrant of the left breast in the area of the surgical scar. The mass was poorly demarcated within the generally indurated breast.

Sonography

Figure **a**: sagittal scan over the palpable mass.

Readability: good.

The scan shows thickening of the skin line, which is interrupted by a discontinuity (* = scar) above a focal lesion, 30×22 mm. The lesion is located within the hyperechoic (fibrotic) breast parenchyma.

Interpretation

All the sonographic criteria suggest a recurrence. The sharp contrast of the almost anechoic recurrence with its echogenic surroundings is particularly noteworthy.

X-ray Mammography

Comparative views of both breasts in the craniocaudal projection.

Figure **b**: normal-appearing mammogram of the nonirradiated right breast.

Figure **c**: the left breast, which shows extensive radiation-induced change with no discernible focal abnormality.

Histology

Extensive local recurrence (3 cm in diameter) with nodular tumor infiltration of the pectoral muscle.

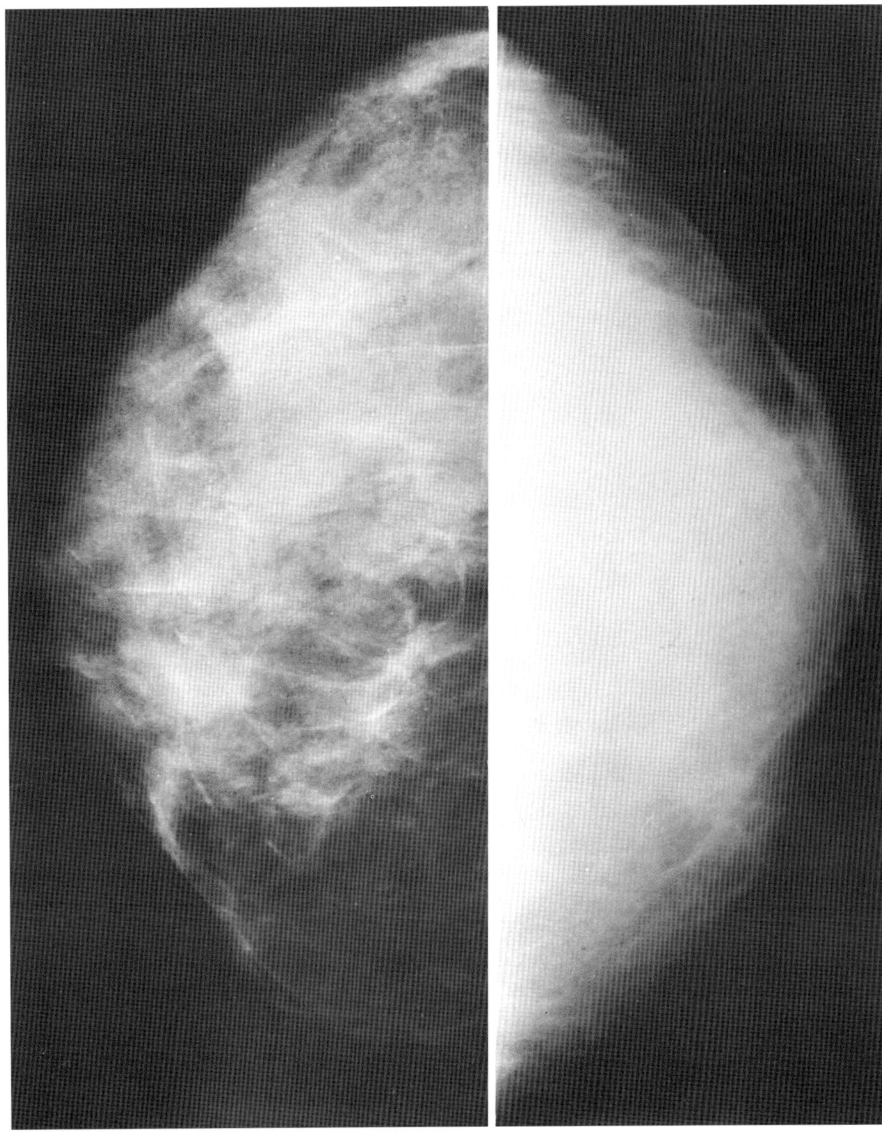

b c

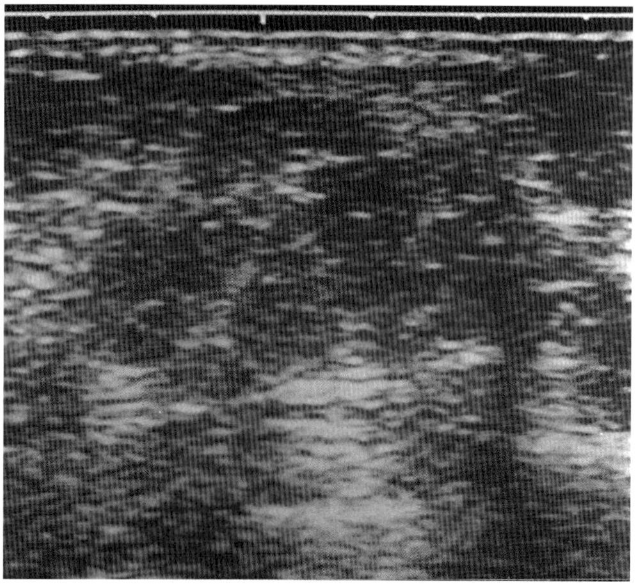

a

Analysis

1. Margins	sharp, jagged
2. Retrotumoral acoustic phenomena	alternating posterior enhancement and slight shadowing
3. Internal echo pattern	nonhomogeneous
4. Echogenicity	fat-equivalent
5. Compression effect on **shape**	no deformation
6. Compression effect on **internal echoes**	no change

History

The 56-year-old woman had undergone a breast-conserving resection for carcinoma. Radiotherapy had been terminated 6 months before.

Palpable Findings

A poorly demarcated, indurated area the size of the ball of the thumb, examined repeatedly with ultrasound, had been present since shortly after surgery. Recently that area increased in size and firmness, warranting biopsy.

Sonography

Figure **a**: sagittal scan over the focal lesion.

Readability: good.

Hypoechoic focal lesion with scalloped margins.

Interpretation

The sonographic criteria are inconsistent and do not permit a prediction of benignancy or malignancy. The overall impression is of a benign process.

X-ray Mammography

Figure **b**: mediolateral projection demonstrating a spiculated area of scar fibrosis. Below it is a circular radiolucency with well-defined margins. The radiographic impression, too, is that of a benign process.

Histology

Extensive fat necrosis with degenerative changes of mammary lobules and duct epithelium. No evidence of a recurrence.

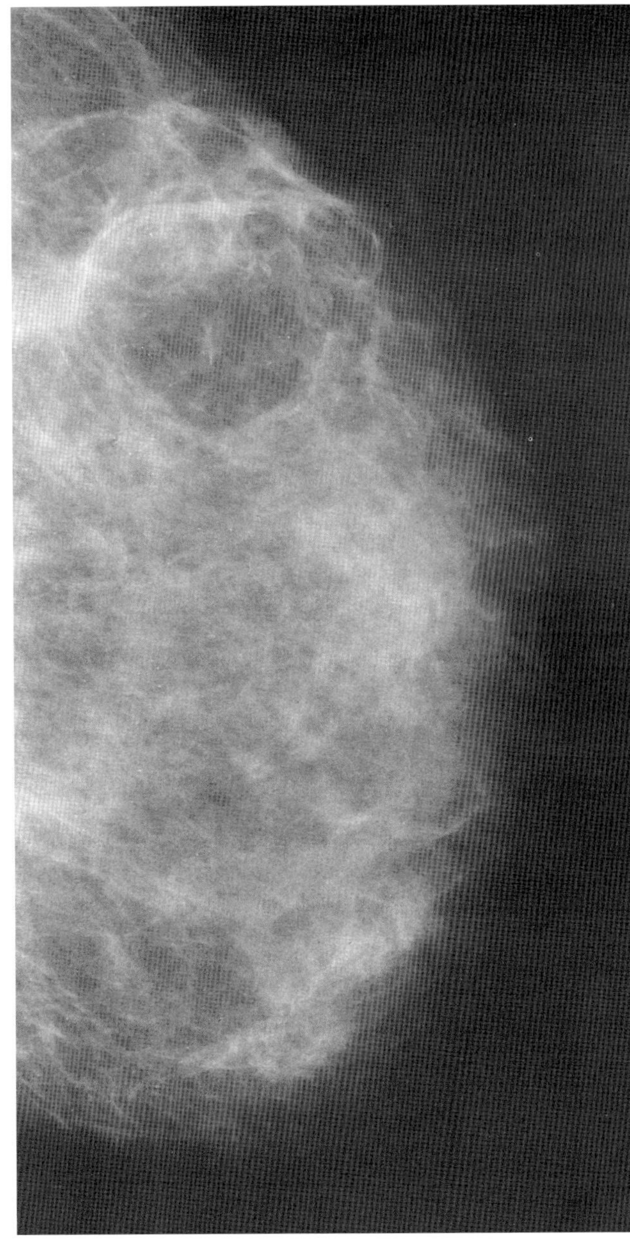

b

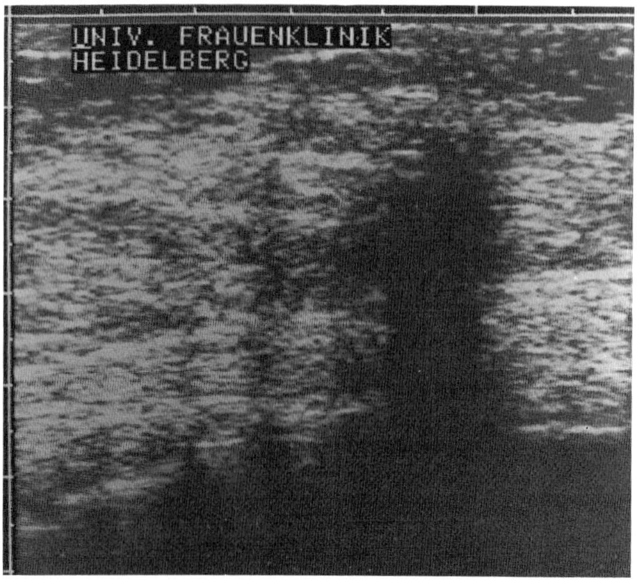

a

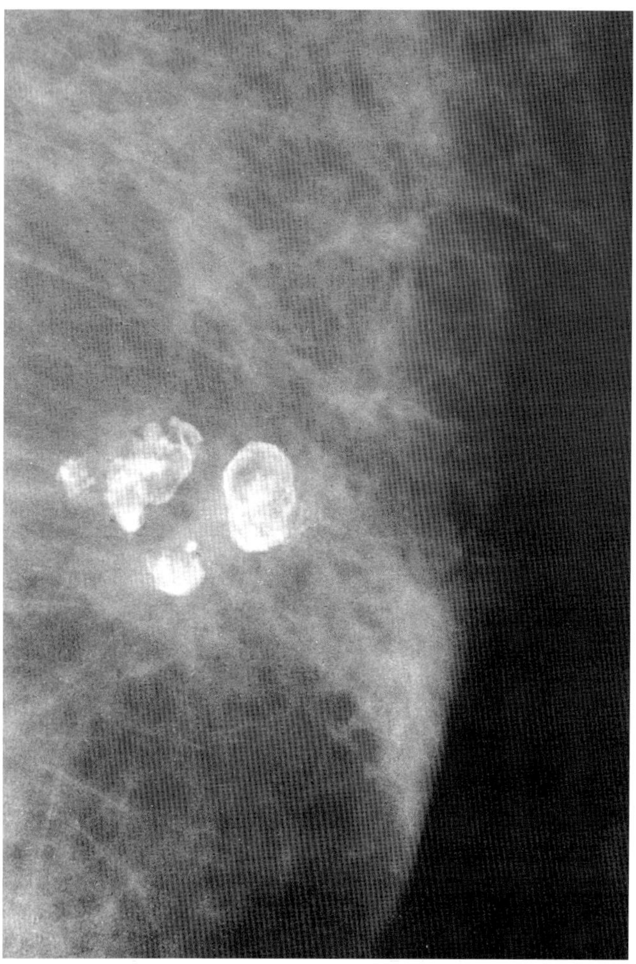

b

History

The 56-year-old woman had undergone a breast-conserving resection for carcinoma. Her radiotherapy had been terminated 7 years ago.

Palpable Findings

For years, an indurated area as large as the ball of the thumb had been palpable in the region of the old scar. The area appeared clinically innocent.

Sonography

Figure **a**: transverse scan over the indurated area showing very dense shadowing apparently unassociated with a true focal lesion. This shadowing so obscures the region that analytic criteria cannot be applied.

X-ray Mammography

Figure **b** (magnified view): typical appearance of multiple calcified foci of fat necrosis.

Histology

The area was not investigated histologically.

Postoperative Follow-Up

Ultrasound is a valuable aid in the detection and monitoring of hematomas and seromas during the immediate postoperative period. It is especially valuable for guiding punctures in patients who have had a prosthesis inserted as part of a reconstructive procedure. Damage to the prosthesis can be largely avoided by performing needle aspirations under sonographic guidance.

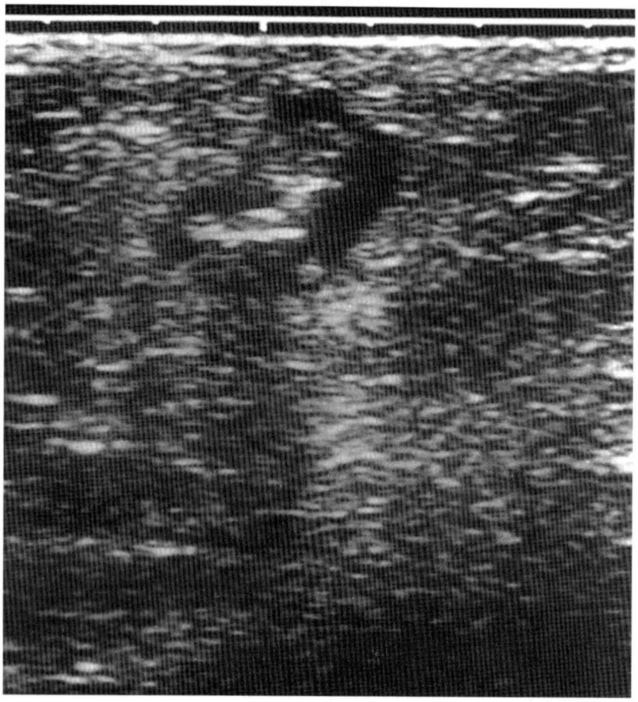

Analysis

1. Margins	sharp, jagged
2. Retrotumoral acoustic phenomena	slight posterior shadowing
3. Internal echo pattern	nonhomogeneous
4. Echogenicity	ranges from hyperechoic to anechoic
5. Compression effect on **shape**	shape distortion
6. Compression effect on **internal echoes**	no change

History

The 43-year-old woman's 13th postoperative day after a right breast biopsy, which indicaded a benign histology. Clinically there was abscess formation in the region of the biopsy cavity.

Palpable Findings

Tense, fluctuant mass with mild erythema in the biopsy area.

Sonography

Figure: transverse scan over the palpable mass.

Readability: good.

Focal sonographic lesion, 20×20 mm, conspicuous by its high contrast.

Interpretation

Criteria 1, 4 and 5 suggest a benign process, while criteria 2 and 3 imply malignancy. Sonographic image interpretation without knowledge of the clinical course is imprecise. But when the postoperative clinical occurrence of abscessation is known, the lesion is easily interpreted as an abscess. The bright echoes originate from necrotic areas within the abscess cavity, which also may cast shadows.

Subsequent incision of the abscess confirmed the diagnosis.

History

The 35-year-old woman underwent breast-conserving resection of mammary carcinoma. Swelling was noted in the area of the segmentectomy scar on the 5th postoperative day.

Sonography

Figure: sagittal scan over the swelling showing an extensive echo-free area that can only represent a fluid-filled space.

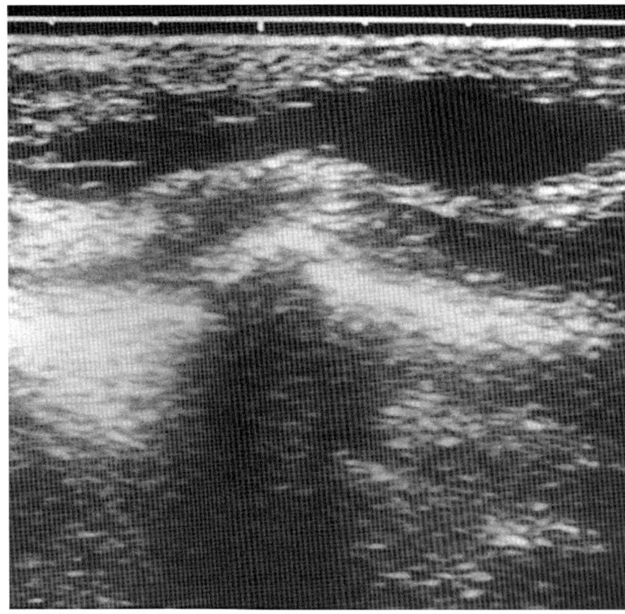

Analysis

The analytic criteria cannot be meaningfully applied.

Interpretation

The extent, aspiration, and further course of hematomas and seromas can be evaluated by ultrasound in the immediate postoperative period. In this case the lesion was an extensive, shallow hematoma that was percutaneously aspirated.

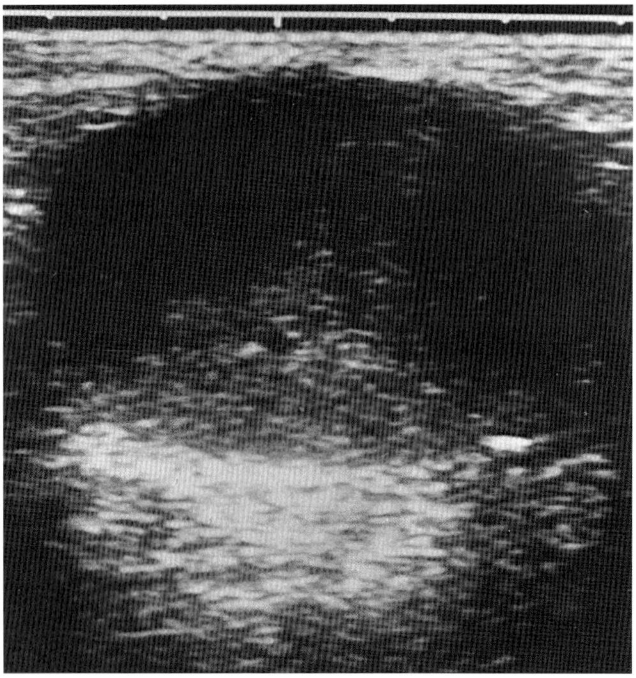

Analysis

1. **Margins**	sharp and smooth
2. **Retrotumoral acoustic phenomena**	posterior enhancement
3. **Internal echo pattern**	mostly anechoic, with an area of homogeneous echogenicity
4. **Echogenicity**	anechoic (density assessment is unnecessary in the uniformly echogenic area)
5. **Compression effect** on **shape**	shape distortion
6. **Compression effect** on **internal echoes**	no change

History

The 37-year-old woman underwent breast-conserving surgery elsewhere 2 weeks ago for breast carcinoma. The recently noticed an egg-sized lump in the region of the axilla, that had been operated on.

Palpable Findings

Tense, egg-sized mass in the axilla, that had been operated on.

Sonography

Figure: longitudinal scan over the palpable mass demonstrating a focal lesion, 45×32 mm.

Interpretation

This is a classic cystic pattern made unusual by the "ingrowth" of a uniformly echogenic structure into the echo-free cavity. The clinical presentation implies that the structure is most likely a hematoma or seroma. It may represent a partially organized hematoma.

Aspiration yielded 25 mL of a serosanginous fluid that was not investigated cytologically.

History

The 44-year-old woman underwent a tumor-adapted reduction mammoplasty of the right breast for breast carcinoma and severe macromastia. Postoperatively a hematoma formed in the region of the primary tumor cavity, and a firm induration subsequently developed in that area. On postoperative day 48, an ultrasound examination was performed.

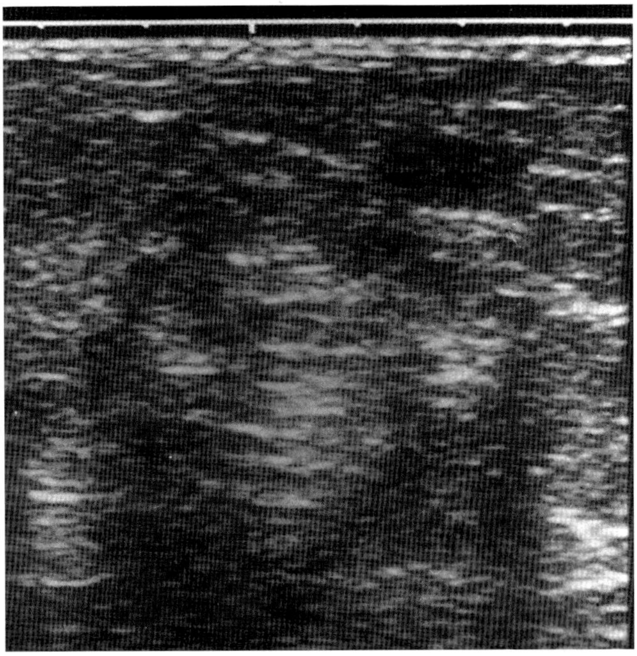

Palpable Findings

Approximately tangerine-sized, poorly demarcated, indurated area.

Sonography

Figure: sagittal scan over the indurated area not demonstrating a focal lesion in the true sense, but only a hyperechoic area with bilateral shadows. The sonographic picture is consistent with an organized hematoma.

Analysis

Not possible due to the absence of a focal lesion.

Histology

(drill biopsy)

Fibrosed connective tissue. No evidence of malignancy or specificity.

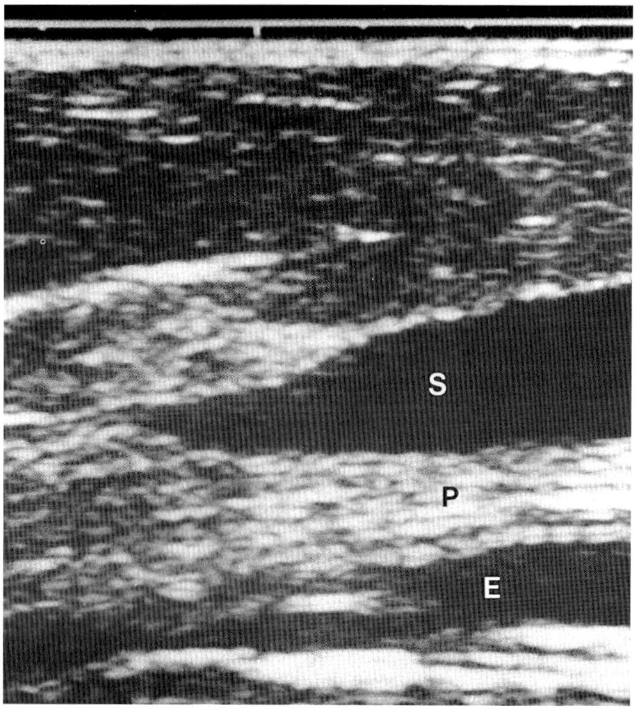

History

The 52-year-old woman underwent mastectomy and first-stage reconstruction with a subpectoral tissue expander that was filled intraoperatively with 100 mL of saline. On the 14th postoperative day, extreme swelling was noted over the left chest wall.

Palpable Findings

A fluctuant fluid collection was palpable over the entire left chest wall.

Sonography

Figure: transverse scan over the fluctuant mass showing no focal abnormality. Deep to the subcutaneous fat is a relatively broad, anechoic area representing a subcutaneous seroma (S). Beneath the well-defined pectoral muscle (P) is a relatively echo-free band representing the partially inflated, subpectorally placed tissue expander (E).

Interpretation

The point of ultrasound visualization of this seroma, which was easily diagnosed clinically, is that it permits the seroma to be localized to a specific layer and percutaneously aspirated under sonographic guidance without damaging the prosthesis.

History

The 43-year-old patient underwent mastectomy and first-stage reconstruction with a tissue expander. Extensive postoperative seroma formation was noted on the 10th postoperative day.

Palpable Findings

The inflation valve of the expander could not be located due to extensive postoperative seroma formation, so ultrasound was performed.

Sonography

Figure: scan over the lateral chest wall demonstrating the inflation valve (*) and the initial portion of the tube connecting it to the expander *(arrow)*. The tube and valve are surrounded by an extended shallow area representing the seroma.

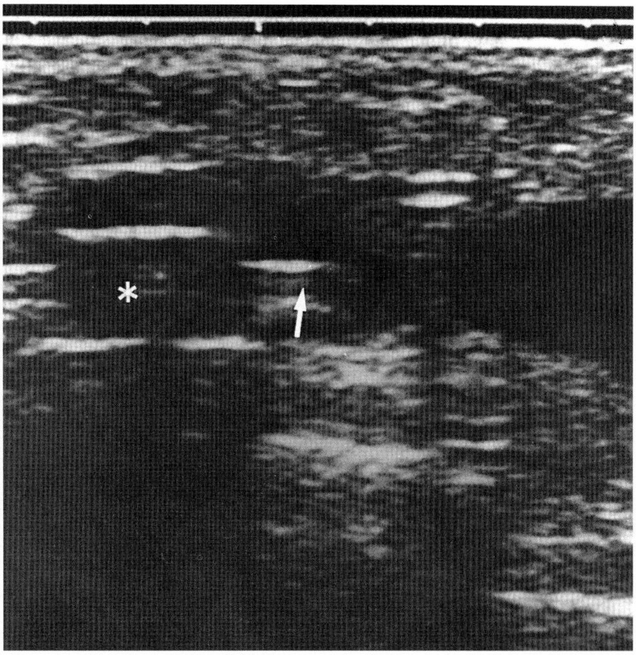

Interpretation

In cases where the fill system of a tissue expander is difficult to detect because of postoperative seroma, it can be easily located with ultrasound, which also avoids inadvertent puncture of the implant.

Aspiration under ultrasound vision yielded 70 mL of seromatous fluid.

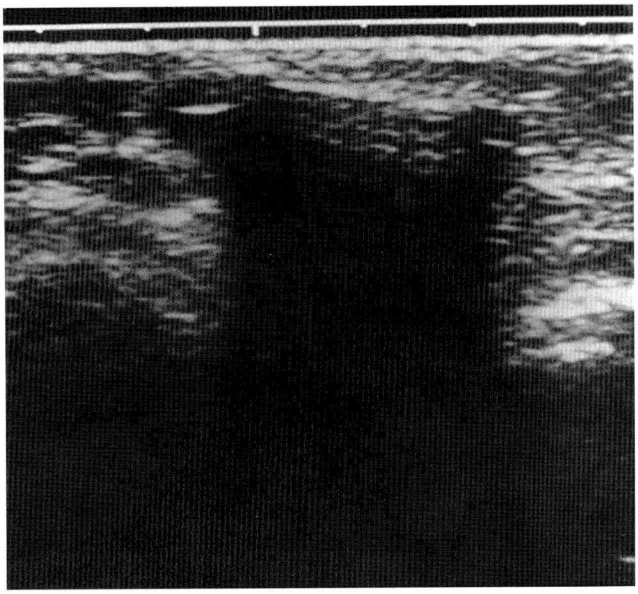

History

The 50-year-old woman underwent right mastectomy and first-stage reconstruction with a tissue expander.

Palpable Findings

Though the valve was easily palpated on the left chest wall, it could not be pierced with a percutaneous needle to inflate the expander. Sonography was performed to locate the valve.

Sonography

Figure: sagittal scan over the palpable structure presumed to be the valve, demonstrating an area with marked posterior shadowing.

Analysis

The analytic criteria cannot be meaningfully applied.

Interpretation

Below the skin is a hyperechoic structure with cone-shaped indentations on its right and left sides. There is complete shadowing deep to the structure. A repeated attempt to inflate the implant under ultrasound vision showed that the needle was unable to pierce the hyperechoic structure. The logical interpretation of this finding is that the valve became inverted, placing the impenetrable backing of the valve uppermost. Further inflation of the expander was accomplished by passing the needle tangentially into the valve under sonographic guidance.

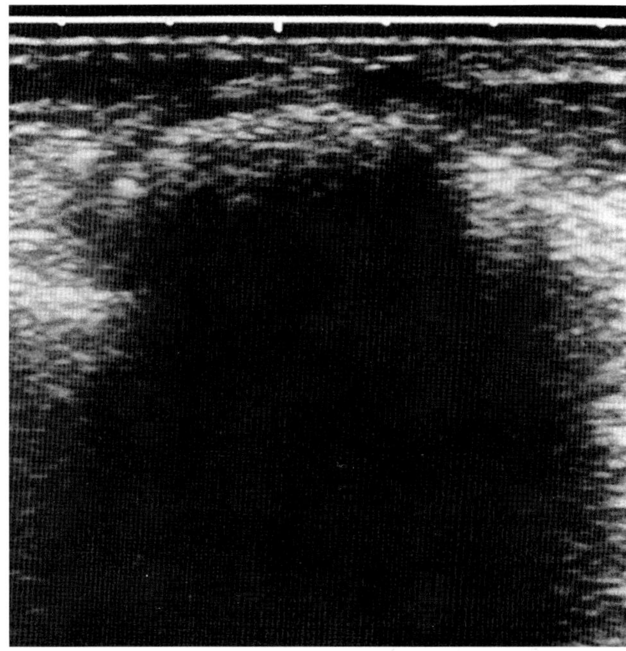

History

The 43-year-old woman underwent bilateral subcutaneous mastectomy for lobular carcinoma in situ and a secondary left axillary lymphadenectomy for occult carcinoma in the removed left mammary gland. Afterward there was persistent inflammatory infiltrate in the left axillary region.

Palpable Findings

Palm-sized area of infiltrate in the left axilla with erythema and tenderness to pressure.

Sonography

Figure: sonogram of the left axilla on the 20th postoperative day showing a subcutaneous, hyperechoic area demarcated from its surroundings by a narrow hypoechoic rim. Behind this area there is complete shadowing for a distance of 50 mm.

The analytic criteria cannot be applied.

Interpreted in the context of the patient's history, the sonographic findings are strongly suggestive of a foreign body.

Intraoperative Findings

Retained surgical sponge.

Interpretation

Foreign bodies frequently cause complete posterior shadowing.

Ultrasound-Guided Aspirations

Real-time ultrasound is helpful not only in the evacuation of cysts but also in the precision aspiration of solid lesions. When the operator sees the tip of the aspirating needle at the center of the lesion on the ultrasound monitor, he or she can be certain that the center of the mass has been impinged. Although a negative cytologic diagnosis is not definitive, a positive cytologic result can obviate the need for frozen section in breast-conserving operations. The preoperative needle or wire localization of a nonpalpable lesion can be performed more quickly and accurately under sonographic guidance, assuming that the lesion can be imaged with ultrasound.

History

The 41-year-old woman presented with premenstrual tension in both breasts and carcinophobia linked to a family history of breast cancer.

Palpable Findings

Both breasts coarsely nodular and tender to pressure; no definite masses.

Sonography

Systematic survey ot the breast reveals a very dense parenchyma with multiple hypoechoic areas of varying size.

Figure: sagittal scan over one focal lesion (13×4 mm).

Readability: good.

Interpretation

Criteria 1, 2, 3, 5, and 6 suggest a benign lesion, while the low echogenicity is more characteristic of malignancy. Nevertheless, the overall sonographic impression is not entirely typical of a benign process! Lesions such as these should be aspirated under sonographic guidance. In this case, aspiration yielded 0.8 mL of an extremely viscous secretion. This high viscosity is responsible for the internal echoes. Following aspiration, the lesion was no longer demonstrable. If the lesion were found to be solid, however, biopsy would definitely be indicated.

Aspiration Cytology

Papanicolaou grades I/II.

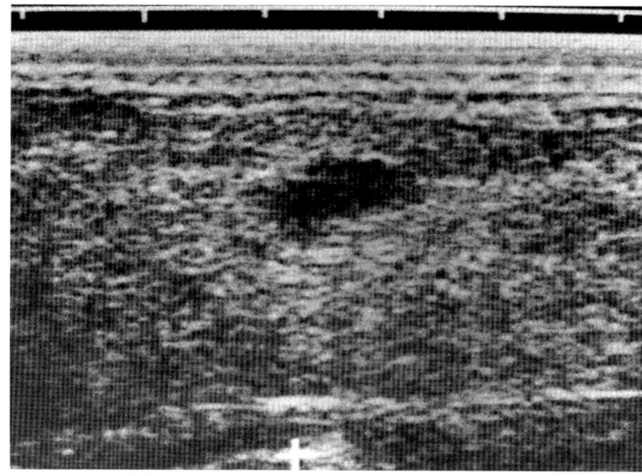

Analysis

1. **Margins**	sharp, jagged
2. **Retrotumoral effect**	faint posterior enhancement
3. **Internal echo pattern**	homogeneous (but very few echoes)
4. **Echogenicity**	almost anechoic
5. **Compression effect** on **shape**	shape distortion
6. **Compression effect** on **internal echoes**	no change

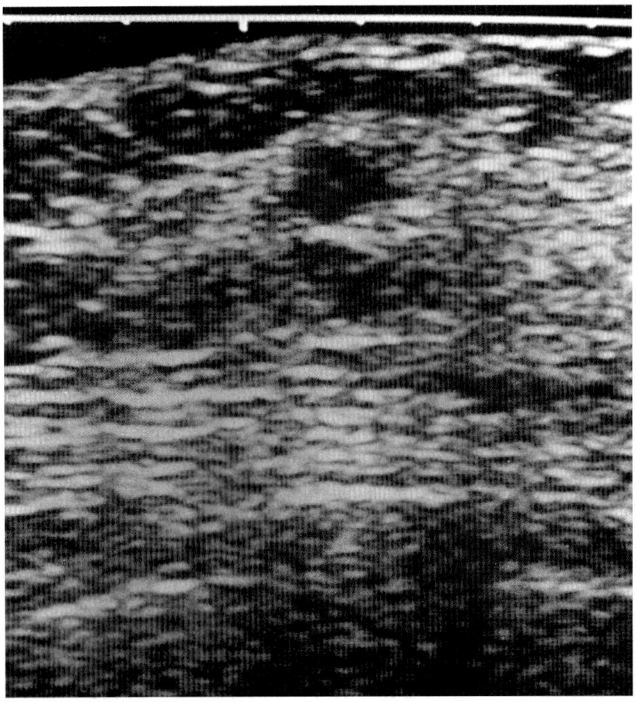

a

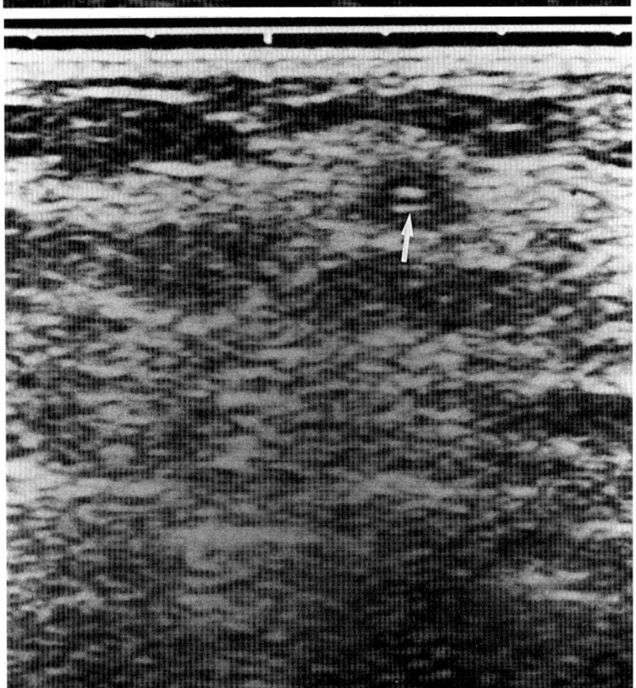

b

Analysis

1. Margins	indistinct, jagged
2. Retrotumoral effect	unchanged echoes
3. Internal echo pattern	few echoes, nonhomogeneous
4. Echogenicity	almost anechoic
5. Compression effect on **shape**	no deformation
6. Compression effect on **internal echoes**	no change

History

The 32-year-old woman had a metastatic large-cell carcinoma discovered during a right axillary lymphadenectomy. Prior to that time there had been no evidence of a primary breast tumor.

Palpable Findings

No palpable masses in either breast.

Sonography

(with water path)

Figure **a**: one of a series of transverse scans through the right breast demonstrating a focal lesion, 7×8 mm, in the upper outer quadrant.

Readability: good.

Figure **b**: same focal lesion with the needle tip at its center *(arrow)*.

Interpretation

Sonography was performed because the patient had a lymph node metastasis but no palpable or radiographic evidence of a focal breast lesion. Ultrasound then disclosed the focal lesion shown here. The lesion was aspirated for cytologic analysis, and a localizing wire was passed into the mass through the aspiration needle.

This case demonstrates that breast carcinoma can be detected using ultrasound alone. The lesion can then be aspirated and marked with a localizing wire under sonographic guidance.

X-ray Mammography

Radiographically dense breast, edematous mastopathy. No focal abnormality.

Aspiration Cytology

Papanicolaou grade V.

Histology

Extensive infiltrating duct carcinoma with a predominantly intraductal component (pT2 pN1 M0).

History

A faint stellate density was noted in the breast of this 49-year-old woman having her first screening mammogram.

Palpable Findings

Pronounced bilateral fibrocystic disease with no palpable abnormalities.

Sonography

Figure **a**: transverse scan through the upper outer quadrant of the right breast.

Readability: good.

A focal lesion, 3×5 mm, with a posterior shadow is seen within the residual glandular tissue of a predominantly involuted breast. A wire guide was inserted into the lesion *sonographically* prior to excision. The target pattern in the focal lesion is produced by the localization wire *(arrow)*.

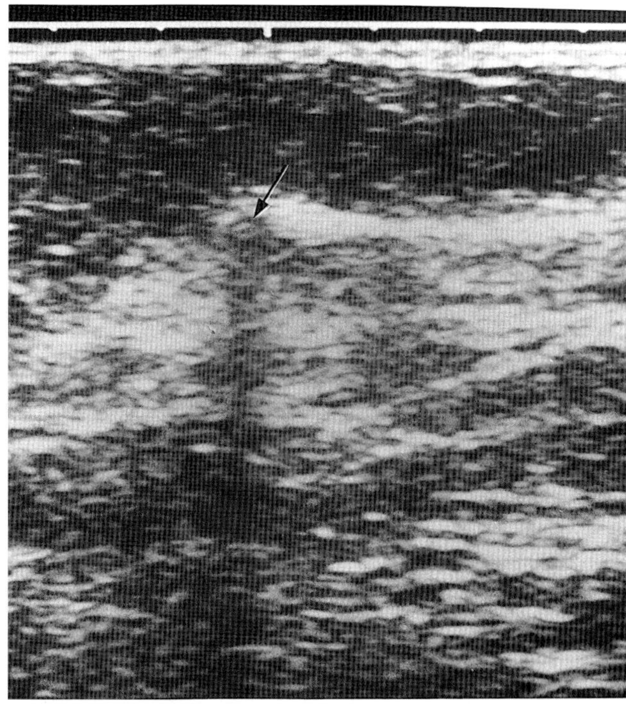

a

Analysis

The lesion is too small for a criteria analysis.

Interpretation

The lesion was first detected by X-ray mammography, and that finding enabled the visualization and localization of a sonographic equivalent. The size of the mass is at the very limit of detectability of focal sonographic lesions. Without the posterior shadow, the lesion would very likely have been undetectable by ultrasound.

X-ray Mammography

Figure **b**: craniocaudal projection showing a lateral, faintly spiculated, 3-mm density in an otherwise predominantly involuted breast.

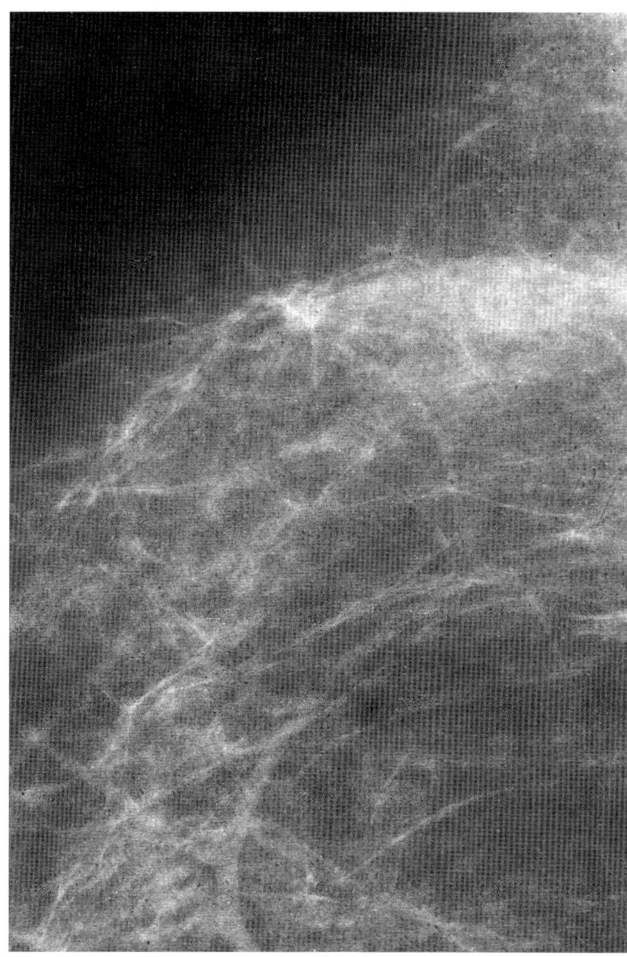

b

Histology

Tubular carcinoma, 5 mm in diameter, with disseminated intraductal extensions.

Axillary, Supraclavicular, and Infraclavicular Lymph Nodes

The value of axillary sonography for the preoperative staging of breast carcinoma is disputed, especially since it does not influence therapeutic decision making. On the other hand, ultrasound has an indispensable role in the search for recurrent disease. The diagnostic accuracy of ultrasound in these cases is enhanced by the postoperative improvement of imaging conditions provided by the removal of lymphatic and fatty tissue during the primary operation.

Sonography can be helpful in the investigation of palpable lymph nodes with no demonstrable disease in the ipsilateral breast, especially when it comes to establishing the topography of the mass in relation to neighboring structures (vessels).

The criteria for the evaluation of breast tumors are *not* useful for predicting the benignancy or malignancy of sonographically demonstrable lymph nodes.

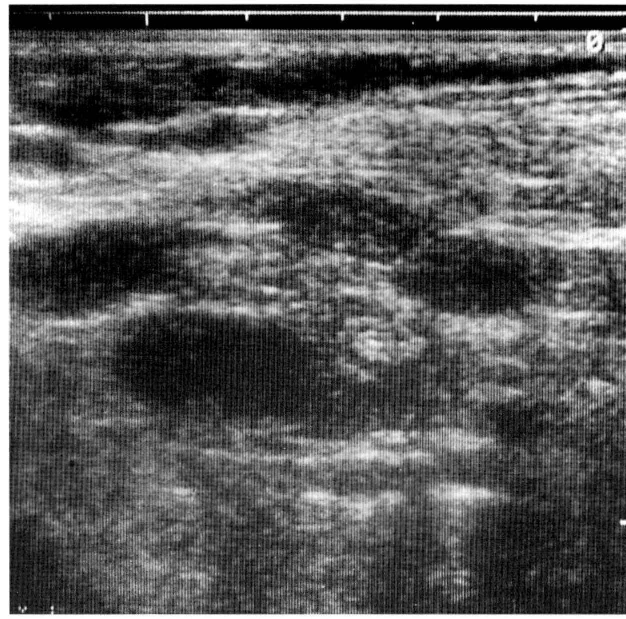

History

The 63-year-old woman, who had undergone bilateral reduction mammoplasty 6 years before, presented with large palpable lymphomas in the left axilla.

Palpable Findings

Neither breast had palpable abnormalities. Large, mobile lymphomas as large as 3–4 cm were palpated in the left axilla.

Sonography

Figure: sonogram of the left axilla.

Readability: good.

Four focal sonographic lesions of varying echogenicity.

We do not feel that our analytic criteria should be applied to axillary lymph nodes due to the relatively low diagnostic confidence of this analysis in the axillary region.

Interpretation

The focal lesions in the axilla represent four enlarged lymph nodes that cannot be categorized as benign or malignant by ultrasound. Of course, a coexisting suspicious breast mass would suggest that the axillary lymphadenopathy is probably malignant.

Histology

Based on their morphology, the lesions could represent giant follicular lymphoblastoma (Brill–Symmers disease), i.e., a non-Hodgkin lymphoma of low-grade malignancy. A more likely interpretation, however, is follicular lymphatic hyperplasia.

Histochemical investigation furnished a definitive diagnosis of chronic lymphadenitis. Malignant lymphoma was excluded.

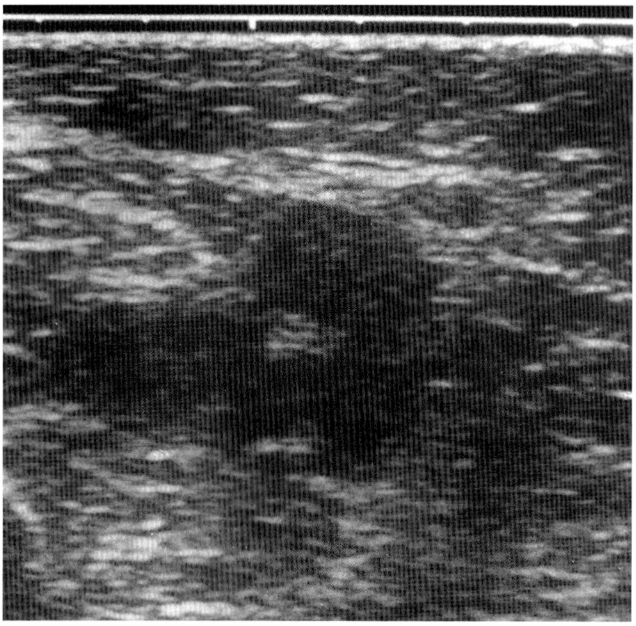

Analysis

1. **Margins**	sharp, jagged
2. **Retrotumoral effect**	unchanged echoes
3. **Internal echo pattern**	nonhomogeneous
4. **Echogenicity**	almost anechoic
5. **Compression effect** on **shape**	not tested
6. **Compression effect** on **internal echoes**	not tested

History

The 32-year-old woman was referred for intermittent, painful lymph node swellings in the left axilla. Ipsilateral arm motion was markedly restricted.

Palpable Findings

Soft, painful swellings in the left axilla.

Sonography

Figure: scan over the axillary swelling demonstrating a focal lesion of varying echogenicity.

Interpretation

The sonographic criteria do not permit a definitive assessment of benignancy or malignancy. In connection with the clinical presentation, the constellation of sonographic findings is consistent with a sudoriparous abscess, especially in view of the bright central echoes.

The suspicion of sudoriparous abscess was confirmed by incision.

History

The 54-year-old woman had undergone left mastectomy and axillary lymphadenectomy 2 years before. During subsequent follow-up, a mass was discovered in the left axilla.

Palpable Findings

Firm, mobile, approximately 2.5-cm mass on the posterior axillary line, directly overlying the latissimus dorsi muscle.

Sonography

Figure: sagittal scan over the palpable mass.

Readability: good.

Focal sonographic lesion, 28×27 mm.

Interpretation

All sonographic criteria suggest a malignant process.

Sonographic findings are equivocal with regard to latissimus dorsi infiltration.

Histology

Soft-tissue metastasis from known breast carcinoma; diameter 25 mm.

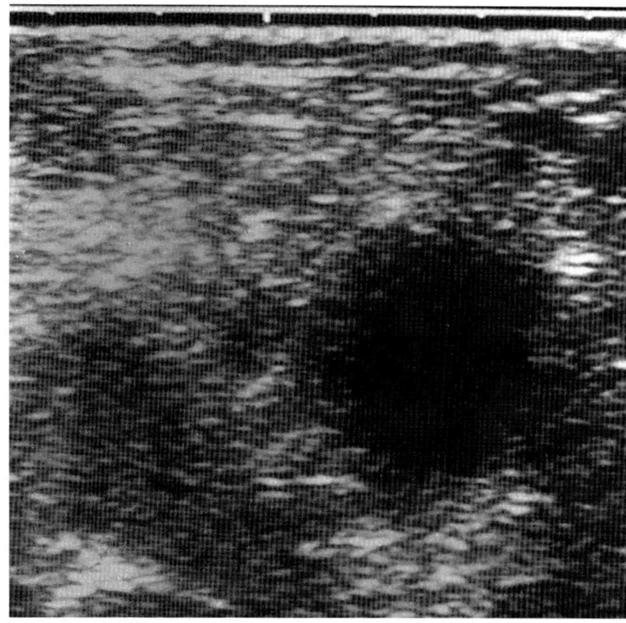

Analysis

1. Margins	indistinct, jagged
2. Retrotumoral effect	unchanged echoes
3. Internal echo pattern	few echoes, nonhomogeneous
4. Echogenicity	almost anechoic
5. Compression effect on **shape**	no deformation
6. Compression effect on **internal echoes**	no change

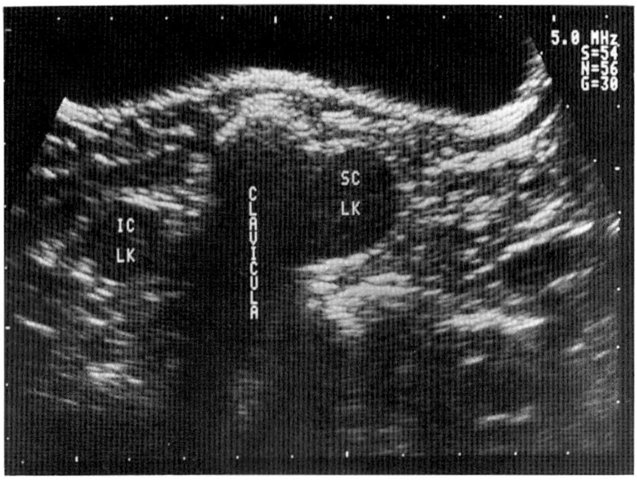

a

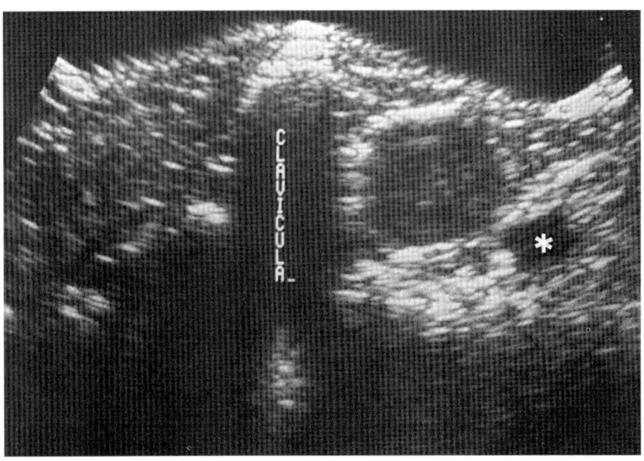

b

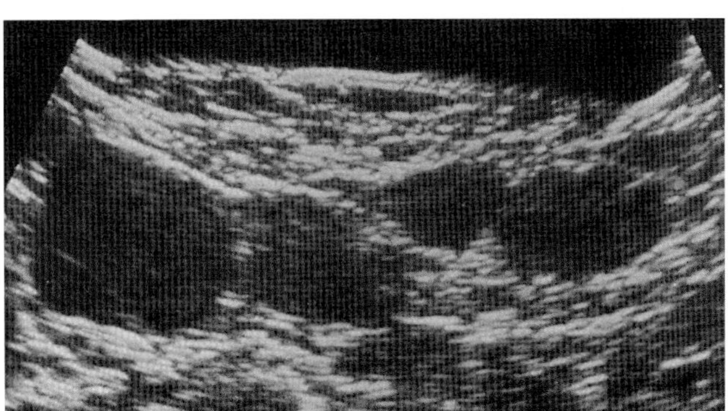
c

History

The patient herself noticed palpable masses in the supraclavicular and infraclavicular region.

Palpable Findings

Multiple fixed lymphomas in the left supraclavicular and infraclavicular region.

Sonography

(with standoff)

Figure **a**: sagittal scan on the midclavicular line demonstrating a smoothly marginated infraclavicular lymph node (IC LK) and supraclavicular lymph node (SC LK).

Figure **b**: sagittal scan slightly medial to the plane in Figure **a** showing a large, smoothly marginated lymphoma in close proximity to an artery (*).

Figure **c**: multiple left axillary lymph nodes.

Interpretation

The sonographic picture of enlarged lymph nodes usually does not permit a confident assessment of benignancy or malignancy.

X-ray Mammography

Involuted breasts, no findings suspicious for malignancy or warranting biopsy.

Histology

Extensive infiltration of all infraclavicular and supraclavicular lymph nodes by a solid, undifferentiated tumor showing extensive necrosis. The primary may be 1) a primary breast carcinoma (not supported by palpable, sonographic, or roentgen findings), 2) undifferentiated bronchogenic carcinoma, or 3) amelanotic malignant melanoma.

History

The 36-year-old woman had undergone breast-conserving resection of a left mammary carcinoma 4 years before.

Palpable Findings

At follow-up a firm and infiltrate, 2.5×2 cm, adherent to the chest wall, was palpated in the left infraclavicular area.

Sonography

Figure: sagittal scan over the palpable mass demonstrating a focal lesion, 34×20 mm. At the base of the lesion is a conspicuous round structure *(arrow)*, identified as a blood vessel by its pulsations on real-time ultrasound.

Interpretation

The sonographic criteria suggest a malignant process. The close proximity of the metastasis to a large arterial vessel is of particular interest.

Histology

Infraclavicular lymph node metastasis from an undifferentiated carcinoma with extensive necrotic foci and infiltration of the paranodal fibrofatty tissue.

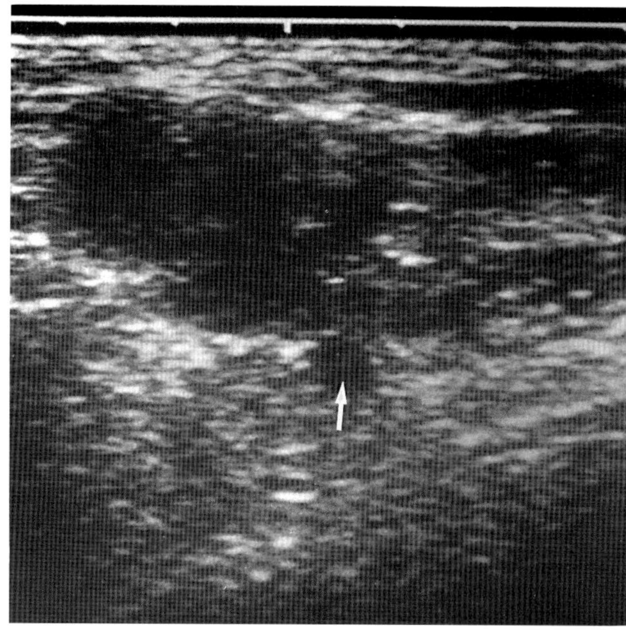

Analysis

1. Margins	sharp, jagged
2. Retrotumoral effect	unchanged echoes
3. Internal echo pattern	few echoes, non-homogeneous
4. Echogenicity	almost anechoic
5. Compression effect on **shape**	no deformation
6. Compression effect on **internal echoes**	no change

Microcalcifications in Sonography

At present, ultrasound cannot reduce the need for excisional breast biopsy when used adjunctively to evaluate suspicious microcalcifications noted on X-ray mammograms.

When a focal sonographic lesion is detected which corresponds to the roentgen location of microcalcifications, the ultrasound analytic criteria can be applied to predict the benignancy or malignancy of the lesion (e.g., "malignant calcification correlate"). Calcific correlates not associated with a focal sonographic lesion are not accessible to benign/malignant differentiation, although our experience indicates that these changes most likely represent benign or preinvasive disease.

Nevertheless, the general preoperative use of sonography is advantageous, for it permits the immediate planning of a one-stage surgical procedure in women who are found to have a "malignant calcification correlate" on their breast sonogram (flowchart in Fig. 6.**9**). The preoperative needle localization of clinically occult areas of microcalcification on the X-ray mammogram can be accomplished much more quickly and easily when the area is visualized with ultrasound (Leucht et al. 1987).

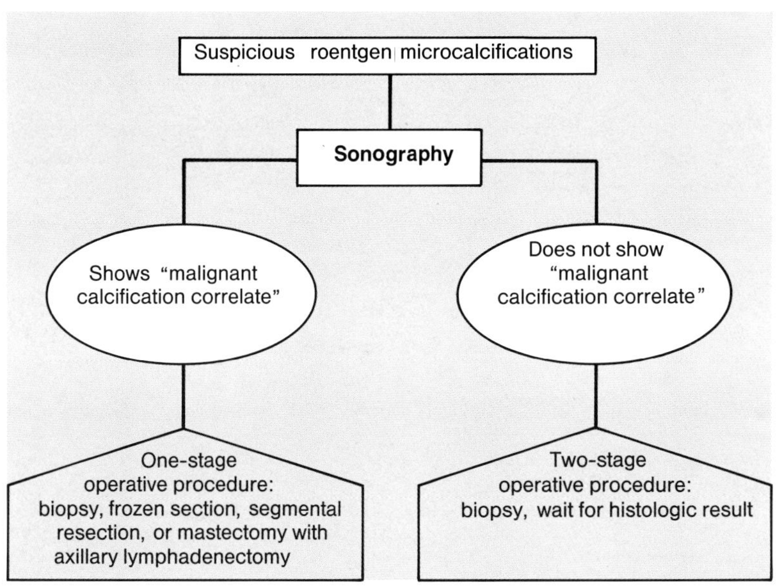

Fig. 6.**9** Flowchart

History

The 46-year-old woman was found to have intramammary, clustered microcalcifications in a screening examination.

Palpable Findings

Neither breast had palpable abnormalities.

Sonography

(7.5 MHz)

Figure **a**: transverse scan over roentgen microcalcifications.

Readability: good.

Scan demonstrates focal sonographic lesion *(arrows)*, 10×7 mm, with streaklike internal echoes.

Interpretation

Knowledge of the roentgen findings identifes the striate echoes within the focal sonographic lesion as microcalcifications. The sonographic criteria are inconsistent, so a benign/malignant differentiation is not possible by ultrasound.

Figure **b**: specimen radiograph showing a region with typical carcinoma microcalcifications and a subtle focal density.

Histology

Infiltrating ductal carcinoma, 12 mm, with predominantly intraductal spread and sites of comedo necrosis.

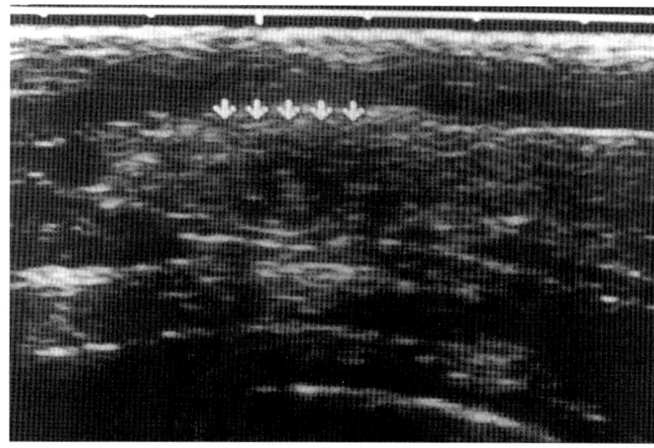

a

Analysis

1. Margins	indistinct but smooth
2. Retrotumoral effect	unchanged echoes
3. Internal echo pattern	few echoes, nonhomogeneous
4. Echogenicity	almost anechoic
5. Compression effect on shape	no deformation
6. Compression effect on internal echoes	no change

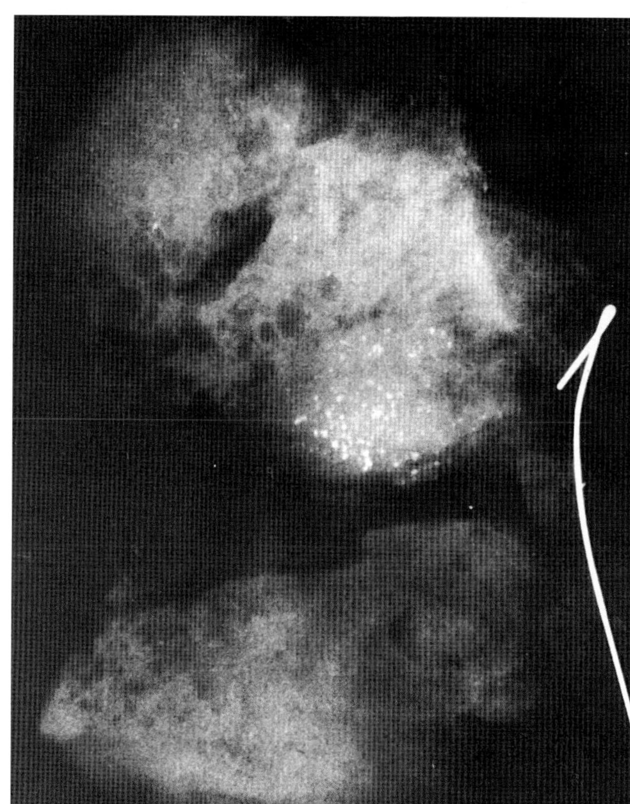

b

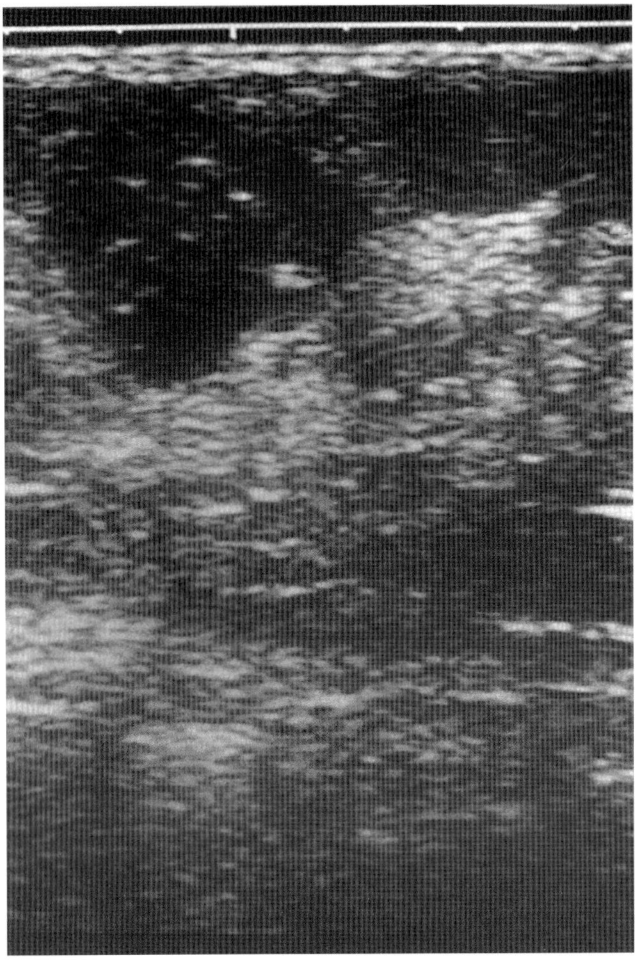

a

Analysis

1. Margins	sharp, jagged
2. Retrotumoral acoustic phenomena	unchanged echoes
3. Internal echo pattern	few echoes, nonhomogeneous
4. Echogenicity	almost anechoic
5. Compression effect on **shape**	no deformation
6. Compression effect on **internal echoes**	no change

History

The 52-year-old woman noticed a lump in her breast 2 weeks before.

Palpable Findings

Relatively fixed, walnut-sized mass in the upper outer quadrant of the right breast.

Sonography

Figure **a**: sagittal scan over the palpable mass.

Readability: good.

Focal sonographic lesion, 29×28 mm, with irregular, high-level internal echoes.

Interpretation

Except for margination, all the analytic criteria suggest a malignant process. The bright internal echoes, representing calcifications, are particularly striking.

X-ray Mammography

Figure **b** (magnified view): large, focal density with microcalcifications typical of carcinoma.

Numerous calcifications coalesce to form larger aggregates.

Histology

Partly solid, partly papillary 22-mm infiltrating ductal carcinoma with pronounced sites of comedo necrosis.

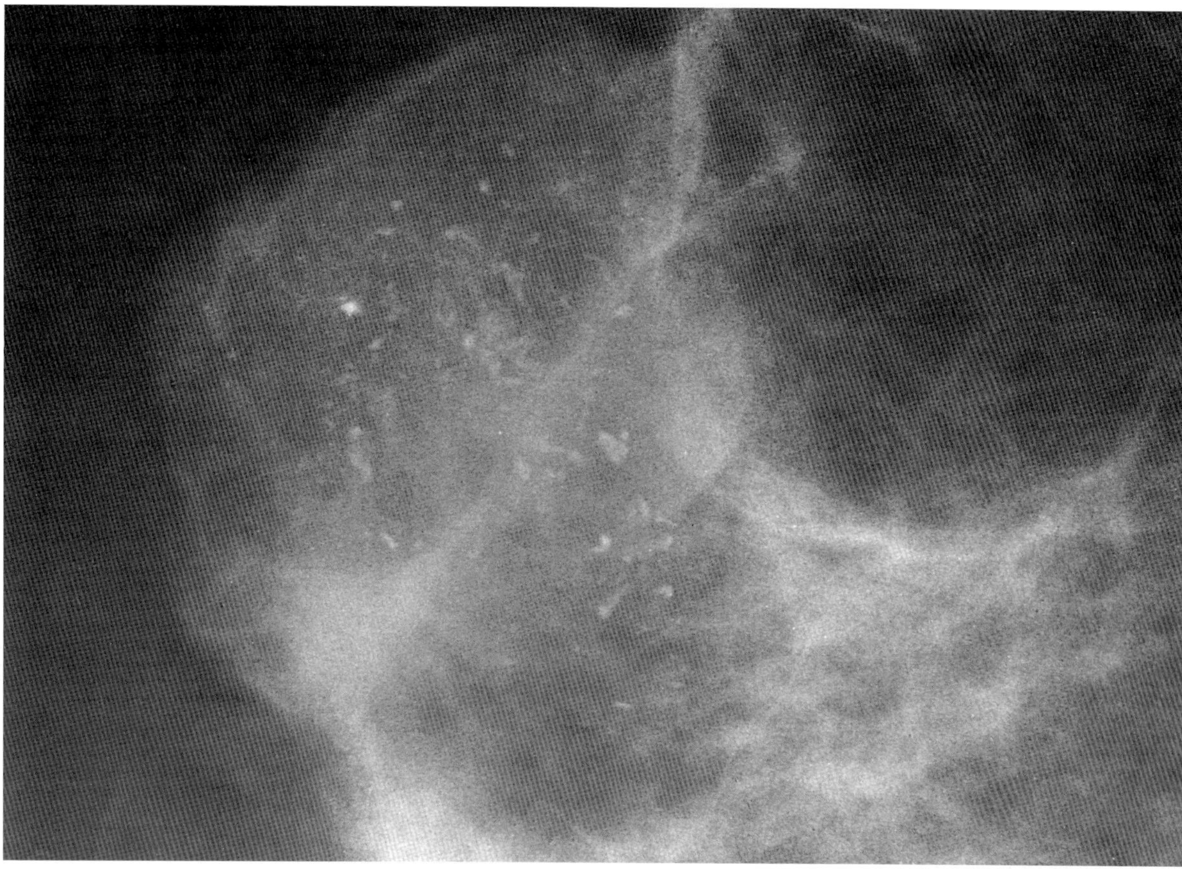

b

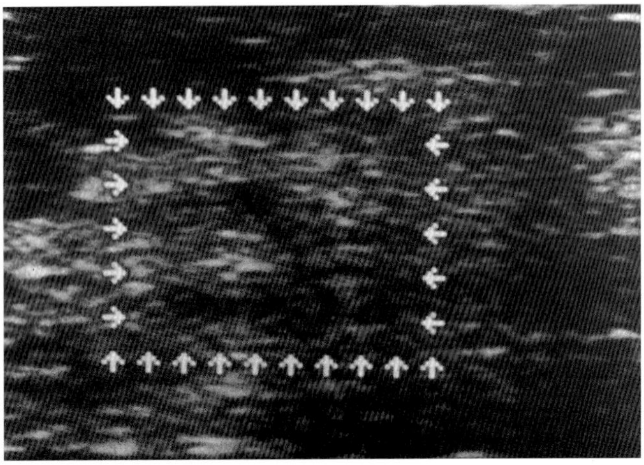

a

Analysis

1. Margins	sharp, jagged
2. Retrotumoral acoustic phenomena	unchanged echoes
3. Internal echo pattern	nonhomogeneous
4. Echogenicity	fat-equivalent
5. Compression effect on **shape**	no deformation
6. Compression effect on **internal echoes**	no change

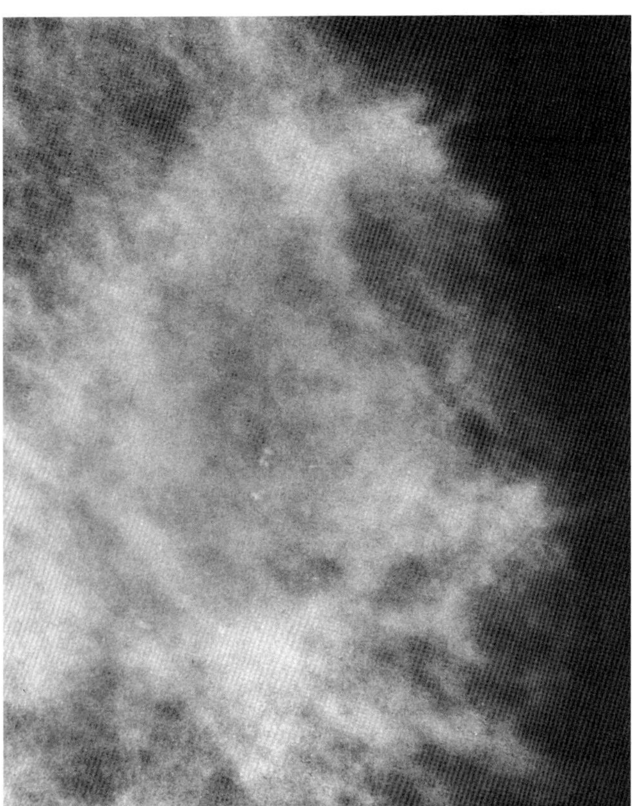

b

History

The 60-year-old woman, who had a family history of breast cancer, had an intramammary roentgen density with faint microcalcifications.

Palpable Findings

Neither breast had palpable abnormalities.

Sonography

Figure **a**: sagittal scan over the microcalcifications (7.5 MHz) showing a 16-mm focal lesion with high-level punctate and striate echoes *(arrows)*.

Interpretation

Although the analytic criteria do not suggest a malignant process, the roentgen microcalcifications and their sonographic correlate within the focal mass create a high index of suspicion for carcinoma.

X-ray Mammography

Figure **b** (magnified view): density with faint microcalcifications of indeterminate nature.

Histology

Infiltrating ductal carcinoma, 25 mm, with predominantly intraductal spread and sites of comedo necrosis.

Figure **c**: area of intraductal carcinoma with intraluminal calcification (H&E stain, × 22.5).

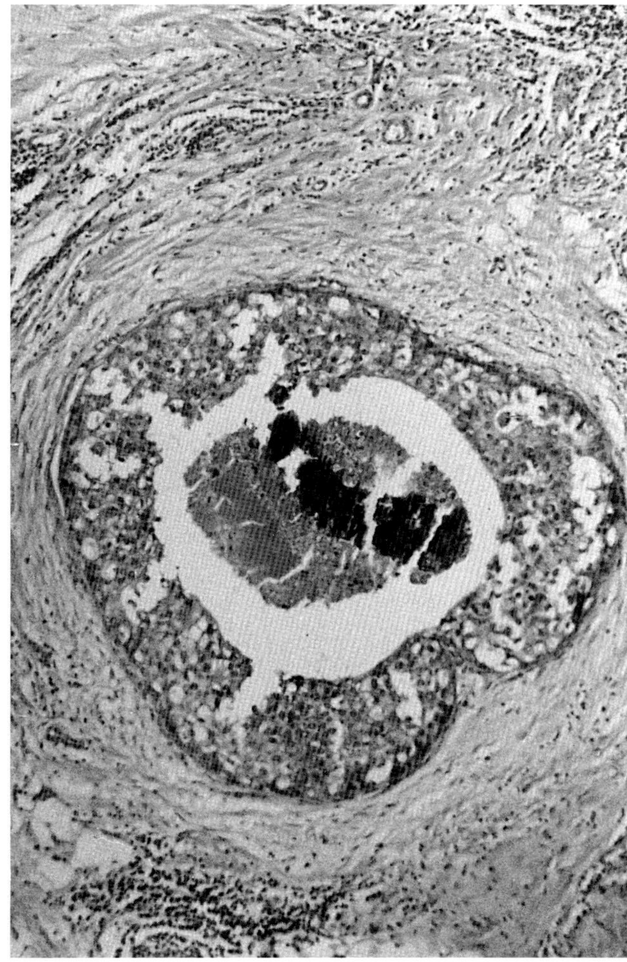

c

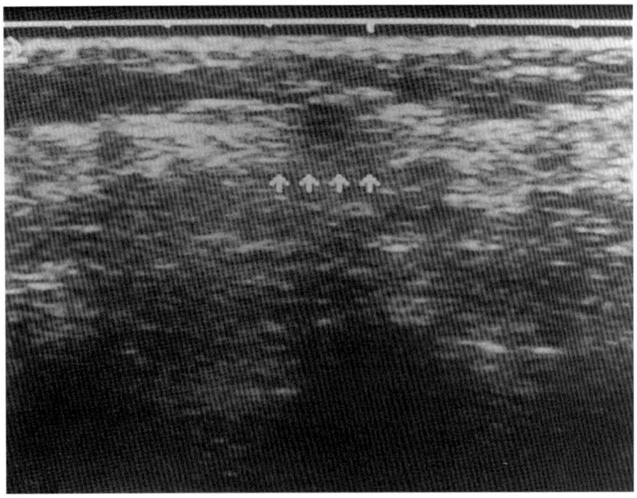

a

Analysis

1. Margins	indistinct, jagged
2. Retrotumoral acoustic phenomena	unchanged echoes
3. Internal echo pattern	few echoes, nonhomogeneous
4. Echogenicity	almost anechoic
5. Compression effect on **shape**	no deformation
6. Compression effect on **internal echoes**	no change

History

During a routine mammography, the 49-year-old woman was found to have clustered microcalcifications.

Palpable Findings

Both breasts were finely nodular with no definite masses.

Sonography

(7.5 MHz)

Figure **a**: transverse scan over the roentgen area of microcalcifications.

Readability: good.

Sonographic round lesion, 8 mm, with low-level striate echoes *(arrows)*.

Interpretation

The systematic search for a known area with clustered microcalcifications revealed a focal sonographic lesion with malignant criteria.

X-ray Mammography

Figure **b** (magnified view): irregular density containing clustered microcalcifications of varying density and size, some granular and some of the cast type. Preoperative mammogram following *sonographic* needle localization.

Histology

Infiltrating ductal carcinoma, 10 mm, with comedo-like foci of necrosis.

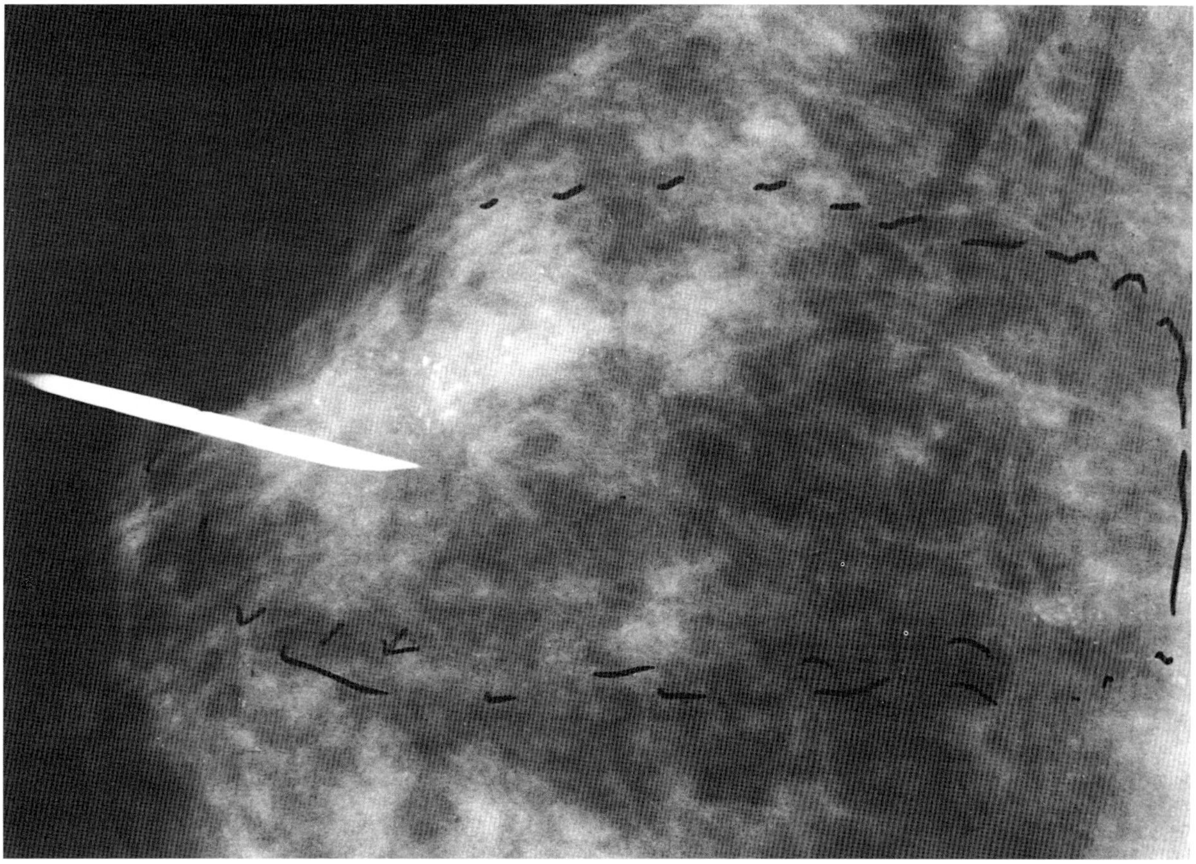

b

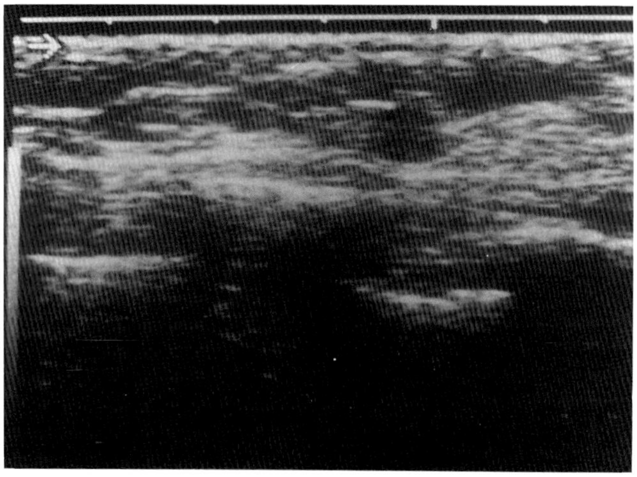

a

Anaysis

1. Margins	indistinct, jagged
2. Retrotumoral acoustic phenomena	unchanged echoes
3. Internal echo pattern	few echoes, nonhomogeneous
4. Echogenicity	almost anechoic
5. Compression effect on **shape**	no deformation
6. Compression effect on **internal echoes**	no change

History

During screening mammography, 46-year-old woman was found to have clustered microcalcifications.

Palpable Findings

No palpable masses in either breast.

Sonography

(7.5 MHz)

Figure **a**: sagittal scan over the roentgen area of microcalcifications.

Readability: good.

Focal sonographic lesion, 8 mm, with faint internal echoes.

Interpretation

The sonographic criteria suggest a malignant process. Knowledge of the roentgen findings guided the ultrasound examination, which disclosed a conspicuous focal lesion having the features of invasive carcinoma.

X-ray Mammography

Figure **b** (magnified view): preoperative mammogram following *sonographic* needle localization of the mass. The needle tip is adjacent to very fine microcalcifications typical of carcinoma, some of which have coalesced into a larger calcification.

Histology

Infiltrating ductal carcinoma with predominantly intraductal spread and extensive comedo necrosis.

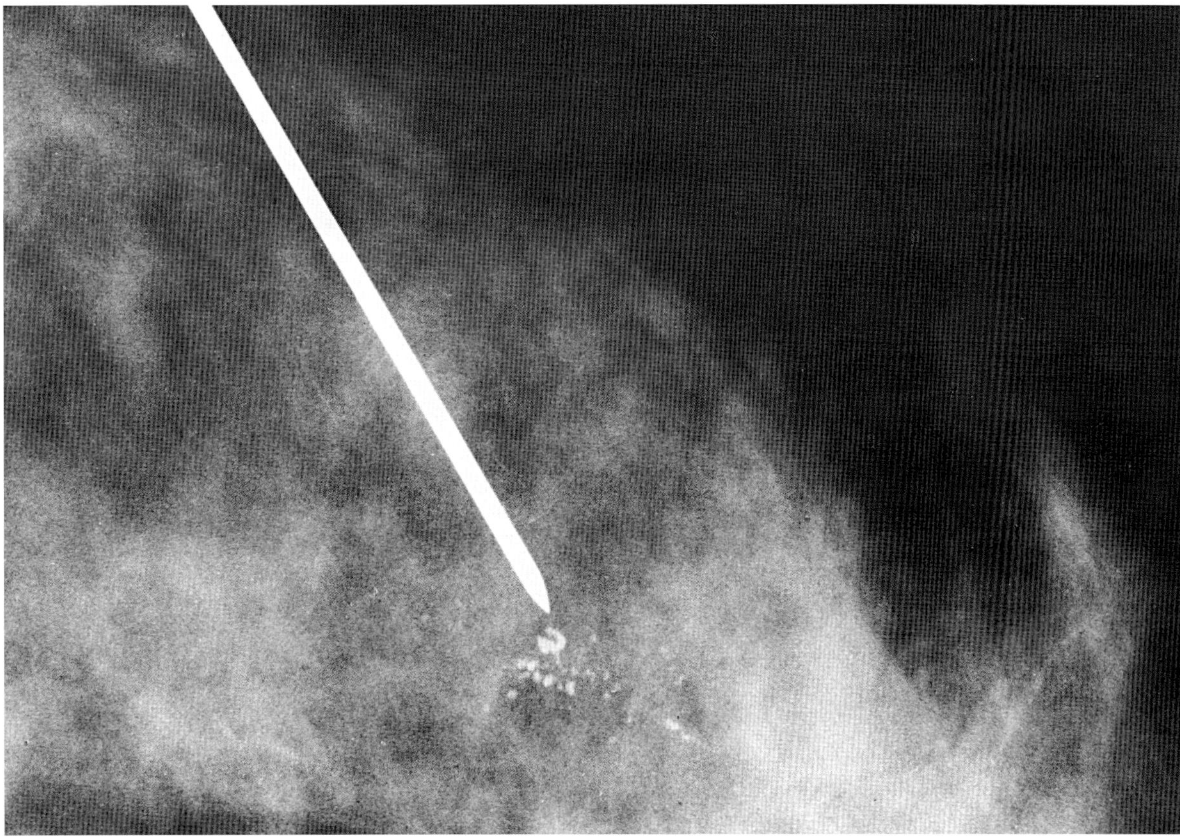

b

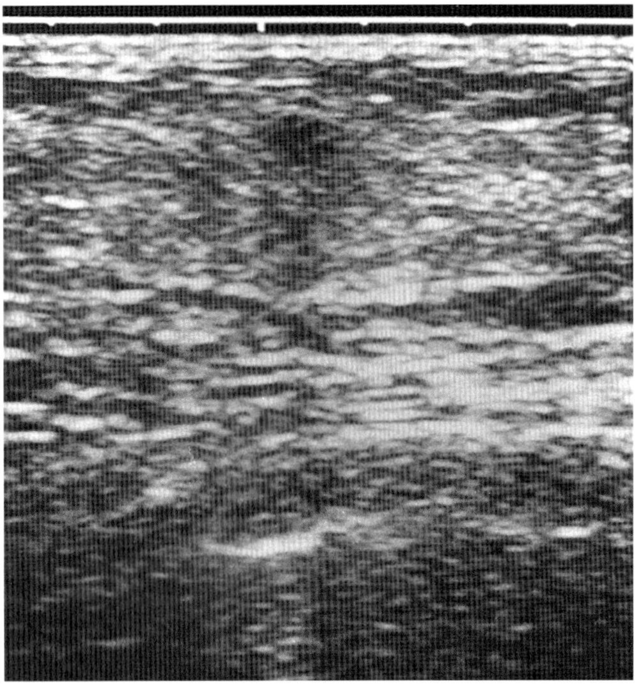

a

Analysis

1. **Margins**	indistinct, jagged
2. **Retrotumoral acoustic phenomena**	slight posterior shadowing
3. **Internal echo pattern**	few echoes, nonhomogeneous
4. **Echogenicity**	almost anechoic
5. **Compression effect** on **shape**	no deformation
6. **Compression effect** on **internal echoes**	no change

History

The 37-year-old woman, who had a family history of breast cancer, was found to have clustered microcalcifications in her left breast during a routine mammography.

Palpable Findings

No palpable masses in either breast.

Sonography

Figure **a**: oblique scan over the roentgen area of microcalcifications.

Readability: good.

Small focal sonographic lesion, 6×7 mm, with slight posterior shadowing.

Interpretation

The sonographer was aware of the X-ray location of the clustered microcalcifications and interpreted the small focal lesion as a malignant process.

X-ray Mammography

Figure **b**: craniocaudal projection of the left breast showing suspicuous clustered microcalcifications with no focal abnormality. Same on mediolateral view.

Histology

Infiltrating lobular carcinoma measuring 10 mm.

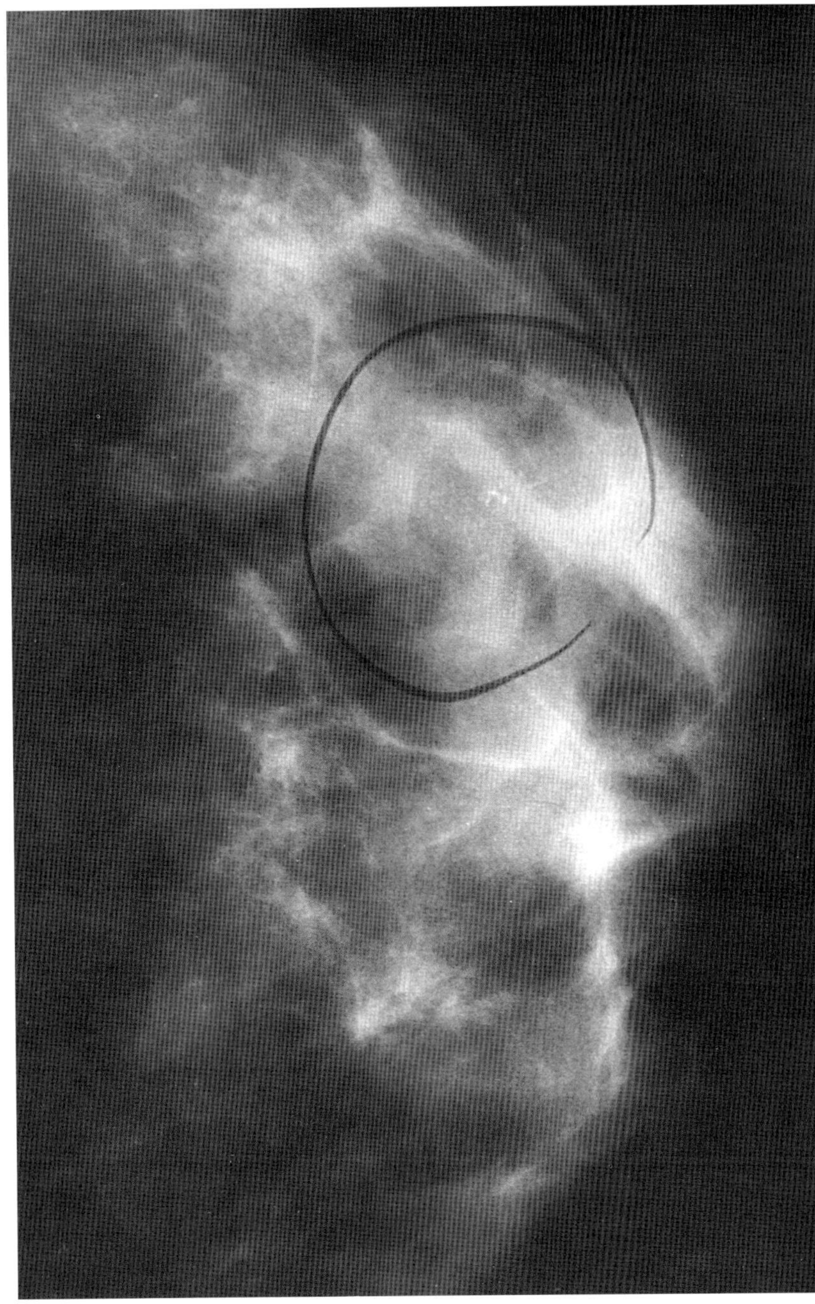
b

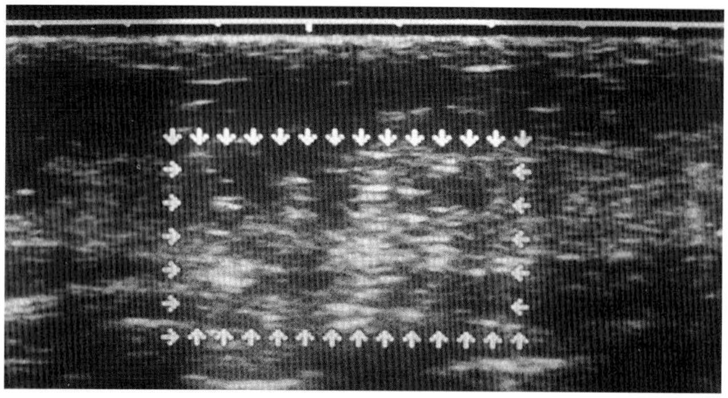

a

History

During a routine mammography, the 66-year-old woman was noted to have diffuse flecks of calcifications scattered over a large area in the upper outer quadrant of the right breast.

Palpable Findings

Both breasts nodular and fibrocystic with no definite palpable masses.

Sonography

Figure **a**: sagittal scan over the suspicious area (7.5 MHz).

Readability: good.

High-level punctate to striate echoes with no focal sonographic lesion (within area outlined by *arrows*).

Analysis

Not possible in this case.

Interpretation

Sonographic correlate of the roentgen microcalcifications with no focal lesion. Benignancy or malignancy cannot be evaluated.

X-ray Mammography

Diffuse flecks of calcification, not typical of carcinoma, scattered over a large area.

Histology

Intraductal tissue proliferation with cellular atypia. Ductal carcinoma in situ identified at some sites.

Figure **b**: polarization microscopic appearance of birefringent crystalline substances (H&E stain, × 15.8).

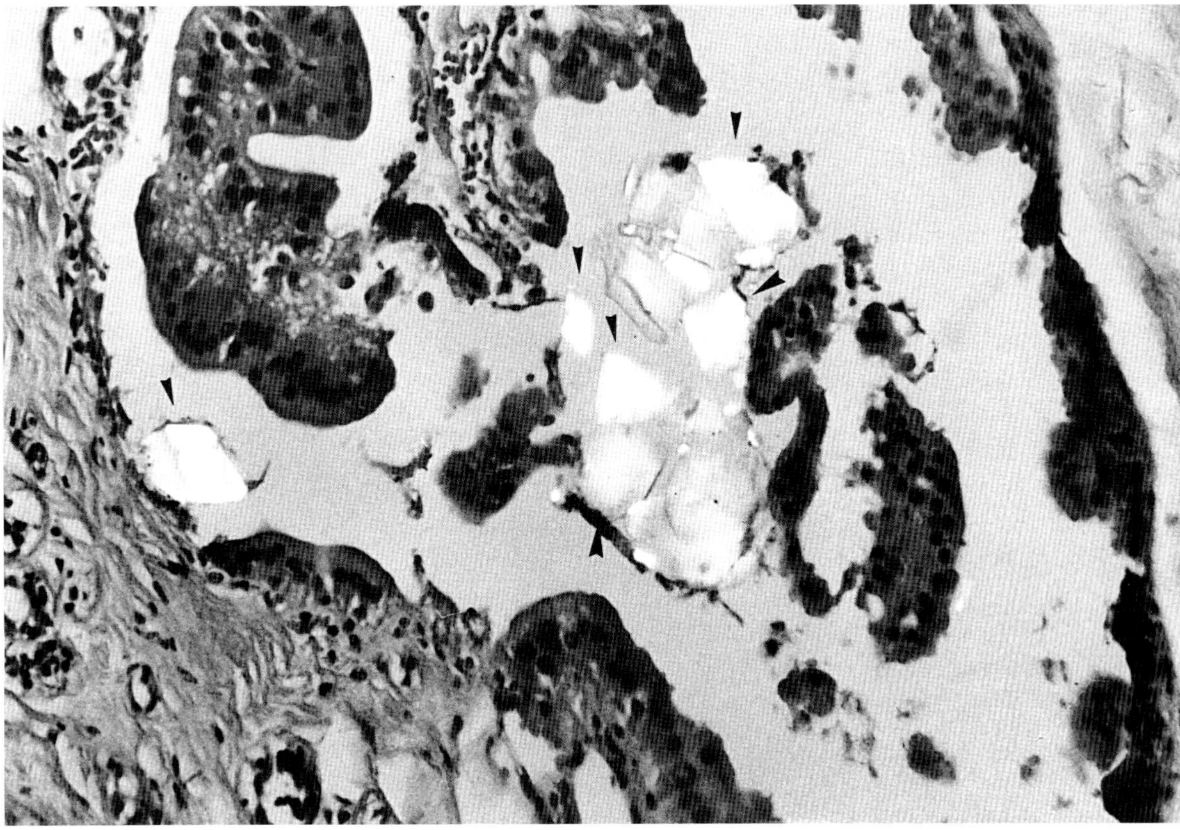

b

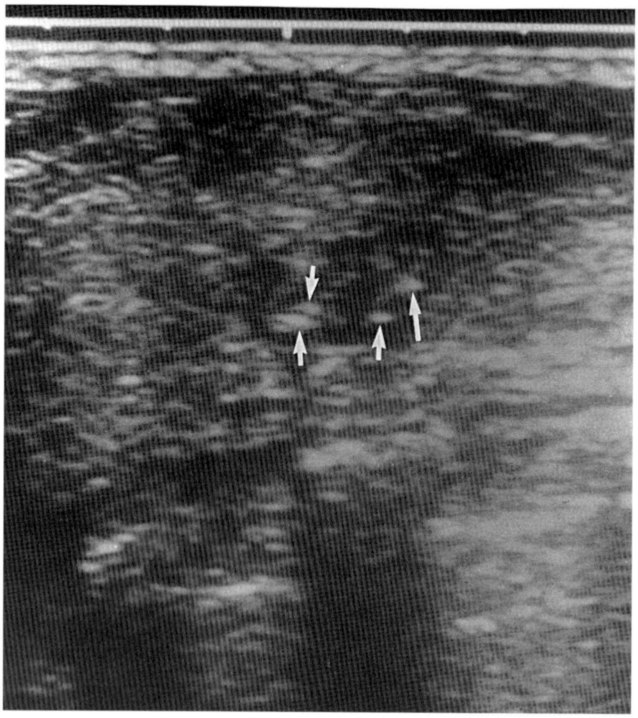

Analysis

1. **Margins**	sharp and smooth
2. **Retrotumoral acoustic phenomena**	unchanged echoes
3. **Internal echo pattern**	nonhomogeneous
4. **Echogenicity**	fat-equivalent
5. **Compression effect** on **shape**	no deformation
6. **Compression effect** on **internal echoes**	no change

History

The 49-year-old woman was noted to have calcifications in her left breast during a screening study.

Palpable Findings

No palpable masses were detected in either breast.

Sonography

Figure: sagittal scan through the upper outer quadrant of the left breast.

Readability: good.

Scan shows 4 or 5 high-level echoes within a well-circumscribed lesion *(arrows)*.

Interpretation

The bright echoes are easily detected, their approximate location having been established by X-ray mammography. On closer scrutiny, the echoes are seen to lie within a focal lesion with benign-appearing analytic criteria. The nonhomogeneous internal echo pattern in this case is caused by the calcium particles. Sonographic diagnosis: calcified fibroadenoma. The sonographic detection of calcium particles associated with a focal lesion not demonstrated by mammography led to the diagnosis of fibroadenoma.

X-ray Mammography

Both projections demonstrate coarse calcifications that were not present on the previous films (5 years before). A focal mammographic abnormality is not seen.

Histology

Calcified fibroadenoma with regressive change.

Differential Diagnostic Problems

As in any diagnostic procedure, problems of differential diagnosis will arise in breast sonography. This may occur when the analytic criteria "let the examiner down," or when "experience" proves to be of little help in patients with uncommon disorders.

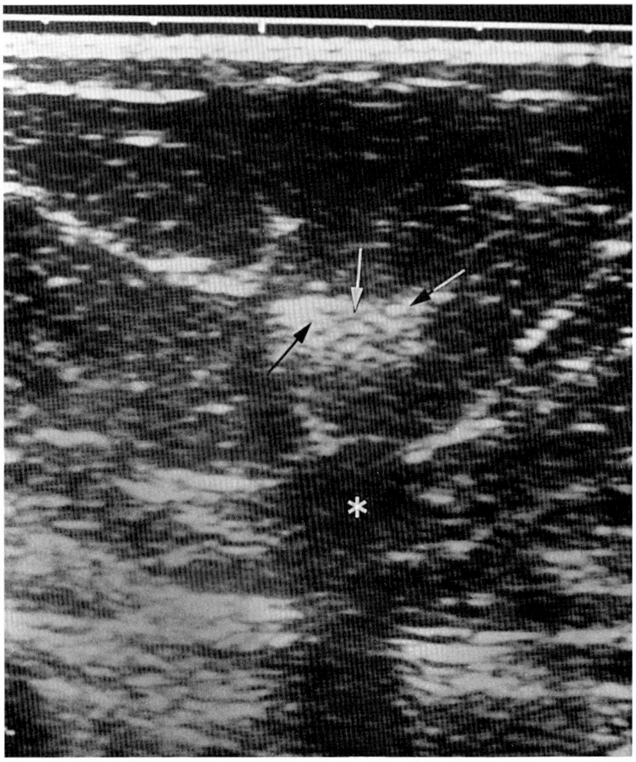

a

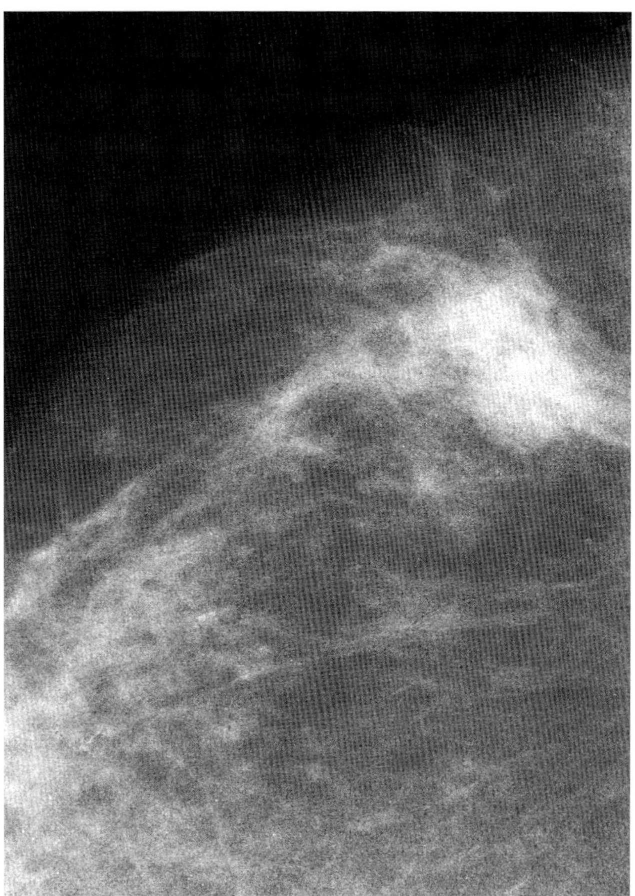

b

History

The 65-year-old woman was referred for ultrasound evaluation of a mammographically indeterminate round lesion within an area of increased density.

Palpable Findings

Large, soft, ptotic breasts with no definite palpable masses.

Sonography

Figure **a**: involuted breast. Hyperechoic area in the upper outer right breast quadrant at the site of the mammographically indeterminate lesion, with a circumscribed posterior shadow. The analytic criteria cannot be applied because a definite focal lesion is not seen.

Interpretation

The first notable finding in the fatty, involuted breast is a hyperechoic area *(arrows)*, 15×7 mm, which, however, displays no suspicious features. Separate from it is a hypoechoic area (*) with moderate posterior shadowing. It is unclear whether this shadow emanates from the hyperechoic feature or from the area beneath it.

Sonographic findlings are equivocal, and biopsy is warranted following sonographic wire localization.

X-ray Mammography

Figure **b** (magnified view): craniocaudal projection showing an approximately 1-cm round lesion in the right lateral portion of the breast. This lesion is difficult to localize on the mediolateral view. Sonographic localization was checked by X-ray mammography.

Histology

Biopsy specimen shows focal ductal papillomas, microcalcifications, and focal duct ectasia. No evidence of epithelial atypia or malignant growth.

History

The 45-year-old woman complained of mastodynia and breast hardening, predominantly left-sided, relating to her menstrual cycle.

Palpable Findings

Firm, mobile, approximately walnut-sized mass in the upper outer quadrant of the left breast.

Sonography

Figure **a**: transverse scan over the mass demonstrating a hypoechoic focal lesion.

Figure **b**: sagittal scan over the palpable mass.

Readability: good.

Size: 31×20×13 mm.

Interpretation

The criteria for this lesion vary within the transverse scan plane and in relation to the sagittal plane. The finding of several different patterns within the same mass should always raise suspicion of medullary carcinoma, especially when posterior enhancement is noted behind an otherwise "malignant"-appearing process.

Histology

Solid undifferentiated breast carcinoma with a focal medullary component.

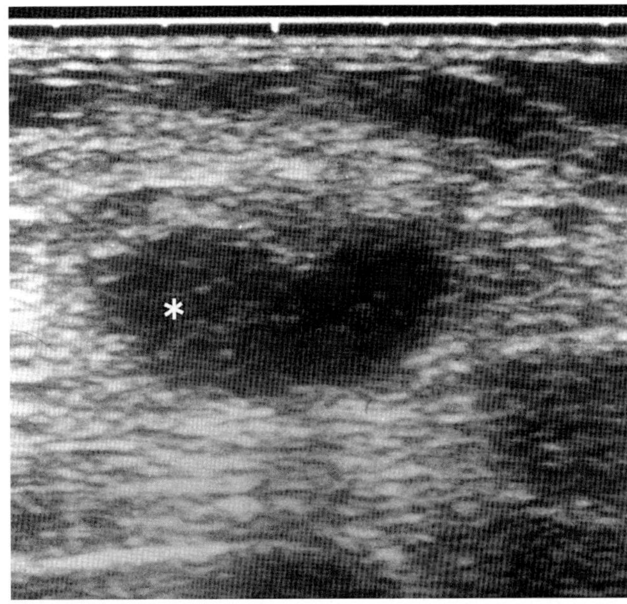

a

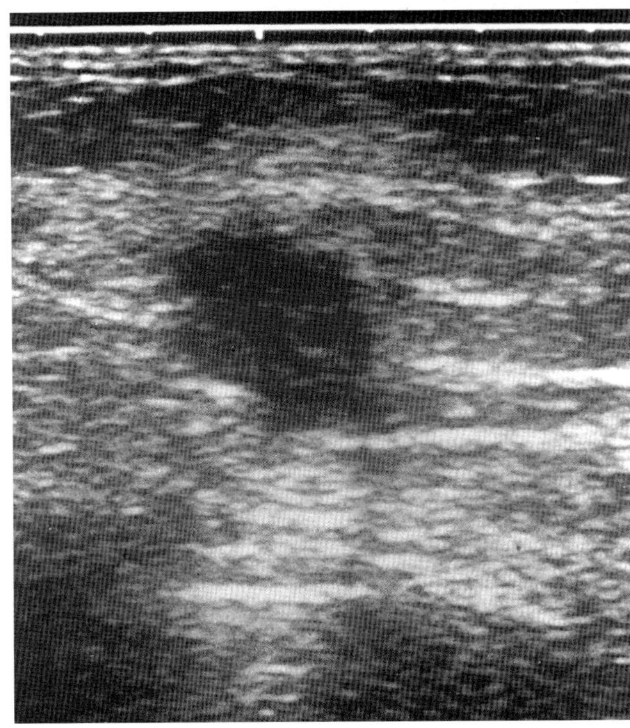
b

Analysis

	a	**b**
1. **Margins**	indistinct but smooth	sharp, jagged
2. **Retrotumoral acoustic phenomena**	enhancement	enhancement
3. **Internal echo pattern**	partly homogeneous (*); partly few echoes, nonhomogeneous	few echoes, nonhomogeneous
4. **Echogenicity**	hypoechoic to fat-equivalent	almost anechoic
5. **Compression effect** on **shape**	no deformation	no deformation
6. **Compression effect** on **internal echoes**	no change	no change

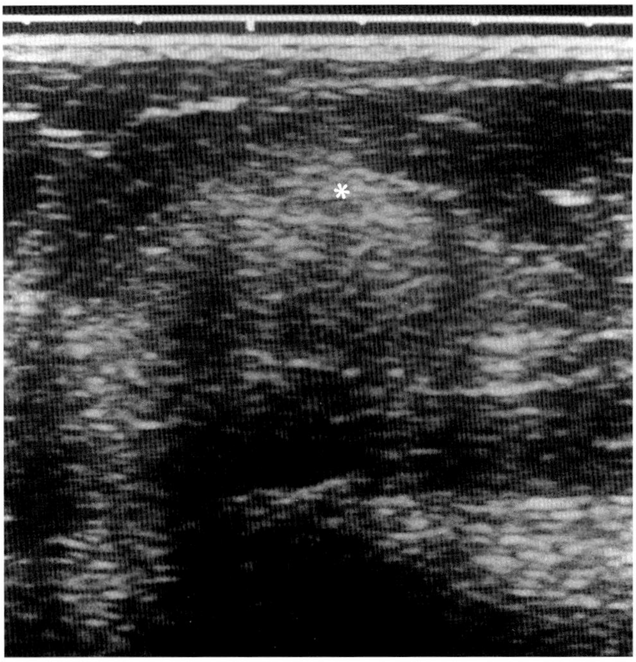

Analysis

1. **Margins**	indistinct but smooth
2. **Retrotumoral acoustic phenomena**	moderate posterior shadowing
3. **Internal echo pattern**	homogeneous
4. **Echogenicity**	hyperechoic
5. **Compression effect** on **shape**	no deformation
6. **Compression effect** on **internal echoes**	no change

History

The 42-year-old woman felt a lump in her right breast 1 week before.

Palpable Findings

Suspicious 2-cm mass at 12 o'clock in the right breast.

Sonography

Figure: sagittal scan over the palpable mass.

Readability: good.

Hyperechoic focal lesion (*), 25×20 mm.

Interpretation

The posterior shadowing suggests a malignant process. This case involves the very rare sonographic finding of a hyperechoic malignant tumor.

Intraoperative findings: grossly no circumscribed focus. The lesion most closely resembles a cyst filled with polypous tissue masses.

Histology

Infiltrating ductal carcinoma with extensive tumor cell necrosis and dystrophic calcification. The tumor stroma shows lymphoplasmocytic infiltration (diameter 15 mm).

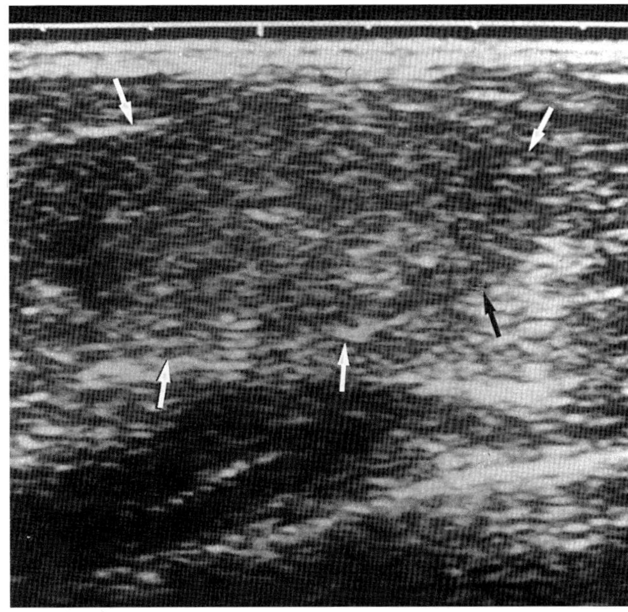

History

During a screening mammography, the 47-year-old woman was noted to have a new round lesion in the upper outer quadrant of her right breast. Presumptive diagnosis: fibroadenoma.

Palpable Findings

Both breasts dense. Mobile, approximately almond-sized mass in the upper outer quadrant of the right breast. No other suspicious clinical findings.

Sonography

Figure: transverse scan over the palpable mass.

Readability: good.

Focal lesion *(arrows)*, 42×20 mm.

Interpretation

All the sonographic criteria suggest a benign process. Isoechoic lesions are very rare on the whole, and they are difficult to distinguish from their surroundings. Both factors supported the ultrasound diagnosis of a circumscribed area of fibrocystic disease.

Histology

Fibrocystic mastopathy with mammary fibrosis and apocrine metaplasia with low epithelial proliferative tendency. No evidence of malignant or premalignant change.

Analysis

1. **Margins**	sharp and smooth
2. **Retrotumoral acoustic phenomena**	unchanged echoes
3. **Internal echo pattern**	homogeneous
4. **Echogenicity**	isoechoic
5. **Compression effect** on **shape**	no deformation
6. **Compression effect** on **internal echoes**	no change

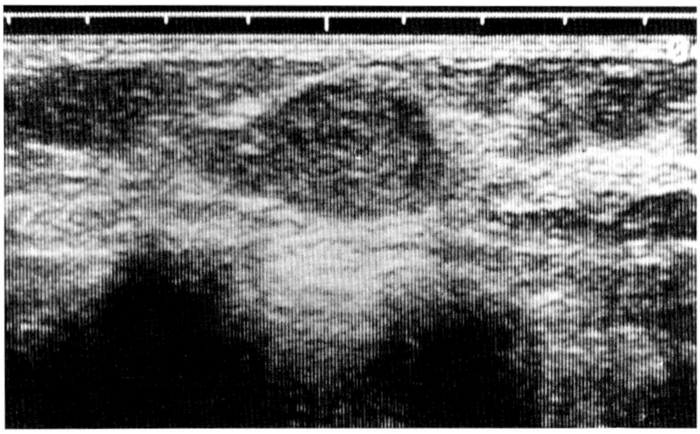

Analysis

1. Margins	sharp and smooth
2. Retrotumoral acoustic phenomena	posterior enhancement
3. Internal echo pattern	homogeneous
4. Echogenicity	hypoechoic
5. Compression effect on **shape**	no deformation
6. Compression effect on **internal echoes**	no change

History

The 44-year-old woman felt a lump in her left breast 2 weeks before. She had a family history of breast cancer.

Palpable Findings

Mobile, smooth-bordered, approximately walnut-sized mass in the lower outer quadrant of the left breast.

Sonography

Figure: sagittal scan over the palpable mass.

Readability: good.

Well-cirumscribed, focal sonographic lesion, 32×20 mm.

Interpretation

All the sonographic criteria suggest a benign process, most likely fibroadenoma. However, retrospective analysis following the histologic diagnosis (see below) indicates that the left side of the lesion is not smoothly marginated but appears to infiltrate adjacent tissues. Colloid carcinomas often produce acoustic enhancement by virtue of their relatively fluid components. This is a rare entity that illustrates how the analytic criteria can overlap.

X-ray Mammography

Both projections demonstrate a smoothly marginated round lesion.

Histology

Colloid carcinoma.

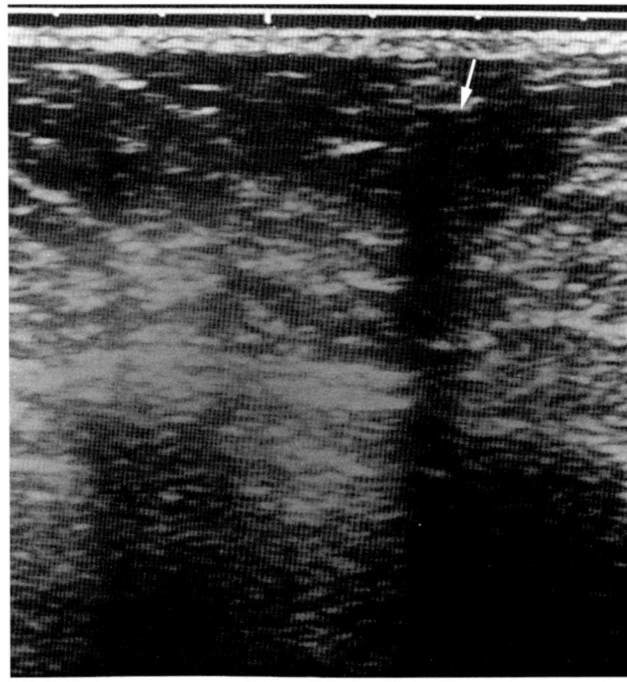

History

The 56-year-old woman was referred with a palpable mass in the periareolar region of the right breast. The unanimous diagnosis of the previously attending physicians was fibroadenoma.

Palpable Findings

Small palpable nodule at the perioareolar border.

Sonography

Figure: sagittal scan over the palpable mass.

Readability: good.

Scan shows a prominent, well-defined posterior shadow that does not emanate from a true focal lesion but from a hyperechoic structure *(arrow)* whose width equals that of the acoustic shadow.

Analysis

Not possible.

Interpretation

A well-defined posterior shadow arising from a hyperechoic area rather than a focal lesion should always direct suspicion toward a calcification, like that occurring at sites of fat necrosis (oil cyst).

Histology

Fat necrosis with central calcifications and a resorptive response. No evidence of malignant growth.

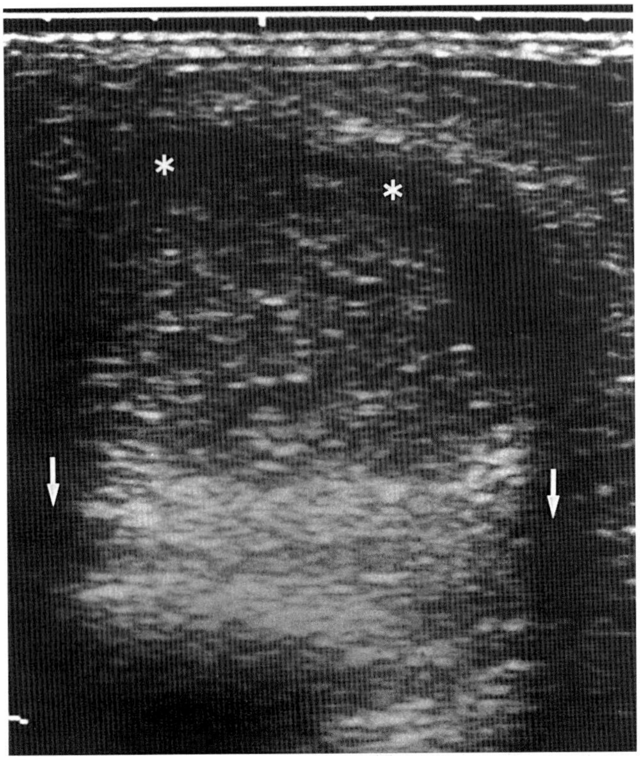

Analysis

1. Margins	indistinct, smooth
2. Retrotumoral acoustic phenomena	posterior enhancement, bilateral shadowing (*arrows*; very faint on the left side)
3. Internal echo pattern	homogeneous
4. Echogenicity	hypoechoic (lesion is bounded anteriorly by an almost anechoic rim [**])
5. Compression effect on **shape**	(slight) distortion
6. Compression effect on **internal echoes**	no change

History

The 47-year-old woman had noted a rapidly enlarging mass in the upper inner quadrant of her left breast in recent months. Initial mammographic findings appeared innocent.

Palpable Findings

Freely mobile, smooth-bordered mass, approximately the size of a Ping-Pong ball, located in the upper inner quadrant of the left breast.

Sonography

Figure: sagittal scan over the mass.

Readability: good.

Focal lesion, 46×34 mm.

Interpretation

Criteria 1, 2, 3, and 5 imply benignancy. The echogenicity of the focal lesion is not uniform.

A rapidly enlarging mass should always be excised regardless of the results of paraclinical studies.

Histology

Fibroadenosis of the cystosarcoma phylloides pattern. No evidence of malignant growth.

History

During a routine examination, the 46-year-old woman was found to have a density in the left breast. Mammography also showed microcalcifications in that area.

Palpable Findings

Fixed, poorly demarcated mass in the upper outer quadrant of the left breast.

Sonography

Figure **a**: sagittal scan over the palpable mass.

Figure **b**: oblique scan over the palpable mass.

Readability: good.

Focal sonographic lesion, 21×15×10 mm.

The mass in Figure **a** appears to infiltrate the chest wall (*), and the pectoralis major fascia is disrupted.

In Figure **b**, the pectoral fascia still appears intact *(arrow)*.

Important: Always image a lesion on two planes!

Interpretation

All the ultrasound criteria suggest a malignant tumor.

Histology

Infiltrating ductal carcinoma, 20×15 mm, with tubular differentiation and comedo elements. Chest-wall infiltration was not demonstrated by histology.

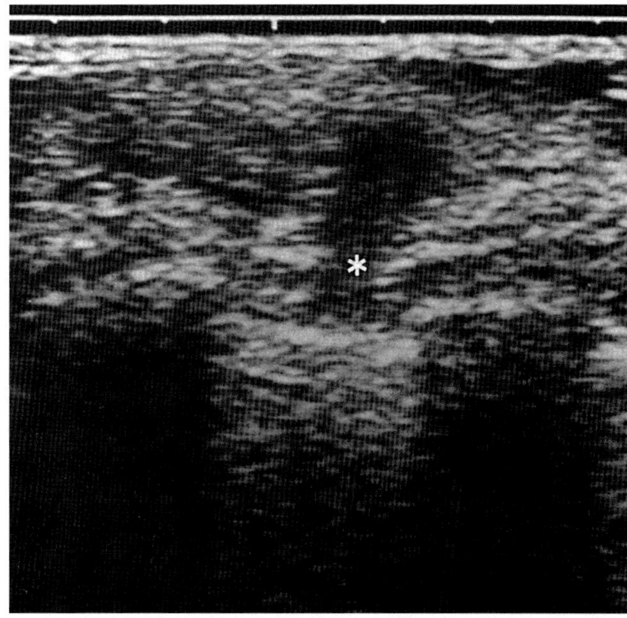

a

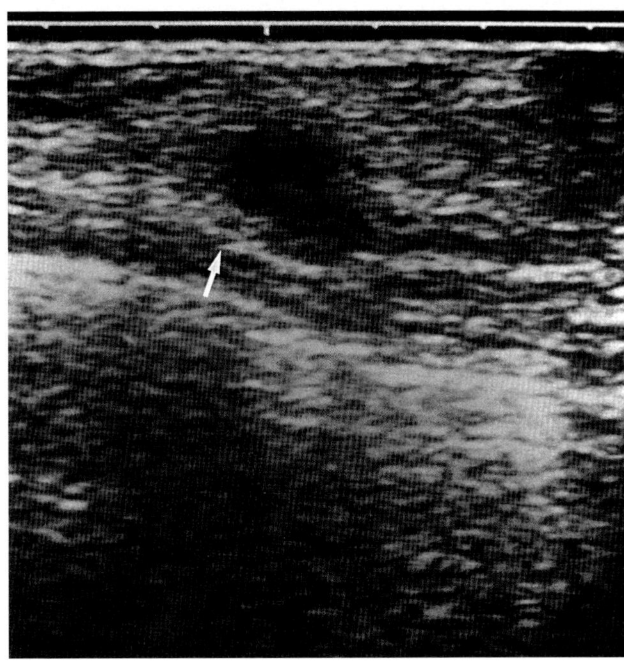

b

Analysis

1. **Margins**	indistinct, jagged
2. **Retrotumoral acoustic phenomena**	unchanged echoes
3. **Internal echo pattern**	few echoes, nonhomogeneous
4. **Echogenicity**	almost anechoic
5. **Compression effect** on **shape**	no deformation
6. **Compression effect** on **internal echoes**	no change

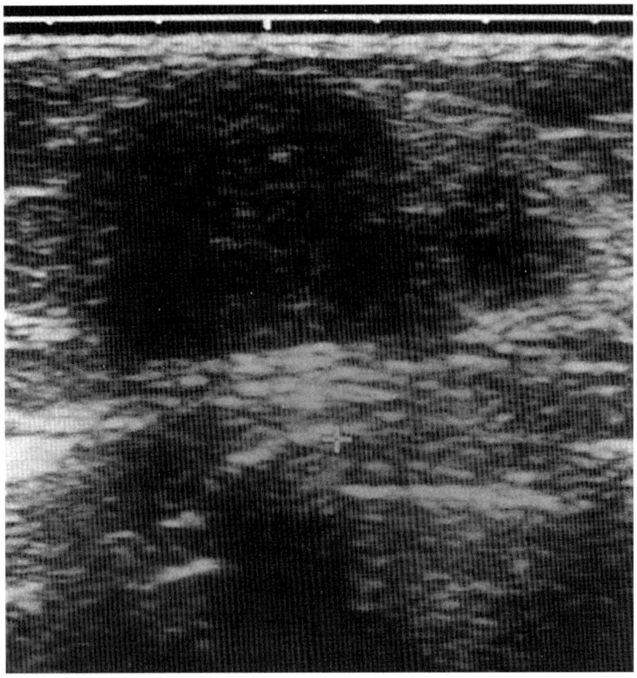

Analysis

1. **Margins**	sharp and smooth (right margin sharp and jagged)
2. **Retrotumoral acoustic phenomena**	unchanged echoes
3. **Internal echo pattern**	nonhomogeneous
4. **Echogenicity**	almost anechoic
5. **Compression effect** on **shape**	no deformation
6. **Compression effect** on **internal echoes**	no change

History

A 54-year-old woman had been aware for 6 months of a slowly enlarging lump in her right breast.

Palpable Findings

Well-demarcated, approximately chestnut-sized, mobile mass at the junction of the upper and lower outer quadrants of the right breast.

Sonography

Figure: sagittal scan over the palpable mass.

Readability: good.

Scan demonstrates a large focal lesion with scalloped borders.

Interpretation

The sonographic criteria are inconsistent, so it is difficult to predict benignancy or malignancy. A striking feature is the lobular projection of the mass toward the right side of the image; the lobulation itself, though, has sharp margins.

With regard to internal echo pattern, it is important to consider that fibroadenomas may appear nonhomogeneous. This is especially true of larger tumors.

Histology

Fibroadenoma with predominantly fibrous components.

History

The 15-year-old girl with a "birthmark" below the left nipple noted an occasional brownish (possibly hemorrhagic) discharge from the lesion. She presented now with a very high suspicion of malignant melanoma.

Palpable Findings

An approximately quarter-sized pigmented nevus was noted below the left areolar border. There was no palpable breast abnormality.

Sonography

Figure: transverse scan over the pigmented nevus.

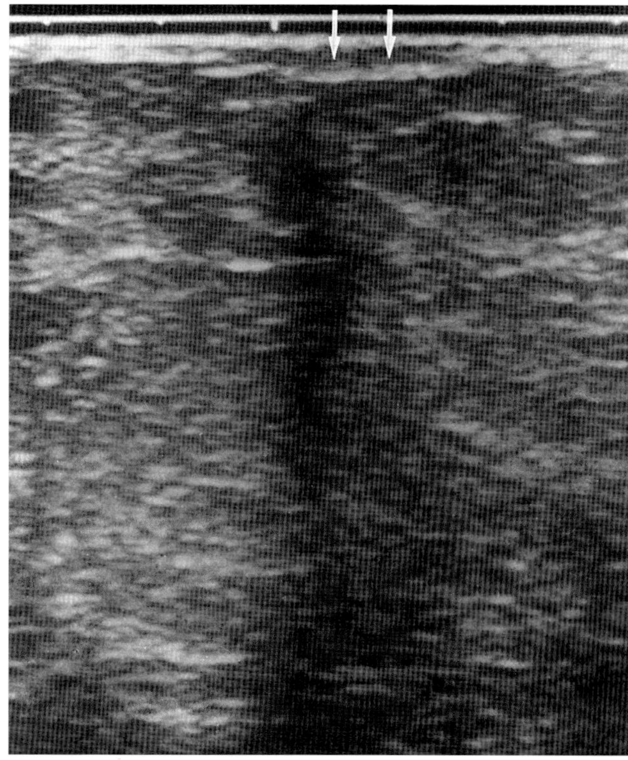

Readability: good.

Scan demonstrates a double skin contour *(arrows)* with posterior acoustic shadowing (intradermal lesion: 20×15×2 mm, vertical).

Interpretation

The normal cutaneous structure on the right and left sides of the image is disrupted by a marked separation of the skin lines at the center. This area corresponds to the pigmented nevus (whose intradermal location is thus documented by ultrasound).

Deep to the lesion is a shadow whose origin remains unclear even after histologic study. It may be an artifact, or it may in fact relate to the melanoma.

X-ray Mammography

Both breasts mammographically normal.

Histology

Verruciform, highly pigmented grade III malignant melanoma. Vertical tumor diameter 2 mm. At the base of the tumor is a pronounced infiltrate composed of histiocytes and lymphocytes surrounding dilated, thin-walled vessels. At the periphery is a spherical area containing whorls of cells with spindle-shaped nuclei.

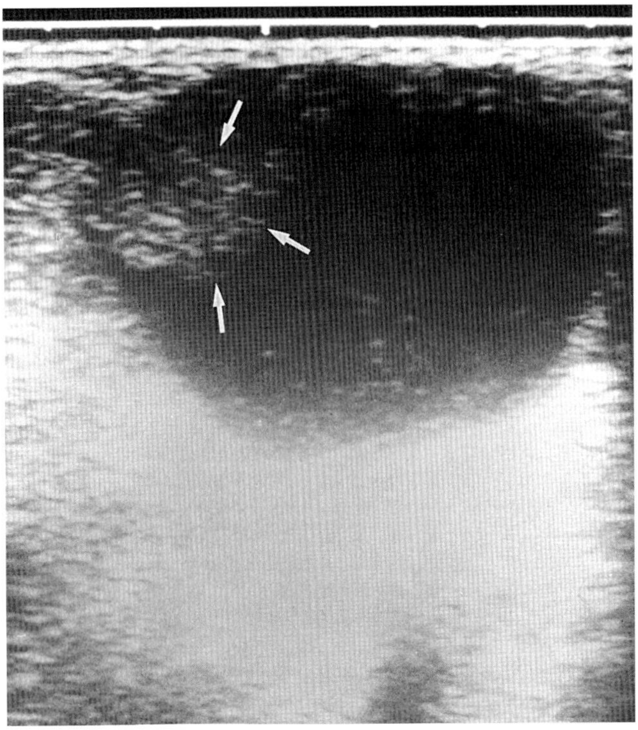

a

Analysis

1. **Margins**	sharp and smooth
2. **Retrotumoral acoustic phenomena**	strong posterior enhancement
3. **Internal echo pattern**	no echoes aside from an echogenic structure projecting into the cyst lumen
4. **Echogenicity**	anechoic
5. **Compression effect** on **shape**	shape distortion
6. **Compression effect** on **internal echoes**	no change

History

The 50-year-old woman had had a known history of bilateral breast cysts for some years. She underwent 3 cyst extirpations on the left side, the most recent 1 year before. Later she noticed a left breast discharge, which had been bloody for 14 days. Cyst aspiration 1 week ago showed a suspicious, Papanicolaou grade III cytology.

Palpable Findings

Tense mass, approximately 5×5 cm, with irregular borders in the upper outer quadrant of the left breast.

Sonography

Figure **a**: sagittal scan over the palpable mass.

The image is dominated by a large anechoic mass.

Interpretation

The mass is a very large cyst made striking by an intraluminal vegetation *(arrows)* of indeterminate nature.

X-ray Mammography

Galactography showed duct termination with an intraductal space-occupying lesion.

Figure **b**: Pneumocystography shows a large, partially evacuated cyst (>>> = air bubbles) with a suspicious peripheral intracystic mass (*).

Aspiration Cytology

Aspiration yielded a clear, amber-colored fluid. Papanicolaou grade III. Fluid expressed from the nipple was Papanicolaou grade V.

Histology

Malignant cystosarcoma phylloides. At the periphery of the cyst are poorly marginated tissue defects, some showing villous-polypoid expansion. These deformations are cherry-sized. Tumor expansion is generally nodular within the approximately 10-cm cyst, and there is no skin infiltration.

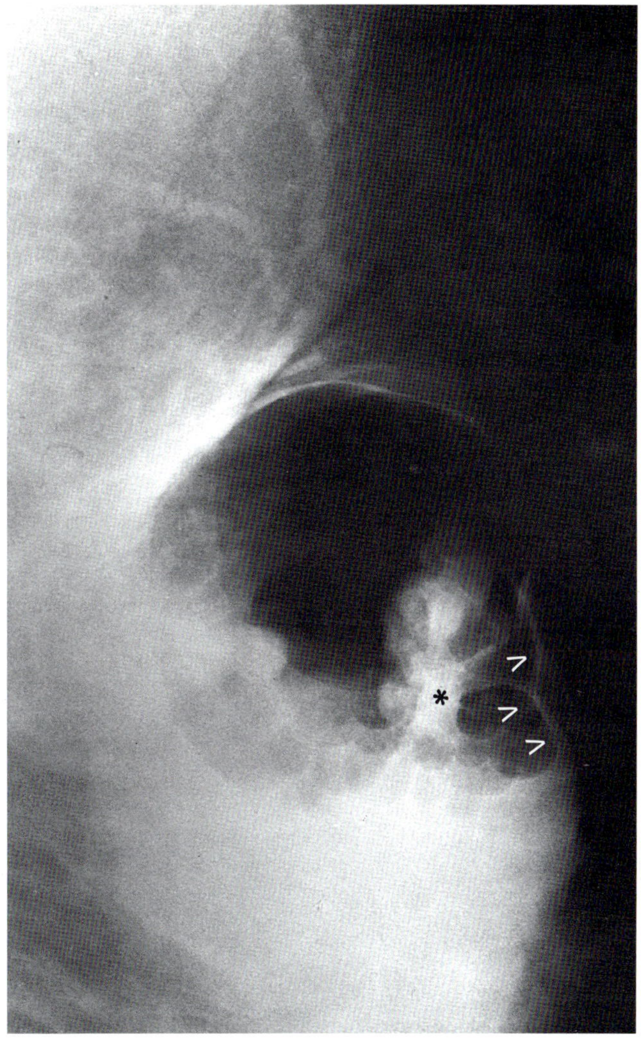

b

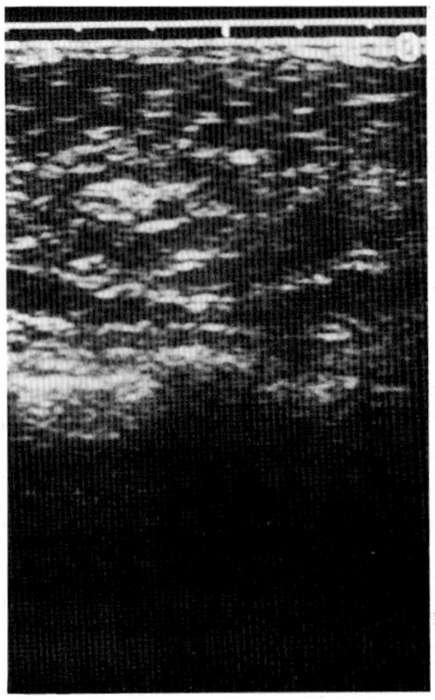

a

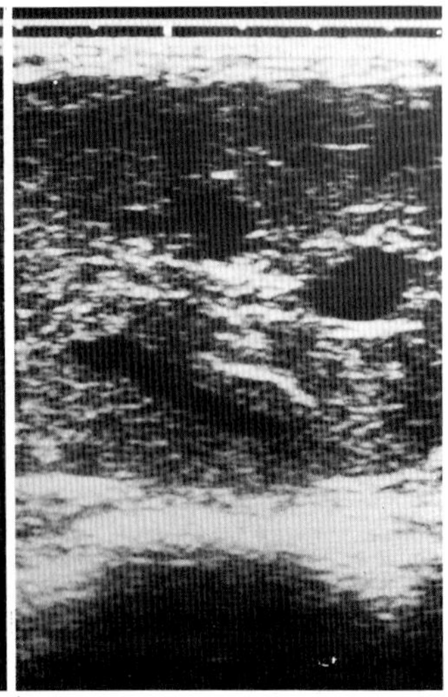

b

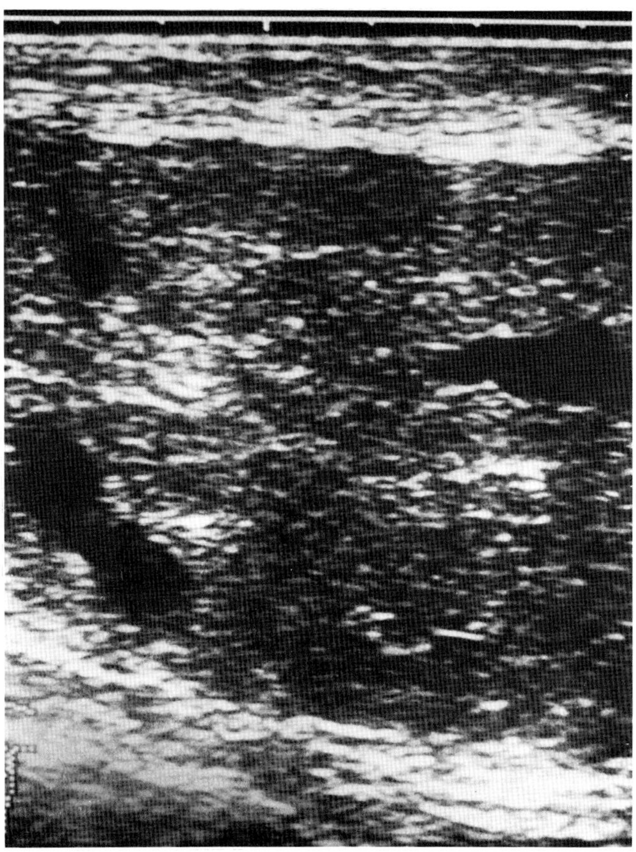

c

History

The 32-year-old primigravida presented in her 36th week of pregnancy with a greatly enlarged, warm, erythematous left breast.

Palpable Findings

A marked size discrepancy was noted between the two breasts. The left breast was reddened and felt significantly warmer than the right. The initial clinical impression was mastitis or severe galactostasis, although the patient reported no pain or fever. From that time until about 2 months postpartum she was treated with bromocriptine and scheduled for regular clinical and ultrasound follow-ups. The clinical presentation remained constant through delivery and afterward showed little change. At the last follow-up, 5 months postpartum, a fist-sized, well-demarcated infiltrate was palpated within the markedly enlarged left breast.

Sonography

Sagittal scans over the right breast (Fig. **a**) and an identical site in the left breast (Fig. **b**) in 36th week of pregnancy.

Readability: good.

The right breast manifests the pregnancy-specific changes of a loose-textured parenchyma and dilated milk ducts. The left breast is markedly enlarged in its anteroposterior dimension. A combination of round and oblong cystic masses are visible within a homogeneous area.

Figure **c** (36th week of pregnancy): zoom image of the left breast showing an echogenic streak below the normally configured skin that may represent subcutaneous fat or original glandular tissue. Below it is a very homogeneous zone permeated by cystic structures of varying configuration. The pectoral fasciae at the bottom of the image.

Figure **d** (1 week postpartum): though somewhat smaller, the abnormal area shows no significant structural change. Its boundary with normal glandular tissue is on the left side of the image.

Figure **e** (6 weeks postpartum): area unchanged in size and structure. The cystic masses are still present.

Figure **f** (5 months postpartum): still no change.

Analysis

The analytic criteria cannot be applied due to the absence of a true focal lesion.

Interpretation

The sonographic presentation of this case is unusual. On the one hand, it suggests a peculiar form of fibrocystic disease (cystic lesions in an otherwise homogeneous tissue). But because the mass arose in pregnancy, the differential diagnosis must also include severe galactostasis or mastitis.

Aspiration Cytology

Aspiration of a cystic area in week 36 yielded a milky fluid, Papanicolaou grades I/II.

Histology

Histologic examination was performed on tissue obtained by drill biopsy at 6 weeks postpartum. Besides changes typical of a lactating breast, examination revealed marked hyalinosis of the mammary connective tissue. This finding is most consistent with fibrocystic disease.

Unfortunately, the patient has consistently refused excisional biopsy. Follow-up is stil being continued with her.

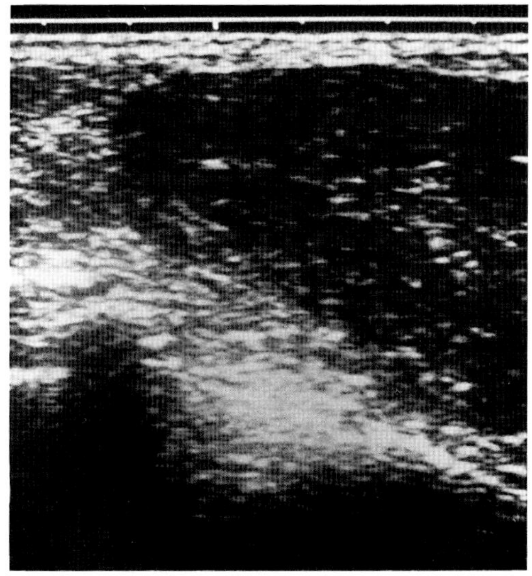

d

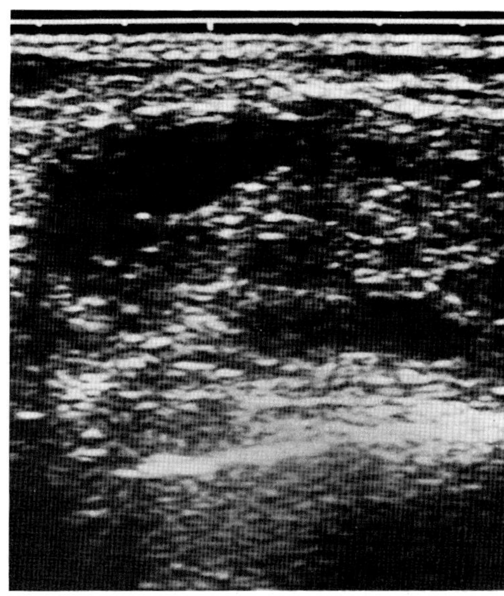

e

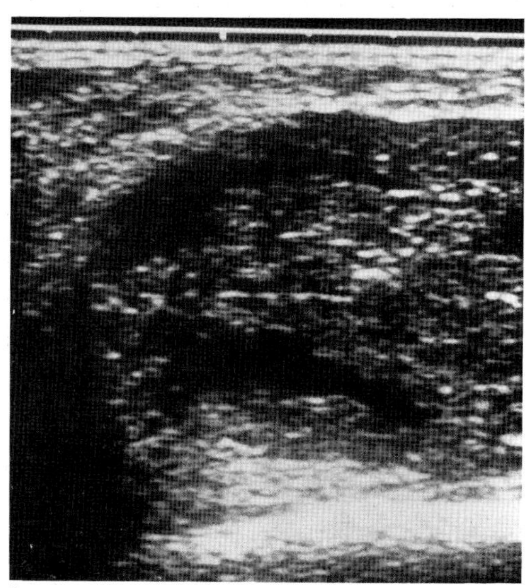

f

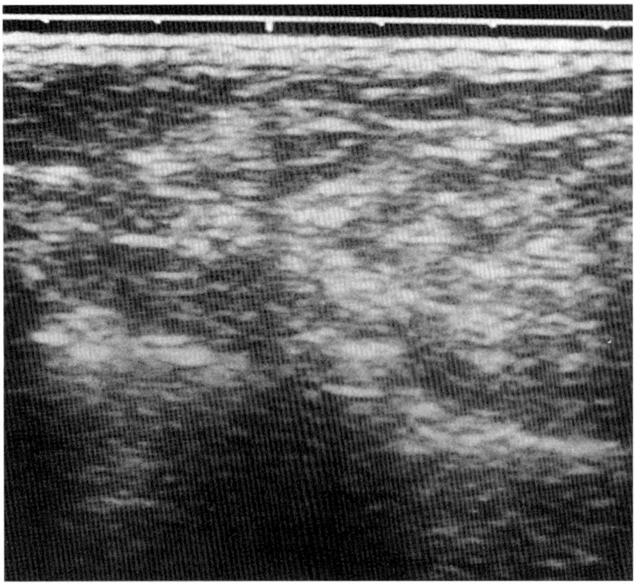

a

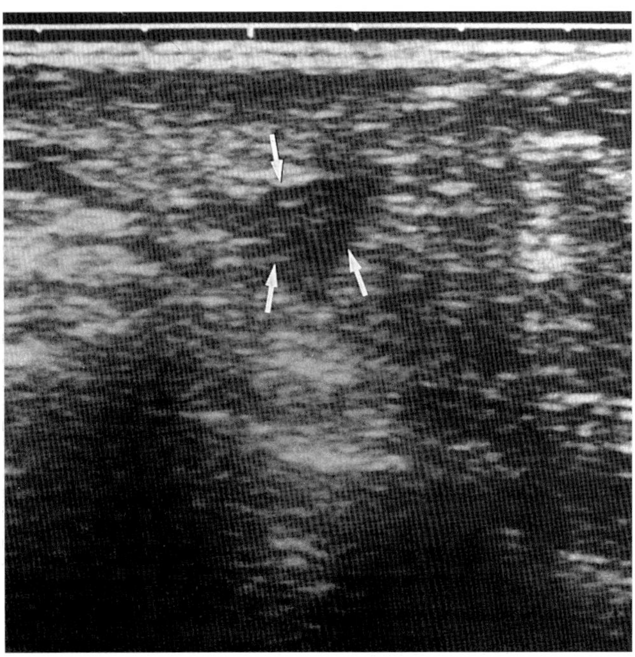

b

History

The 34-year-old woman had undergone five right breast biopsies for recurrent bilateral nonpuerperal mastitis. She also underwent a left biopsy for mastitis 2 months before. She presented now with a recurrence of abscessation in the left breast.

Palpable Findings

Moderate edema of the left breast, no discharge. Slight induration in the upper outer quadrant separate from the fresh periareolar scar.

Sonography

Figure **a**: sagittal scan over the indurated area of the left breast.

Readability: good.

Relatively chaotic architecture of the breast parenchyma, whose boundaries with the subcutaneous and retromammary fat are obscured.

Figure **b**: sagittal scan over the same area 4 days later after high-dosage antibiotic therapy. At the center of the image is a triangular area with partially sharp margins that appears hypoechoic to its surroundings *(arrows)*. This represents incipient liquefaction of the inflammatory infiltrate.

Analysis

A meaningful criteria analysis cannot be made.

Interpretation

Mastitis involving an extended area of the breast parenchyma usually presents a chaotic sonographic picture, although this type of finding does not necessarily signify the presence of mastitis. Incipient absceccation or a fully developed abscess appears as a focal sonographic lesion.

Histology

(taken at the time of abscess incision)

Duct ectasia with subacute to chronic galactophoritis.

History

The 35-year-old woman was admitted with suspicion of nonpuerperal mastitis with abscessation.

Palpable Findings

Somewhat poorly demarcated, fluctuating mass palpable beneath an erythematous area over the upper quadrants of the right breast.

Sonography

Figure: transverse scan over the reddened area.

Readability: good.

Shallow focal lesion with polygonal boundaries, 36×9 mm.

Interpretation

All sonographic criteria except 3 (internal echoes) suggest a benign process. The predominantly horizontal extent and shallow depth of the lesion also can be interpreted as a benign feature (L/T ratio < 0.5). The clinical picture and ultrasound findings are strongly suggestive of abscessation.

Incision of the abscess confirmed the suspicion.

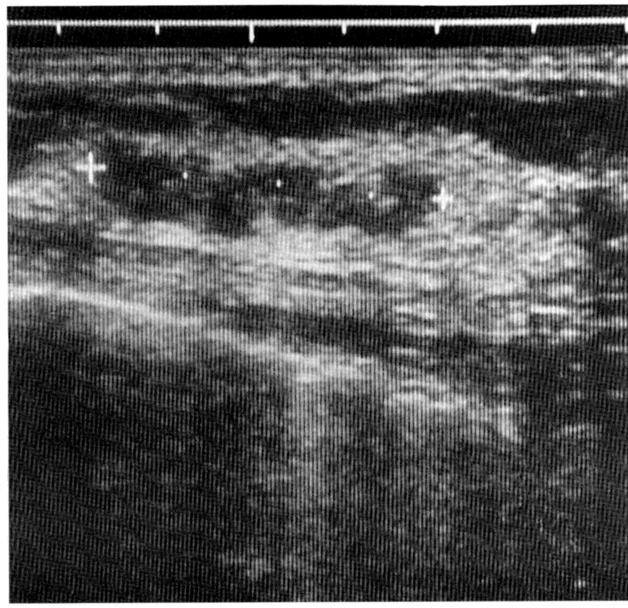

Analysis

1. **Margins**	sharp, jagged
2. **Retrotumoral acoustic phenomena**	unchanged to faint posterior enhancement
3. **Internal echo pattern**	few echoes, non-homogeneous
4. **Echogenicity**	fat-equivalent
5. **Compression effect** on **shape**	shape distortion
6. **Compression effect** on **internal echoes**	echoes become more homogeneous

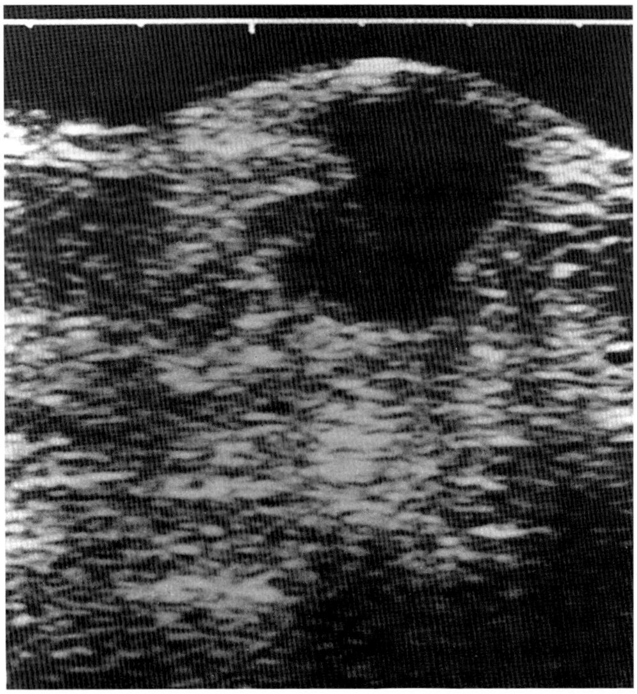

Analysis

1. **Margins**	sharp, jagged
2. **Retrotumoral acoustic phenomena**	faint posterior enhancement
3. **Internal echo pattern**	no echoes except for a few nonhomogeneous echoes at the left border
4. **Echogenicity**	almost anechoic
5. **Compression effect** on **shape**	shape distortion
6. **Compression effect** on **internal echoes**	no change

History

The 46-year-old woman had been aware of a milky discharge from her right nipple for 15 years (!).

Palpable Findings

Erythematous area overlying a centrally fluctuant mass in the inner quadrants of the right breast. Slight nipple retraction in the medial side.

Sonography

(with water path)

Figure: sagittal scan over the palpable mass.

Readability: good.

Well-demarcated focal sonographic lesion, 20×20 mm.

Interpretation

The overall impression is of a benign cystic process, although criteria 3 and 4 are not inconsistent with malignancy. When the clinical findings are known, the sonographic diagnosis of abscess is very likely, especially since particulate components can always be found in an abscess.

Aspiration Cytology

Papanicolaou grades I/II.

Histology

Acute inflammatory, partially necrotizing connective-tissue changes with glandular elements showing epithelial proliferation.

History

For several months, the 29-year-old woman had been aware of a clear discharge from the left nipple.

Palpable Findings

Normal-appearing breasts with no palpable masses. Left nipple compression elicited discharge of a clear, slightly greenish fluid.

Cytology of nipple discharge: Papanicolaou grades I/II.

Sonography

Figure: sagittal scan over the nipple region.

Readability: good.

A focal sonographic lesion is visualized.

Interpretation

Although nipple discharge is not a primary indication for sonography, ultrasound is well able to demonstrate ectatic milk ducts. In this case a papillomatous structure is seen projecting into the duct lumen from the left side of the image. Although the sonographic criteria indicate a benign prognosis, a histologic examination is mandatory even with negative cytology of nipple smears.

X-ray Mammography

Galactography showed duct ectasia with an irregular wall structure.

Histology

Milk duct papillomatosis.

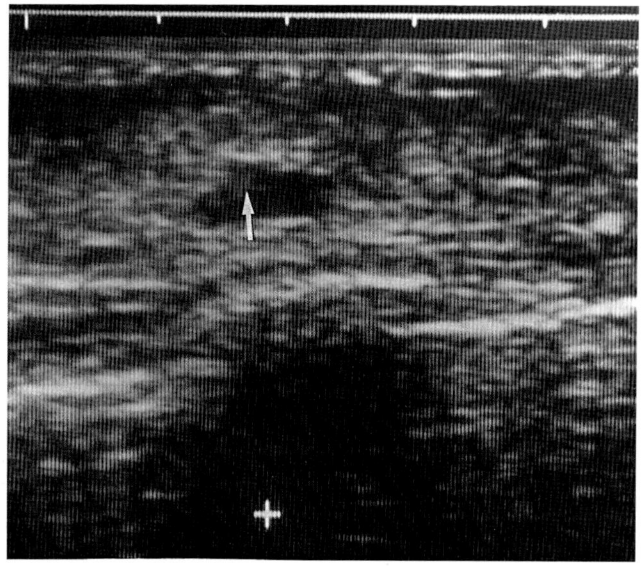

Analysis

1. **Margins**	sharp and smooth
2. **Retrotumoral acoustic phenomena**	unchanged echoes
3. **Internal echo pattern**	no echoes except for a small intraluminal vegetation on the left side *(arrow)*
4. **Echogenicity**	anechoic
5. **Compression effect** on **shape**	shape distortion
6. **Compression effect** on **internal echoes**	no change

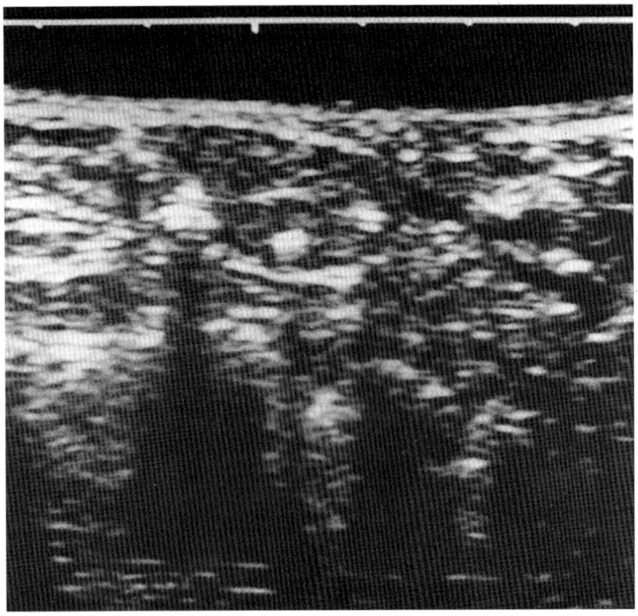

a

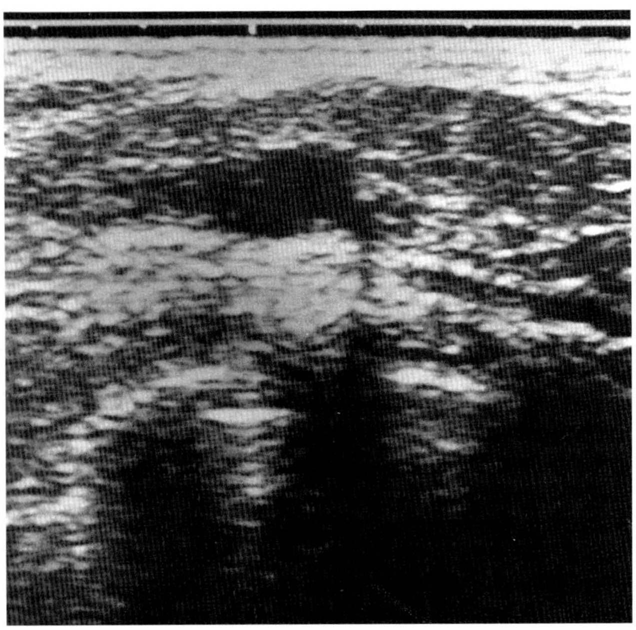

b

History

The 47-year-old woman underwent excision of a left axillary lymph node elsewhere, and histology showed a metastasis of solid undifferentiated carcinoma. As part of the primary tumor search, X-ray mammograms were taken which showed coarse calcifications in the right breast. Otherwise breasts were dense and difficult to evaluate.

Palpable Findings

A firm, circumscribed mass was palpated in the right breast. The left breast parenchyma was dense and difficult to evaluate. A large postbiopsy infiltrate was found in the left axilla.

Sonography

Figure **a**: sagittal scan over the palpable mass in the right breast.

Readability: good.

Focal sonographic lesion, 25×15 mm, with large hyperechoic particles.

Figure **b**: sagittal through the lower outer quadrant of the left breast.

Readability: good.

Focal sonographic lesion, 20×10 mm.

Analysis

	a	b
1. Margins	sharp and smooth	sharp, jagged
2. Retrotumoral acoustic phenomena	shadowing behind the hyperechoic particles	unchanged echoes
3. Internal echo pattern	homogeneous (with large hyperechoic foci)	few echoes, nonhomogeneous
4. Echogenicity	hypoechoic	almost anechoic
5. Compression effect on **shape**	no deformation	no deformation
6. Compression effect on **internal echoes**	no change	no change

Interpretation

The right-sided focal lesion with its coarse, high-level internal echoes has the appearance of a calcified fibroadenoma. The lesion in Figure **a** is somewhat difficult to categorize by the standard analytic criteria, but in conjunction with the patient's history it definitely warrants biopsy. The lesion in the left breast was localized preoperatively with a sonographically inserted wire.

X-ray Mammography

Figure **c**: mediolateral localization of the left breast showing dense parenchyma with no discernible focal lesion. The tip of the localization wire, which was well visualized by sonography, is not visible on the mammogram due to the proximity of the lesion to the chest wall.

Note: The carcinoma near the chest wall would have been missed if the tumor had been sought by X-ray mammography alone.

Histology

Right breast biopsy: intracanalicular fibroadenoma with regressive change.

Left breast biopsy: 16-mm, moderately to poorly differentiated infiltrating ductal carcinoma with intraductal tumor extensions.

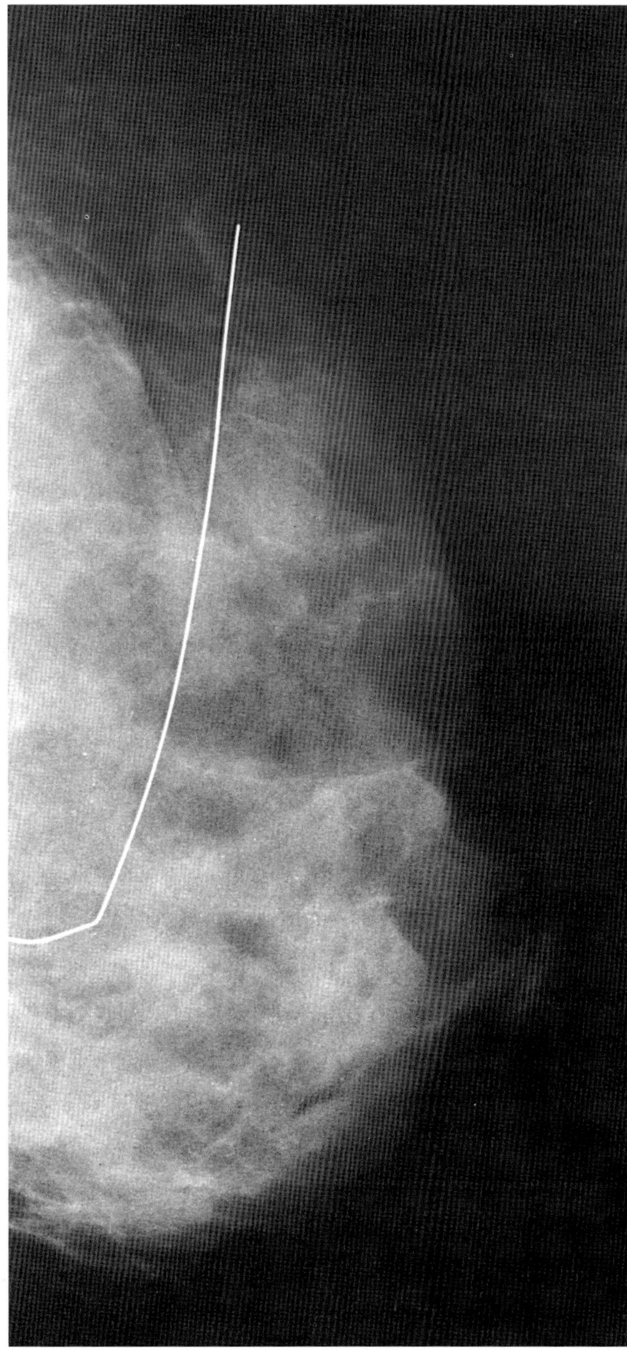

c

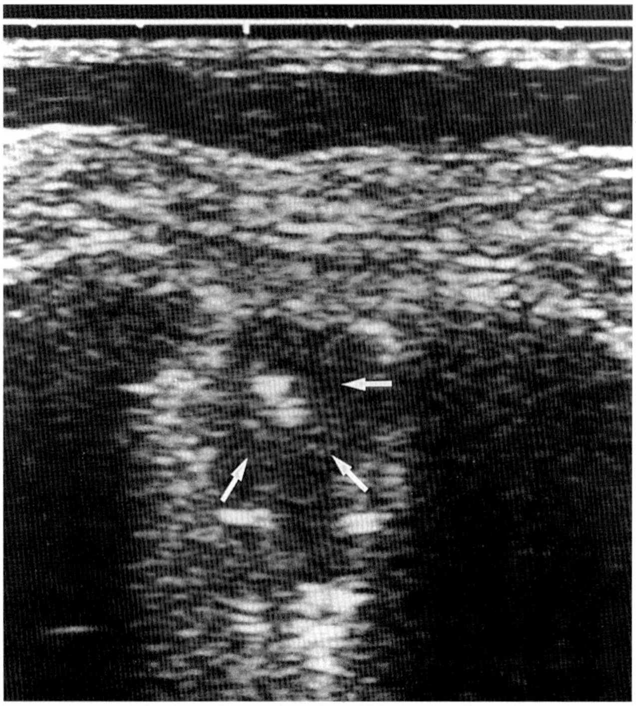

History

The 65-year-old woman was reffered for ultrasound evaluation of a radiographically dense breast.

Palpable Findings

No palpable abnormalities were noted in the parenchyma or axillary lymphatic drainage of either breast.

Sonography

Figure: oblique scan over the upper inner quadrant of the right breast demonstrating a circumscribed, intrathoracic focal lesion with hyperechoic structures.

The breasts themselves were sonographically normal.

Analysis

Not possible as there is no intramammary focal lesion.

Interpretation

Ultrasound demonstrated no breast abnormalities but incidentally revealed a mass within the chest cavity *(arrows)*. The patient was referred for thoracic surgical evaluation. Following an inconclusive transbronchial biopsy, the patient was advised to undergo thoracotomy for the suspected tumor. She refused the operation. Following a 3-week course of high-dosage antibiotic therapy, the roentgen correlate—initially represented by a dense, tangerine-sized, vascular-conducted infiltrate—was almost gone. It is very likely that the mass was a chronic inflammatory process (e.g., chronic segmental pneumonia). Sonographic follow-up showed no further evidence of the lesion.

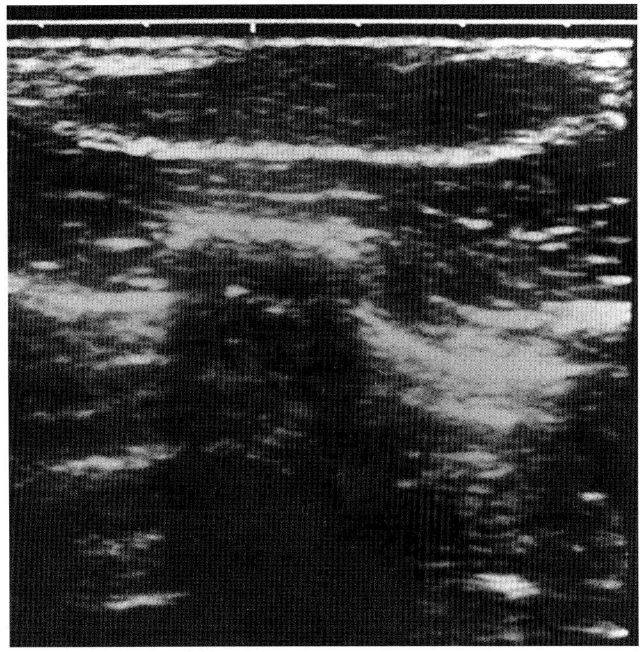

History

This 17-year-old boy was referred with gynecomastia.

Palpable Findings

Both breasts were mildly enlarged and had a relatively soft consistency; no isolated palpable abnormality.

Sonography

Figure: sagittal scan over the nipple.

The entire gland is visible on the image. There is no focal lesion.

Analysis

Not possible in the absence of a focal lesion.

Interpretation

The spindle-shaped breast parenchyma shows homogeneous echoes with no subcutaneous fat. Retroareolar fat is also absent. The discontinuity in the skin outline is from the nipple and areola. Deep to the breast bud are the pectoral muscle, a rib with posterior shadow, and the chest wall.

The last case, involving the sonographic examination of a male breast, could represent a new indication for breast ultrasound. Our experience to date in this area is very limited, however.

The illustrations in this atlas are based on current state-of-the-art imaging technology. While it is unclear how the rapid development of electronics with influence our technical capabilities, our present-day insights and discoveries will form the basis for the advancement of breast imaging in the future.

Careful, repeated viewing of the illustrations will train the eye for the images seen on the monitor and can help to fill gaps even for the experienced examiner.

The list of references is presented at the end of chapter 5 on p. 31.

Index